From reviews of *New Approach to Headache and Migraine*

"A well-researched, holistic overview of all the elements of life that impact on headaches and their management, this book is a passionate and comprehensive discussion of what can be done to reduce and prevent headaches for the long term."

DR ANGELA WEBB MBBS, MS, FRACS
Peter MacCullum Hospital – Surgeon and Head of Plastic Surgery

"I strongly commend this exceptional and comprehensive book to medical professionals and patients alike. A beautiful balance of text and illustrations, based on decades of medical and applied health research, this book is a guide for everyone who deals with headaches and migraines."

DR JASON D. WINNETT MB, BS, FRACS
Winnett Specialist Group – Surgeon

"I couldn't be more excited by this book – credible, understandable information on the many causes of headaches, as well as actionable, sustainable solutions for symptoms reversal and reduction – WITHOUT medication. Pablo explains formal and complex scientific research using clear, simple language, while acknowledging and answering nearly all of the hallmark questions that arise for headache sufferers."

EVE PERSAK MS RDN CNSC CSSD
Nutritional Counselor, Consultant, Speaker and Writer
COMO Group – Nutrition Advisor

"Pablo is the voice of authority. All his years of working with the body and various modalities have uncovered the many tools and solutions that you can now empower yourself with to overcome headaches forever."

MUKTI Author Truth in Beauty; Mukti Organic Skincare - Founder

"An invaluable, user friendly book for anyone who suffers regular headaches. It has been an enormously helpful resource to both educate and assist clients in better understanding the individual nature of their headaches, identify their triggers and feel empowered to naturally manage their symptoms and outcomes."

JACQUI LOUDER MAPS
Olympic Park Sports Medicine Centre – Psychologist
'The Science of Sport' SEN (116AM) – Co- Host

"This book is packed with detailed yet easy-to-read medical and practical information, that I have been able to apply straightaway to my daily life. In the past, I would reach by default for painkillers, thinking they were my only option. Now, I have been introduced to a whole host of strategies for preventing and managing headaches, and I am equipped with much more comprehensive knowledge for understanding, preventing, and managing headaches. This one is a keeper!"

KARINA WILKIE PhD; Monash University - Senior Lecturer, Faculty of Education

A New Approach to Headache and Migraine

Published by Linked2Health

All enquiries should be made to the author
Info@pablotymoszuk.com

NATIONAL LIBRARY OF AUSTRALIA

A catalogue record for this book is available from the National Library of Australia

ISBN 978-0-9943758-1-0

DISCLAIMER

The information about headaches and their treatment provided in this book is for educational purposes only. It is not intended to be medical or professional advice. It should not be used to diagnose or treat headaches or any other medical condition.

You should talk to your doctor or other licensed healthcare professional so that you get a proper diagnosis and the sort of treatment that is right for you personally.

Do not alter the dose or stop taking any prescription medication without first consulting your doctor. Consult your doctor before taking over-the counter medications, herbal remedies or dietary supplements.

Similarly, before you make any major changes to your diet or activity levels or start a new form of treatment you should seek the advice of your doctor or other licensed healthcare professional.

A New Approach to Headache and Migraine

Understand, manage and prevent your headaches

Pablo Tymoszuk

About the Author

Pablo Tymoszuk has been driven by one consuming passion during his more than 23 years working as a soft tissue therapist – to empower his patients to manage and conquer their pain.

A natural educator, Pablo has always sought to work closely with his patients, embarking on a journey with them to find the most practical, long-lasting solutions for their pain, and is known for communicating his professional knowledge and insights with clarity and impact.

His tireless pursuit to improve the lives of patients with debilitating conditions has led him to investigate the efficacy of a wide range of drug-free methods and strategies, from which he has built a comprehensive, integrated holistic approach to professional treatment and self-care that has transformed the lives of so many of his patients.

His first book, A New Approach to Headache and Migraine, is representative of his generous, thoughtful and considered approach to treatment. In this book, Pablo offers his unique insights into pain management, his years of research and experience and the practical application of his proven strategies with a clarity that makes his approach readily accessible to medical professionals and laypeople.

Professionally, Pablo has specialized in remedial, sports, myofascial and trigger point release techniques. For 15 years, he worked extensively with elite sporting clubs, including the Collingwood Football Club, Richmond Football Club and Australian Cricket Team. Pablo was also fortunate to gain 19 years of invaluable experience treating musculoskeletal injuries and conditions at Olympic Park Sports Medicine Centre.

He currently works from his own clinic in Melbourne Australia whilst also providing ergonomic consultations and presentations in the workplace, delivering presentations about headache and migraine pain and consulting at numerous wellness retreats in Asia.

Dedicated to
Margaret Scarlett

1946 – 2015

This book would not exist if wasn't for the endless research, editing and guidance of Margaret.
I am forever grateful.

Headache Danger Signs

Most headaches aren't symptoms of a serious illness, but some are.

If you experience a new headache or a change in your usual headache pattern, you should consult your doctor or call for an ambulance.

Danger signs to watch out for:

- A new headache, especially after age 50
- A change in your old pattern of headaches
- A headache that is unusually severe, or that has a very rapid onset.

Additional danger signs include:

- A stiff neck and fever
- Severe nausea or vomiting
- Neurological symptoms such as weakness, difficulty speaking, difficulty walking and vision changes.

References in this book

This book is the result of over 23 years of experience and research. If I have quoted or referred directly to a source, it is cited in the text. A list of all references is at the end of the book.

Overview

Contents

Introduction

Headaches are often trivialised, but they're no laughing matter when you've got one, and so much worse when they're a debilitating part of every week, or perhaps every day. Everything is harder when your head hurts. A relatively mild headache makes it harder to function and a severe headache can stop you in your tracks. If the pain is accompanied by nausea and vomiting, you can end up in bed.

To add insult to injury, in many cases, the very thing you are offered as a solution is probably doing more harm than good, particularly over the long term. The marketing of over the counter (OTC) painkillers makes it seem they're an easy, effective solution – one pill and you're on your way. And sure, they work for some people, some of the time. But painkillers are a bandaid at best. They can mask the symptoms of a headache, but they never treat the underlying causes. Worse, they can start to cause headaches of their own. The long-term use of painkillers is a cause of rebound or 'medication overuse' headaches.

I have been successfully treating people who suffer from frequent, severe headache and migraine for 23 years, and never has 'take more painkillers' been the answer.

The solutions I share with my clients are a range of effective alternatives and strategies that minimise their symptoms, treat the underlying causes of their headaches and improve their overall health. The surprising part for many of my clients is that we treat the whole body. Headaches are not all in your head. You feel the pain in your head, but it is referred pain, from elsewhere in your body. You must treat the body to successfully treat recurring headaches.

I'm excited to share these strategies with you and to hopefully convince you of the importance of treating the musculoskeletal system when you treat your headaches. It isn't something you will find discussed in detail in very many headache books, but I believe it is the key to unlocking a headache-free future.

This book offers you the very opposite of OTC painkillers – this is not about finding a quick fix and moving on. I am about long-term solutions and improvements that will put you in control of your condition. I want to do for you what I've done for so many of my clients – help you understand what's happening when you get a headache, give you the tools to find, treat and manage the cause of your headache and encourage you, over time, to be able to reduce the frequency and intensity of future attacks.

In a Nutshell

I care about your wellbeing now, and I care about how you will be coping with headaches in five years. Most of this book is about working towards long-term, sustained solutions, but there are some things you can do that will bring you immediate relief.

While you're reading this book, I recommend starting with some basic strategies and changes that could deliver a big improvement to the frequency and severity of your headaches:

- Have at least 3–5 professional manual therapy treatments
- Stop sleeping on your stomach
- Don't carry bags over one shoulder
- Do some simple stretching and strengthening exercises for your neck and shoulder muscles
- Don't sit for prolonged periods. Take regular breaks and move around
- Be aware of your posture – avoid rounded shoulders and a protruding chin
- Stay well hydrated by drinking water throughout the day
- Eat regularly spaced meals at about the same time each day and eat a varied, healthy, balanced diet. Avoid sugary drinks and snacks
- Do regular, moderate aerobic exercise
- Get enough sleep so that you don't feel sleepy during the day
- Keep a regular sleep pattern – go to bed and get up at about the same time each day
- If you smoke or take illicit drugs, start a program to stop.

The following chapters are grouped into Parts framed around the subtitle of the book: Understanding, Managing and Preventing Headaches

Part A

Understanding:

Headaches

1

The Integrated Headache Model

Traditionally, tension headaches and migraine have been considered distinct conditions with different underlying causes. Tension headaches were thought to be caused by muscular problems, and migraine headaches were thought to be caused by vascular and/or neurological issues. Both conditions were often treated with medication – usually OTC painkillers for tension headaches and prescribed medications for migraine.

I am not very interested in what type of headache my clients have, or think they have, when they come to see me. Don't get me wrong, I'm concerned they're in pain, I want to know all about their symptoms and I am ready to help them reduce the frequency and severity of their headaches, but I am not interested in giving their headache a label.

Labels can be reassuring, and helpful, but they come with baggage – calling a headache a migraine usually generates more sympathy and consideration than saying you have a tension headache. We tend to think people are afflicted by migraines, where tension headaches are somehow the sufferer's fault.

In my experience, labels get in the way of successful treatment. Attaching symptoms to a label can be deceiving and counterproductive. Classic signs of migraine can actually be the symptoms of a tension headache, so if you keep mistakenly calling your tension headache a migraine, you will never improve it.

Categorising the underlying mechanism of tension headaches as muscular, and migraine as neurovascular is artificial and counterintuitive. There are many similarities between tension headaches and migraines, particularly in their chronic forms, and muscles, joints, blood vessels and nerves don't work in isolation – a malfunction in one system will impact the other systems in the body.

This is not to say I think a migraine is the same as a tension headache. What I am saying is that migraine and tension headaches have more in common than we think. The longer I've worked with clients to lessen the impact of headaches on their life, the more I am convinced that migraine and tension are different points on a headache spectrum, not different conditions.

Many scientists now view tension headaches and migraines as two ends of a spectrum,[1,2,3] rather than as separate entities. They believe tension headache and migraine share a common cause, but progress differently, depending on the unique conditions of the individual headache sufferer.

In 1991, the prominent headache researcher Dr. Jes Olesen presented his three-component model for headache pain, which articulated the three common causes of headache pain as myofascial, supraspinal and vascular. Importantly, for the first time, a model explicitly included a contribution to headache pain from muscular trigger points.

Quoting from Olesen's paper:

> *The model explains much of the complexity of the clinical picture of these disorders as well as their tendency to overlap and to change into one another.*
>
> *[The model also explains] ... why muscles are tender during migraine, why trigger-point injection may cure migraine attacks and why chronic tension-type headache is often associated with episodes of pulsating pain ... It may thus serve a useful purpose in explaining the disorder to patients.*[4]

Over the years of treating headache and migraine sufferers, I have broadened the components of this model to musculoskeletal, emotional and neurovascular.

Let's consider these factors individually first.

Musculoskeletal Factors

Your musculoskeletal system includes all the bones, muscles, joints, tendons, ligaments, cartilage and other connective tissue in your body. All these elements work together to keep you moving and stable. The impact of the musculoskeletal system on headache pain can be felt partly through posture, stiff joints and muscular tension and mostly through the development of muscular trigger points.

Muscular trigger points (not to be confused with headache triggers such as coffee or red wine) are hard nodules within a tight band of muscle fibres that are very painful when pressed.

Muscular trigger points are well recognised as a source of headache pain by both dentists and manual therapists, however, in my experience, very few doctors are aware of muscular trigger points and their role in producing pain in the body, and their impact on headaches in particular.

Emotional Factors

Both tension headache and migraine sufferers identify emotional stress as one of their most common headache triggers. Emotional stress is defined into two broad categories – acute and chronic. Acute stress is the 'fight or flight' sensation brought on by an immediate, unusual or unexpected event, like public speaking or a car accident. Chronic stress is the everyday stress of living – relationships, commuting, kids, work and paying bills.

Both acute and chronic stress can be divided again into eustress – positive events – and distress – negative events. A wedding, a new baby, a promotion, winning money are all examples of eustress and divorce, injury, financial problems and ill health are all distress. All these stresses influence how intensely you feel headache pain.

Neurovascular Factors

'Neuro' refers to the nervous tissue of the brain and 'vascular' to the blood vessels that supply blood to the brain.

In the past, migraines were attributed to either vascular or neurological factors. The vascular migraine was thought to be due to the constriction of blood vessels that supply the brain, reducing oxygen levels in the brain, which leads to a protective reflex in which the blood vessels dilate to increase blood supply.

According to the neurological theory, migraines start within the nervous tissue of the brain. A temporary malfunction within the brain-stem causes it to fire off erratic nerve signals, similar to what happens during epileptic seizures. These signals travel outward along the trigeminal nerve system, the main sensory nerve of the face, which releases inflammatory substances that cause parts of the meninges – the membranes covering the brain – to become inflamed. Pain receptors in the meninges send nerve signals back along the trigeminal nerve system to the brain-stem. This continues to fire off more nerve signals causing more inflammatory substances to be released from the trigeminal nerve endings, in a self-perpetuating cycle.

The neurovascular theory unifies the neurological and vascular theories. It asserts that migraines start in the brain-stem, but dilation of blood vessels and inflammation of the meninges are both important sources of pain, and both contribute to the progression of the attack. This seems to me to be the most sensible theory and the one which matches most people's experience of a migraine.

The Integrated Headache Model

I believe these three factors are always at play in every headache you have. Headaches differ, between people and for each individual, because of the balance between these three factors. Just as the three core ingredients in bread – flour, water and yeast – can be combined in different ratios to make different types of loaves – pita, dinner rolls and a sandwich loaf – so the musculoskeletal, neurovascular and emotional factors combine to make different types of headaches. The same three ingredients, producing the same thing, but each with its own characteristics. And each factor influences the others, for better and for worse.

Emotional stress can affect the neurovascular component of a headache by altering blood flow to and within the brain, increasing the excitability of the nervous system in response to stimuli such as light or sound, and triggering the release of histamine, a potent vasodilator (widener of the blood vessels) and inflammatory substance. Emotional stress contributes directly to musculoskeletal pain by making muscular trigger points more painful (through interference with pain suppression), and indirectly by increasing muscle tension and increasing jaw and neck stiffness by initiating actions like teeth clenching and grinding.

Muscular trigger points and stiff neck joints can impact the neurovascular factors indirectly by constricting blood vessels, mechanically irritating nerves by friction, compressing or stretching, and chemically irritating nerves and blood vessels by releasing inflammatory substances and putting traction on the highly pain-sensitive dural tissues of the meninges.

The Integrated Headache Model considers the amount each of these three factors brings to your headache. The percentage of musculoskeletal, neurovascular and emotional contributions vary from one attack to the next, and so your headaches will vary in severity, and in the extent to which they show typical migraine or tension headache features. If neurovascular pain is the major pain source, your headaches will be migraine-like. If musculoskeletal pain is dominant, you will experience a tension headache.

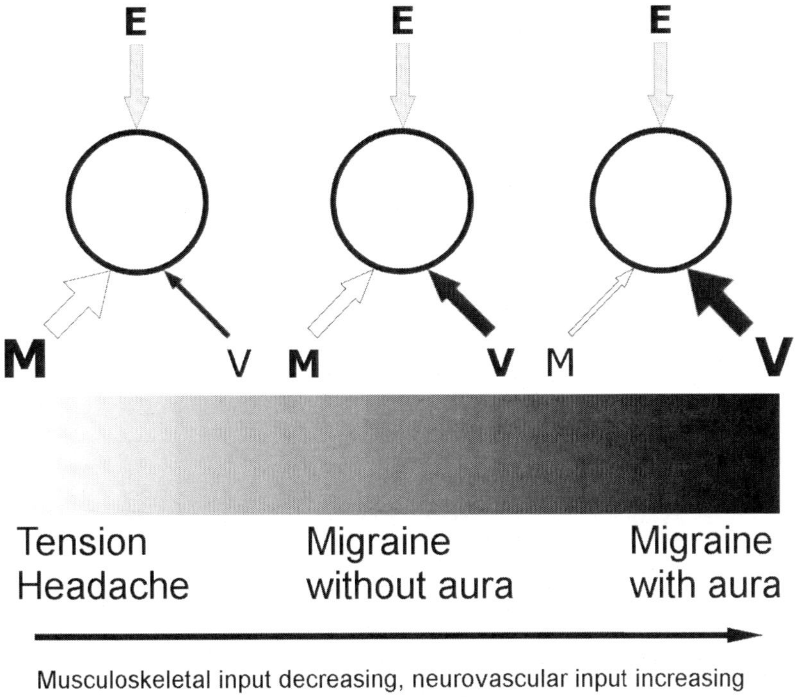

Figure 1.1 – The Integrated Headache Model

The circle represents the trigeminocervical nucleus (headache pain centre). Different arrows represent the musculoskeletal (M), neurovascular (V) and emotional (E) inputs to the trigeminocervical nucleus. The thickness of an arrow indicates whether that contribution is small, medium or large.

You can see the progressive change from tension headache to migraine as pain from neurovascular sources becomes proportionately more important.

The emotional contribution has been kept constant in the diagram to simplify the discussion. If it were to increase or decrease, the resulting headache would have the same features but vary in severity. For example, on the right of the diagram, raising the emotional contribution would lead to a more severe migraine with aura. Lowering the emotional contribution, so pain suppression mechanisms become more effective, may lead to migraine aura without the headache.

The main benefit of the Integrated Headache Model is it gives the appropriate, significant emphasis to the musculoskeletal system as a major factor in producing and intensifying headache pain for both migraine and tension headaches and it allows you to better understand how each of these factors influences the others.

Dealing with one factor will perhaps reduce your pain in the moment, but to manage your headaches successfully over time, you need to deal with all three factors. The Integrated Headache Model also provides insight into why common-sense advice works, and why ignoring it is likely to cause problems in the longer term.

I believe an integrated approach, one that considers and treats the impact of musculoskeletal, neurovascular and emotional factors, is the best approach to diagnosing and treating every kind of headache.

Key Points

- The Integrated Headache Model is an approach to headache diagnosis and treatment that considers all headaches as part of the same continuum, rather than separate conditions.
- The three factors that are part of every headache along the Integrated Headache Model continuum are musculoskeletal, neurovascular and emotional factors.
- Just as three core ingredients in bread – flour, water and yeast – can be combined in different ratios to make different types of bread, so the musculoskeletal, neurovascular and emotional factors combine to make different types of headaches.
- If musculoskeletal factors are dominant, you will experience a tension headache.
- If neurovascular factors are dominant, you will experience a migraine.
- Emotional factors act as a volume control for your pain.
- Musculoskeletal factors are the easiest to treat and the most overlooked in treating headaches.

2

Is It All in My Head?

Although you may feel like your brain is about to explode when you have a headache, it's not your brain that's hurting. Brain tissue (the grey and white matter) doesn't feel pain because it doesn't have any pain receptors. (Which is why most brain surgery can be done using just a local anaesthetic.)

Headache pain is complex. The whole head, neck and upper shoulder region is crammed full of pain sensitive anatomical structures that can cause a headache, as well as an extensive network of sensory nerves that transmit pain signals to the brain. Pain signals come from both chemical receptors stimulated by inflammatory chemicals and from mechanical receptors, particularly stretch receptors, activated by tissue swelling.

Not every anatomical structure in this region causes pain that's perceived as headache, but many do. It depends on the nerve pathway the pain message takes.

The most important structures responsible for headache pain are:

- Neck and jaw muscles
- Neck joints
- Jaw joints
- The meninges – membranes that cover the brain and spinal cord. They are the part of the brain that becomes very painfully infected in meningitis.
- Blood vessels
- Nerves.

The Headache Pain Centre

To make the process more complex, all the pain messages from these structures go through one central transmitter – the trigeminocervical nucleus.

The trigeminocervical nucleus is a small portion of nerve tissue in the lower part of the brain stem, near where the brain stem merges with the top of the spinal cord. It's made up of three different nerves:

- The trigeminal nerve – a very extensive nerve system with multiple branches
- The greater occipital nerve
- The three uppermost cervical (neck) nerves.

These three nerves are wired up so that pain signals from the head and neck are combined before being relayed to the higher parts of the brain for processing. The brain interprets this combination of pain signals as a headache.

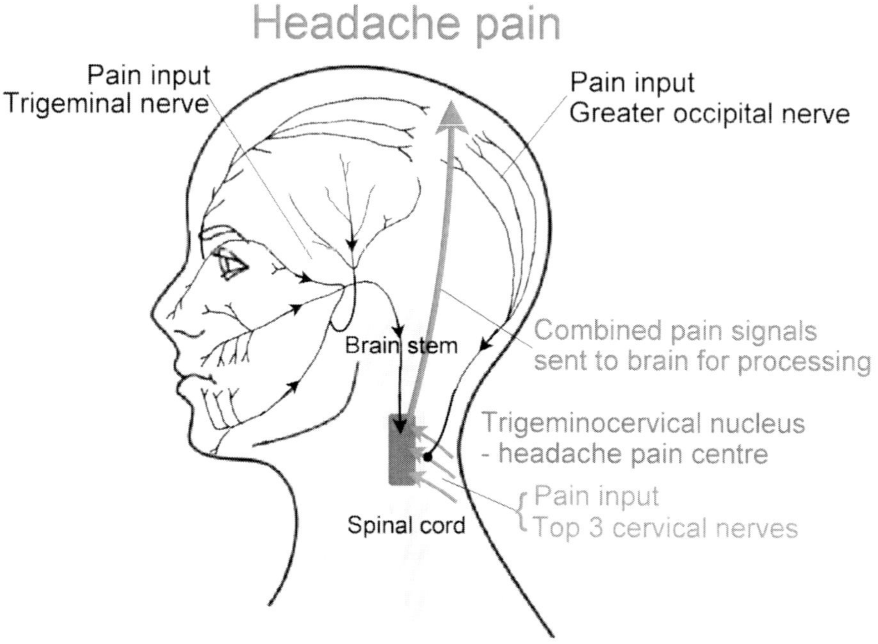

Figure 2.1 – The 'Headache Pain Centre' and nerves which carry headache pain

How It All Works

If you imagine the brain as a cauliflower, then the short stalk it sits on is the brain stem.

The brain stem is a primitive area of the brain that controls the functions for survival, such as breathing, heart rate, blood pressure and digestion, without us having to think about them.

The area of the brain concerned with higher functions, such as thought, memory, language and awareness, is the cerebral cortex. It is the outside layer of the brain and is about 2– 4 mm thick and highly folded.

Below the brain stem and continuous with it, is the spinal cord, protected inside the bones of the spine. Together, the brain and spinal cord make up the central nervous system.

Messages are transmitted between the central nervous system and the rest of the body by a network of peripheral nerves.

The peripheral nerves that serve the head come from the brain stem. The nerves that serve the neck, shoulders and other parts of the body come from different sections of the spinal cord. Peripheral nerves contain large numbers of individual nerve fibres grouped together in bundles.

There are three different types of nerve fibres:

Sensory Nerve Fibres

Sensory nerve fibres carry messages to the central nervous system from sensory receptors located throughout the body.

For example, the eyes and ears gather information about the external environment, and receptors within the body gather information about the internal environment, such as blood pressure, the state of contraction of the muscles and blood glucose levels.

Pain messages are carried to the brain by specialised sensory nerve fibres.

Motor Nerve Fibres

Motor nerve fibres carry messages from the central nervous system to the muscles attached to the skeleton.

Autonomic Nerve Fibres

Autonomic nerve fibres carry messages from the central nervous system to organs such as the heart, lungs and digestive tract and to glands such as tear and sweat glands.

The autonomic nervous system has two divisions – the sympathetic or 'fight or flight' system and the parasympathetic or 'rest and digest' system.

These tend to act in opposition to each other – a bit like an accelerator and a brake – keeping the internal environment of the body constant within its narrow limits, despite changes in the external environment.

Many of the unpleasant symptoms that accompany migraine attacks are the result of increased sympathetic nervous activity as the body goes 'on alert'. These include:

- Nausea, vomiting and diarrhoea
- Delayed emptying of the stomach (which prevents oral medications from being absorbed from the small intestine)
- Re-routing of blood from the skin and gut to the muscles, brain and lungs, leading to pale skin as well as cold hands and feet
- Sensitivity to light and sound, and blurred vision.

On the other hand, several other common migraine symptoms, such as a runny or stuffy nose and watering eyes, are due to increased parasympathetic, or 'resting' nervous activity.

In headache sufferers, and especially those with migraine, the autonomic nervous system seems to be over-reactive. The parasympathetic system tends to over-correct the effects of the sympathetic system, and vice versa. As a result, blood vessels dilate and constrict more readily, and heart rate and blood pressure are more variable.

Pain

Registering Pain

Pain is the way higher regions of the brain are notified of actual or potential tissue damage in the periphery of the body. Pain is detected by special pain receptors, found in most tissues.

There are three types of pain receptors:

- Mechanical pain receptors which respond to direct mechanical pressure when the tissue is squeezed, crushed or stretched, including when it's stretched by the swelling which accompanies inflammation
- Thermal pain receptors which respond to extremes of heat and cold
- Chemical pain receptors which respond to external chemicals like bee venom and to the body's own inflammatory chemicals which are released in response to tissue damage.

A pain receptor won't fire unless it receives a stimulus larger than its threshold value. When this occurs, the receptor produces a nerve signal, a pulse of electrical energy, which travels along a sensory nerve to the spinal cord or brain stem. From there, it goes to the higher areas of the brain, where it's processed.

Processing Pain

Once the pain message is received, it's processed in several of the higher areas of the brain, each performing different functions:

- One area registers the pain and determines its source
- The emotional part of the brain generates the feeling of unpleasantness associated with the pain
- The thinking part of the brain assigns meaning to the pain, and decides what action to take.

The uppermost layers of the skin have lots of pain receptors, which means pain from injuries to the skin is sharp, well-defined, short-lived and highly localised – we can tell quickly and easily where the pain is coming from.

Not all pain is as easy to identify. Deeper tissues such as muscles, bones, blood vessels and organs contain fewer pain receptors. The pain they produce is typically duller, more aching, longer lasting and more diffuse. It is often referred to areas much closer to the surface of the body, with more pain receptors, such as the skin.

Referred pain is pain that is felt in a place other than its origin. It occurs when two sensory nerves join to the same part of the spinal cord or brain stem. The higher area of the brain, whose role is to determine where the pain is coming from, can get confused and misidentify the source of the pain.

Typically, when this happens, one sensory nerve sends a message from a tissue with few pain receptors, like an artery, whereas the other comes from a tissue with many more pain receptors, like the skin. One of the best-known examples of referred pain is when the pain of a heart attack is felt in the left arm rather than in the chest.

Headache Pain is Referred Pain

The most important thing to understand here is that all headache pain is referred pain. Migraines, tension headaches, cluster headaches and sinus headaches – all referred pain. Signals from different pain sensitive areas are combined in the trigeminocervical nucleus and shared along a common pathway to the higher areas of the brain. The brain receives and registers the pain message, but can't distinguish where the messages originally came from.

The location of the pain may be quite distant from the site where it's produced. For example, pain from the muscles at the back of the neck is often felt in the front of the head as pain over the eye. And, to complicate matters, the same spot also registers pain from the inflammation of blood vessels inside the skull.

Any pain sensitive structure in the head, neck and shoulders that transmits pain signals along any of the main nerves can contribute to headache pain. The location of the pain in your head is a poor guide to which anatomical structures are responsible for it.

An 'ice cream' or 'brain freeze' headache is a classic example of referred pain felt as a headache. This brief stabbing headache affects up to a third of people when they quickly consume something very cold. The headache starts after about 10 seconds and may last from 20 seconds to a few minutes. The pain is usually felt in the middle of the forehead, but it can also be behind one eye, or at the side of the head.

Cold food or drink touching the back of the roof of the mouth rapidly cools the blood vessels, causing them to constrict. As the blood vessels warm up again they dilate, triggering nearby pain receptors. These send pain signals through the trigeminal nerve to the brain. However, facial pain also travels via the trigeminal nerve to the brain. Because the skin of the face has many more pain receptors than the blood vessels, the brain misinterprets the source of the pain as the forehead.

What Does This Mean for Treating Your Headache?

To alleviate your headaches, particularly recurring headaches, you need to locate the original source of the pain. You can alleviate the sensation of the pain, with or without drugs, but unless you find the source, your headaches will mysteriously reappear and you will be no closer to freeing yourself of the pain permanently.

It's like a flashlight beamed into the night sky – the light comes from a distant source, and the more flashlights you have on, the brighter the sky is and the harder it is to find the source. You need to locate the source and turn each flashlight off, one by one.

The next chapter discusses the most common sources of referred headache pain so you can start to investigate where your headaches might be originating from. Once you've found the source of the pain, you can begin to treat it, often with surprisingly dramatic improvements.

Key Points

- All headache pain is referred pain.
- Referred pain is pain that originates in one place and is felt in another. An 'ice cream' headache is a classic example.
- If you want to alleviate headache pain, you need to find and treat the original source of the pain.
- It's like a flashlight beamed into the night sky – the light comes from a distant source, and the more flashlights you have on, the brighter the sky is and the harder it is to find the source. You need to locate the source and turn each flashlight off, one by one.

3

If It's Not in My Head, Where Is It?

Muscular trigger points, joints, blood vessels, meninges and nerves are all sources of headache pain, but the main culprit is the muscular trigger point, one of the most common and most neglected sources of headache pain.

Referred Pain from Muscular Trigger Points

What Are They?

A muscular trigger point is a hard nodule within a taut band of muscle tissue. At the microscopic level, the taut band consists of a collection of muscle fibres that are in a highly contracted state. Part of each muscle fibre is contracted into a knot, which is a lot thicker than normal, while the rest of the fibre is stretched thin.

The knot in each muscle fibre restricts blood flow in the immediate area and combines into a collection of knots, acting like a kink in a garden hose. Travell and Simons, in their ground-breaking book, *Myofascial Pain and Dysfunction: The Trigger Point Manual*, describe a muscular trigger point as 'a nest of hornets that contains multiple minute sources of intense trouble.' [5]

A muscular trigger point can feel like a grain of rice or a small pea. It's very painful when pressed, or 'palpated' to use the technical term for the way a manual therapist will press it. In contrast, healthy muscle tissue does not contain tight bands or nodules and it is not overly sensitive to pressure.

When a muscle has muscular trigger points, it contains a number of abnormally tight bands that run parallel to the muscle fibres from one end of the muscle to the other.

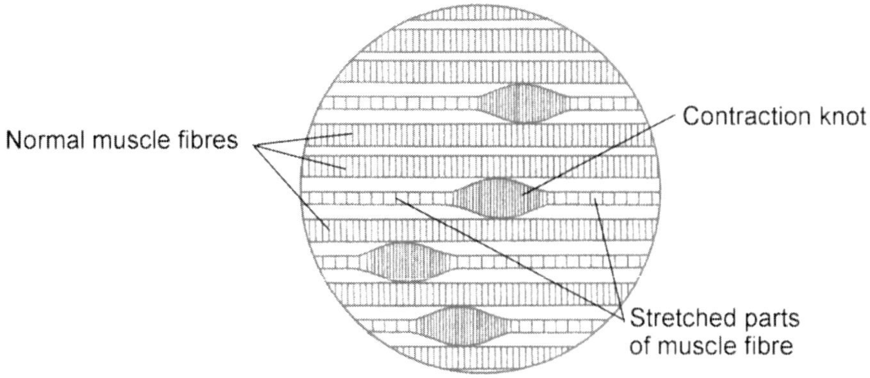

Figure 3.1 – Magnified view of muscle fibres in a Central muscular trigger point

The area of the muscle near a muscular trigger point is starved of oxygen and nutrients. Lactic acid and metabolic waste products accumulate around the trigger point, which causes tissue damage. The damaged tissue sends out pain signals, which release natural inflammatory substances. These further irritate the muscular trigger point, causing swelling on a microscopic scale, and increase the pain, which is why it hurts when a muscular trigger point is pressed.

Where Are They?

Muscular trigger points can be found at the centre of a muscle, at the junction with the motor nerve that carries messages from the brain telling the muscle to contract (Central muscular trigger point). They also tend to form at the end-points of the muscle where it attaches to tendons, as a result of the continual pulling on these areas by the taut band (Attachment muscular trigger points). Attachment muscular trigger points often stop causing pain when the Central muscular trigger point is treated.

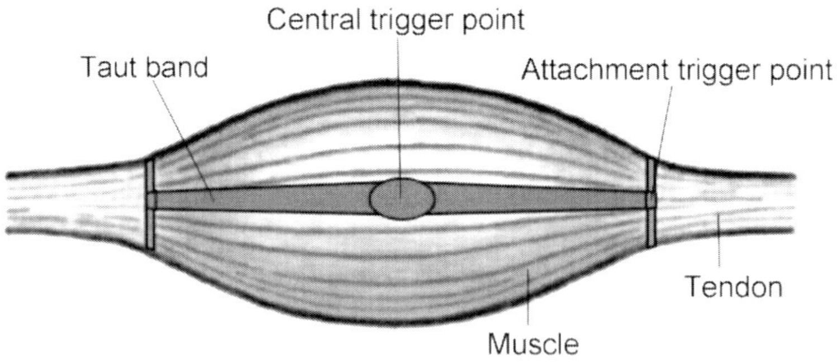

Figure 3.2 – Muscle with taut band and Central and Attachment muscular trigger points

Muscular trigger points are surprisingly common and can be found anywhere there's a muscle, but the ones I'm interested in are those in the following five muscles, which are the muscular trigger points most often involved in producing headache pain and which cause some of the most powerful headache symptoms:

- The SCM (sternocleidomastoid) muscles or 'neck cords' at the front of the neck
- The upper part of the powerful trapezius muscle that extends down the back of the neck across the top of the shoulders to the upper back
- The sub-occipital muscle group at the base of the skull
- The masseter muscle that closes the jaw and is used in chewing
- The temporalis muscle in the temple region above the ear. It also closes the jaw and is used in chewing.

Active, Latent and Satellite Muscular Trigger Points

Muscular trigger points can be either active or latent depending on how irritated they are. Both states cause tightness, weakness, lack of endurance and a restricted range of motion in the affected muscle, and sometimes spasms in other muscles.

Both active and latent muscular trigger points produce pain on palpation, however, only active muscular trigger points produce pain spontaneously.

Latent muscular trigger points tend to increase in number as we age, causing stiffness, altered movement patterns and reduced mobility. They're much more common than active muscular trigger points. Latent muscular trigger points can become active due to factors such as muscle overuse, cold, a viral illness or stress.

Conversely, an active muscular trigger point will occasionally revert to a latent state and stop producing pain. However, it doesn't disappear and it can be reactivated. Although they may change state from active to latent and back again, muscular trigger points won't go away unless they're treated.

In fact, as we get older, muscular trigger points become more irritated. Latent muscular trigger points start to become active and active muscular trigger points become more painful. Before, active muscular trigger points may have only produced pain with certain movements; as we age, they might produce pain constantly, even at rest.

Muscular trigger points also tend to multiply, producing satellite muscular trigger points in other muscles. Satellite muscular trigger points may form in muscles which are in the pain referral zone of the original muscular trigger point or which share the same nerve supply. For example, muscular trigger points in the powerful SCM and upper trapezius muscles tend to produce satellite muscular trigger points in the masseter and temporalis muscles and numerous other muscles in the face and neck. Satellite muscular trigger points may also form in muscles that are overloaded by substituting for muscles containing muscular trigger points and counteracting increased tension in muscles with muscular trigger points.

This is because movement requires muscles to act together in a coordinated fashion. Muscles are organised in pairs with opposite actions. For movement to occur, as the main muscle responsible for the movement contracts, the opposing muscle which reverses the movement must relax. Any 'helper' muscles contract at the same time as the main mover.

A muscle containing either active or latent muscular trigger points is both tighter and weaker than normal. This will cause extra tension on the opposing muscle. It will also place more demand on the helper muscles.

Why Do We Get Trigger Points?

Muscular trigger points are caused by damage to muscle fibres, either directly, because of an injury to the muscle, or indirectly, due to a range of metabolic, environmental and lifestyle factors.

Direct Damage

It's easy to understand how direct damage to a muscle can occur from an acute injury, such as a sporting injury or motor vehicle accident: muscle fibres are overstretched or torn on impact and you know why it's sore.

However, direct damage is much more commonly caused by repeated or on-going overuse of a muscle, or what is a called a chronic injury. When a muscle suffers a chronic injury, its fibres aren't torn. Instead, their internal structure is disrupted.

Muscles in action are muscles that actively contract and relax. A contracting muscle is shorter and fatter than a relaxed muscle. When it contracts, a muscle compresses the small capillaries that pass between individual muscle fibres and supply them with blood. Blood flow to the muscle starts to be restricted when the muscle is only exerting 5% of its full power, and stops completely at 50% of full power. During sustained periods of muscle contraction, groups of muscle fibres work in relays, some groups relaxing while others are working.

Relaxation allows fresh blood to enter the muscle. Fresh blood replenishes depleted supplies of oxygen, fuel and other nutrients, so more energy can be generated. It also removes metabolic waste products.

If a muscle is contracted too strongly or for too long, some of its fibres will start to run low on energy. Eventually, they may not have enough energy left to throw the biochemical switch that releases the contraction, so even when the brain stops telling the fibres to contract, the fibres remain locked in a contracted state, unable to return to their normal resting length. This is how a taut band forms within the muscle.

If the muscle is rested, the taut band may disappear. However, if it continues to be overused, segments of the contracted fibres within the taut band can go into a state of uncontrolled local hypercontraction, like a type of on-going mini-cramp which involves a few muscle fibres rather than the whole muscle. A series of knots form, which are the beginnings of a muscular trigger point.

Indirect Damage

Muscle fibres may also develop muscular trigger points as a result of indirect damage. This can be caused by a range of factors including:

- Getting too cold (the body uses muscle contraction to generate heat)
- Insufficient levels in the body of certain key vitamins and minerals that are essential for the proper functioning of nerves and muscles. The most important are the vitamins C, B1, B6, B12, folic acid and D, and the minerals calcium, magnesium, iron and potassium
- Underactive thyroid
- Fasting
- Drinking insufficient fluid (dehydration reduces blood flow to the muscles)
- Restriction of blood flow by tight clothing
- Non-restorative sleep in which you awake feeling unrested (this means you had insufficient deep sleep – muscle repair takes place during this stage of the sleep cycle)
- Certain prescription medications, especially calcium channel blockers for hypertension and statins for lowering blood cholesterol levels
- Infections and allergies (these cause high levels of inflammatory compounds such as histamine in the blood stream)
- Smoking (this constricts blood vessels causing lower blood flow and reduces the amount of oxygen the blood can hold).

These same factors may also cause previously latent muscular trigger points to become active.

Muscular Trigger Points in Neck and Jaw Muscles

Muscular trigger points in the neck and jaw muscles are one of the most common causes of headache pain. They may occur from a sudden injury or develop over time by bad habits and incorrect posture.

Neck and jaw muscles readily suffer acute injuries in motor vehicle accidents, falls and in playing certain sports. Sudden sharp motion of the head and neck, either backwards and forwards (whiplash) or to the side, causes these muscles to be over-stretched or over-contracted.

The incident doesn't have to be serious. Neck muscles can be injured by excessive or unusual exercise, such as lifting a weight that is too heavy or head-rolling movements in an exercise class. Even the impact of a soccer ball to the head or a minor head-to-tail or side-on vehicle collision may be enough to cause muscular trigger points.

If not recognised and treated, they may cause chronic headaches and neck pain that can last for years, often well after the original injury has been forgotten. Muscular trigger points in the neck and jaw may also irritate nerves, causing symptoms that present as nerve damage, such as numbness and tingling in the arms and hands.

Case Study – Joe and his Undiagnosed Muscular Trigger Points

Joe didn't originally come to see me because of his headaches. He had badly broken his leg and ankle in a fall at work and a metal plate had been inserted in his leg. Ever since his fall, Joe had been in severe and continual pain at the site of his fracture.

He had been advised that an operation to fuse his ankle and shin bone may alleviate his pain. His doctor referred him to me to see if surgery could be avoided.

We were getting some good results. His pain was a lot less and he had more mobility in his leg and ankle. Perhaps it was because of these improvements that he brought up the subject of his headaches. Joe told me he had suffered headaches almost every day for the last 30 years, following a car accident when he was 18.

Joe's headaches were investigated at the time of the accident but no cause was ever found. Nothing would fix the pain. It was there all the time and he had no choice but to put up with it.

When the pain got very bad, Joe would seek medical help. On one of these occasions, he was prescribed a synthetic opioid, Tramadol, which he found dulled the pain, together with Stemetil, an anti-nausea drug. The Tramadol made him feel like 'a total zombie' so he stopped taking it.

Just recently, Joe had been prescribed Maxalt, a triptan used as a migraine abortive, which he put under his tongue to dissolve. This was the only thing that had ever helped his headaches but he was advised against taking it too often.

Since his fall, Joe had still needed to take Maxalt several times for his headaches. The relatively powerful painkillers he was taking for his leg and ankle pain didn't touch his more severe headache attacks.

It turned out that Joe had several very active muscular trigger points in his trapezius and sternocleidomastoid muscles which I immediately treated. The impact was incredible. Even I was amazed at the results of just half a session spent treating these muscular trigger points.

When I saw Joe again after 3 months, he told me he had only experienced one or two mild headaches and he had not needed to take any more Maxalt.

This was the first time in 30 years that Joe had been free of severe headache pain.

Whilst Joe's muscular trigger points were due to his car accident, by far the most common cause of muscular trigger points in the neck and jaw muscles is chronic injury due to overuse of fatigued muscles.

Some of the ways that this typically occurs are:

- Repetitive movements, especially long-term and relatively low-energy movements, such as typing, using a computer mouse, chewing gum, grinding your teeth or sending text messages
- Holding or repeating awkward postures, such as craning your head forward to look at a computer screen, watching TV while slumped on the couch, cradling a phone between your ear and shoulder and continually looking upwards while working above head level
- Emotional stress causing sustained muscular tension. Tensing the muscles of the face, shoulders, neck and upper back is a common response to feeling under stress, as is clenching the jaw and grinding teeth
- Sitting without moving for long periods of time, such as in front of the computer or TV. Movement is needed to make sure fresh blood is kept pumping through the muscles
- Incorrect breathing high into the chest leads to chronic overload of the neck muscles, especially the sternocleidomastoid
- Stiff neck joints which alter your patterns of muscle use, overloading some muscles and under-using others, and pulling on the muscle attachments.

Forward Head Posture

One of the main causes of muscular trigger points in the neck and jaw is sitting in front of a computer for a few hours without moving. It may seem like you haven't been using your muscles at all, but the muscles in your neck and shoulders have been working hard just to hold your head up.

Your head is not perfectly balanced on top of your spine. It has slightly more weight towards the front which is why your head falls forward when you fall asleep – your muscles relax and, unsupported, your head falls forward towards your chest.

Your head weighs around 5kg (10 pounds), about the same as a bowling ball. Think about how long you could hold a 5kg weight stationary before your muscles got tired. Now imagine lowering the weight a small amount and continuing to hold it. The effort involved in counteracting the force of gravity is much greater than before.

Similarly, the stress on your neck and shoulder muscles is much greater if you crane your head forward to look at your computer screen. For every 3cm (1 inch) your head moves forward from a neutral balanced position, the effective weight of your head increases by an extra 5kg.

In this 'forward head posture', which often tends to go with rounded shoulders, you are using muscles to hold up your head that were not designed for that purpose and therefore tire easily.

Forward head posture is a potent cause of muscular trigger points in many muscles of the neck, jaw and upper shoulders, including the trapezius, sub-occipital and SCM muscles.

Projecting your head forwards also compresses the joints and intervertebral discs of your neck, causing pain and accelerating the normal processes of wear and tear, and it alters the alignment of your jaw joint. In fact, computer use in the modern office could be seen as a recipe for producing muscular trigger points and headache pain.

How Do You Get Rid of Muscular Trigger Points?

Muscles with muscular trigger points are chronically contracted, which means they can't relax on their own. Normally, when the signals stop from the brain to a muscle, the muscle stops contracting and starts to relax and lengthen. When a muscle with a muscular trigger point tries to lengthen, the fibres in the taut band are increasingly stretched, pulling on the muscle attachments. This causes pain, which prevents any additional lengthening and the taut band and the muscle are unable to fully relax.

You can find muscular trigger points by applying pressure. Pressure on an active muscular trigger point should produce pain that you recognise as the pain you usually feel, and any other symptoms, such as nausea. In contrast, the pain produced by the palpation of a latent muscular trigger point will not seem familiar to you, and is usually less severe.

Sometimes palpation of a muscular trigger point will lead to what is called a local twitch response, a reflex contraction of the muscle fibres in the tight band only, not the whole muscle.

The twitch, which can be readily felt and seen by both patient and therapist, releases the muscular trigger point. The twitch also confirms the muscular trigger point was accurately located.

Disruption of the tiny knots in the muscular trigger point:

- Restores circulation to the area
- Allows the pain-producing inflammatory substances to disperse
- Allows the taut band to relax so the tight muscle can be stretched and restored to its normal resting length, improving muscle function.

After muscular trigger points are released, the muscle must be stretched to allow it to progressively lengthen. Enabling the muscle to relax and lengthen is an integral part of the treatment of muscular trigger points. It's essential if you want to achieve long-term pain relief.

Referred Pain

Referred Pain from Joints

A joint is a place where two bones meet. Elbows, knees, ankles, wrists, shoulders – joints are everywhere. Almost all joints in the body have the same basic structure, made up of bones, muscles, cartilage, tendons, ligaments and other connective tissue.

Muscles keep the bones in place and move them through contraction or extension. Cartilage, not as rigid as bone, but stiffer than muscle, prevents the bone ends from rubbing on each other and acts as a shock absorber. Tendons are bands of fibrous tissue that connect the muscles to the bones. Ligaments are also bands of fibrous tissue that connect the ends of bones together to form a joint, providing support for the joint as it moves.

The detailed way in which a joint is constructed determines how much and what type of movement can occur around it. However, its range of motion will be less than normal if the muscles attached to it are tight. Restrictions in the other soft tissues discussed above may also contribute to loss of normal joint mobility.

Joints can be affected by illnesses such as arthritis and bursitis, by a sudden impact through extra activity or extra pressure or by repeated impact through exercise or being overweight.

You should take good care of all your joints, but it's the specialised joints of the neck and, to a lesser extent, the jaw that you need to understand when looking at the various referred sources of headache pain.

Neck and Jaw Joints

The three uppermost joints of the neck, located just below the base of the skull, are a common source of headache pain.

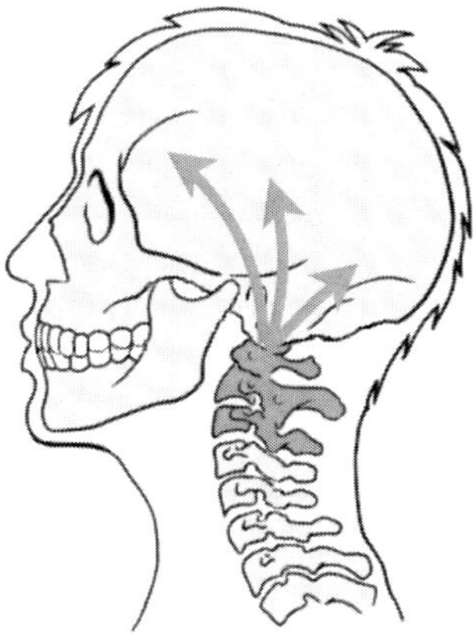

Figure 3.3 – Referred headache pain from stiff upper neck joints

The most common cause of headache pain from these joints is stiffness and restricted range of movement. This is often put down to age-related wear and tear, but usually poor head and neck posture has considerably more impact. Excessive or abnormal movement of the neck joints, and stretching forces on the ligaments can also contribute to headache pain.

The jaw joint is another culprit of headache pain and of referred pain in the face, ear, eye, sinuses, and teeth. Problems can start when the joint is inflamed, immobile or not tracking correctly. It requires careful examination to distinguish whether the pain is coming from the muscles that move the jaw or from the jaw joint itself.

Referred Pain from Blood Vessels

All blood vessels are wrapped in a fine network of nerves that is activated when the vessels dilate (widen), constrict (narrow) or when they pass through inflamed tissues.

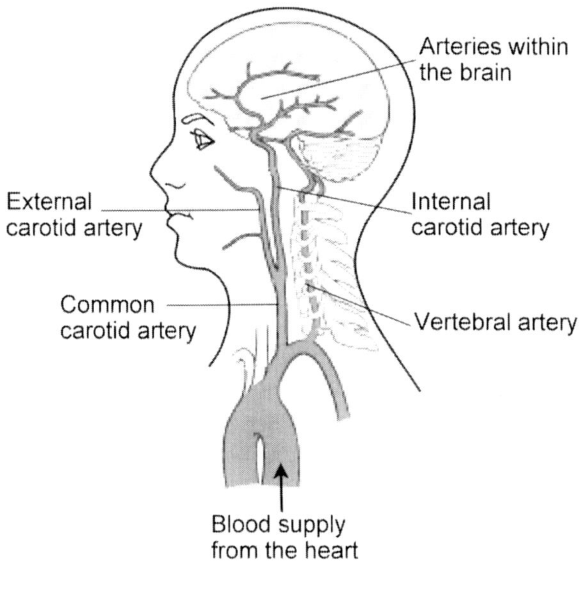

Figure 3.4 – Blood supply to the brain

Blood vessels located outside the skull, just below the surface of the skin, produce pain in the nearby area, whereas the pain from blood vessels within the skull is referred elsewhere. A complex overlapping pain pattern results.

Two pairs of large arteries, the carotid and vertebral arteries, supply blood to the head and neck. These arteries form an extensive highly branched network within the main mass of brain tissue and on its surface. A similarly extensive network of channels and veins drains blood from the brain and directs it into the large jugular veins that run down the neck.

The carotid artery is the artery you can locate by feeling the pulse in your neck. The external branch of the carotid artery outside the skull supplies the face, scalp, skull and meninges and this area can be a significant source of headache pain.

Referred Pain from the Meninges

The meninges are three membranes that cover and protect the brain and the spinal cord.

The outermost layer of the meninges, the dura, is tough and thick to protect the brain from movement within the skull. It has a rich supply of pain receptors, which means any inflammatory substances released by nearby nerves can cause severe head pain.

A band of connective tissue only discovered in 1995 links one of the muscles of the sub-occipital group just below the base of the skull to the dura of the brain stem.[6]

This means that neck movements can put abnormal traction on the dura of the brain stem and this traction can lead to a very severe chronic headache.[7,8]

In much the same way, fine ligaments tether the dura of the spinal cord to the spinal bones and to one of the major ligaments that runs the length of the spine.[9] If the spine is stiff, everyday movements can cause abnormal traction on the dura of the spinal cord which is part of the dura of the brain, and leads to headache.

Referred Pain from Nerves

It's important to remember that nerves are not just passive conductors of electrical signals, like computer cables. Nerves can be injured and so are themselves wrapped in fine sensory nerves. These have pain receptors that respond to chemical and mechanical stimuli, just as in other tissues. Nerves also have their own blood supply.

Sympathetic and parasympathetic nerve fibres – the 'fight or flight' and the 'rest and digest' divisions of the autonomic nervous system – occur in both the peripheral and central nervous system. Mechanical or chemical irritation of these nerves can lead to typical autonomic symptoms, like nausea or a runny nose, in addition to pain.[10] This can occur when nerves pass close by muscular trigger points.

Compression of a cervical nerve root (the first part of the nerve where it exits from the cervical part of the spinal cord) between the vertebrae of the neck can also produce very severe pain. This is usually accompanied by neurological symptoms, such as weakness or pins and needles, and so would normally be diagnosed by neurological testing.

Key Points

- Muscular trigger points are one of the most common and most overlooked sources of headache pain.
- A muscular trigger point is a hard nodule within a taut band of muscle tissue that can cause tightness, weakness, lack of endurance, a restricted range of motion, spasms in other muscles and referred pain.
- The most common cause of muscular trigger points is chronic injury due to forward head posture and the overuse of fatigued muscles.
- Muscular trigger points need treatment to be resolved.
- The three uppermost joints of the neck are a common source of headache pain.
- The jaw joint can cause headache pain and referred pain in the face, ear, eye, sinuses and teeth.

Part B

Understanding:

Causes

4

Headache Triggers

We've discussed muscular trigger points – one of the most neglected aspects of headache management – now let's look at one of the most discussed – headache triggers.

What is a Trigger?

A headache trigger is anything that either initiates a headache or makes an existing headache worse. Headache triggers can range from stress to coffee to dehydration. Most triggers are common to both migraine and tension headache sufferers, although some foods, light, weather, smoke and odours may be more significant for migraine.

There's no such thing as a universal headache trigger, not even stress or red wine. Each headache sufferer responds in their own way to their own personal triggers. Only a small number of triggers are likely to be important for you, and because the effect of triggers is cumulative, sometimes your trigger will start a headache, sometimes it won't.

Not Getting Too Trigger-Happy

While we're investigating triggers, it's important not to get too focused on them. Even though avoiding triggers can lead to a reduction in the severity and duration of headache attacks, it cannot completely prevent them.

The consensus among headache researchers is that avoidance of food triggers is over-emphasised. Food triggers are only of importance for about 20% of migraine sufferers. For a few members of this sub-group, reducing exposure to particular foods can lead to a dramatic reduction in headache frequency, but for most headache sufferers this doesn't apply.[11,12]

The most important dietary headache triggers are:

- Dehydration
- Caffeine withdrawal
- Alcoholic beverages
- Missing meals.

Although it can seem like a solution, excessive avoidance of potential headache triggers, such as rigid elimination diets to remove all likely dietary triggers, offer few real benefits for most headache sufferers. Sometimes, being overly zealous in the search for triggers can be counter-productive. Fear that a trigger will provoke an attack can become a self-fulfilling prophecy, or the so-called 'nocebo effect', the dark side of the placebo effect, where your fears create the symptoms. In the end, correcting your posture, reducing stress, having a regular sleep pattern, staying hydrated and doing regular moderate exercise are likely to have a much greater impact on your headaches and your overall wellbeing than avoiding nitrates.

The Challenges of Finding Your Trigger

The idea of finding your trigger and avoiding it seems like a logical, simple plan. Find the trigger, avoid the trigger. But the reality is more complex. Determining whether a particular factor is a genuine headache trigger can take some real detective work.

Most of the information about headache triggers has come from survey studies, in which people are asked for their opinion about what triggers their headaches. Subjective impressions about headache triggers often turn out to be wrong when put to the test. A 2004 study[13] that matched records from patients' headache diaries with independent weather data found that several patients incorrectly believed the weather triggered their migraines. Other patients whose attacks were triggered by the weather were unaware of it.

When looking for patterns that implicate possible triggers, you need to be on your guard against seeing connections where there aren't any, or seizing upon the wrong factors. Moderate exercise may be incorrectly blamed for triggering a migraine, when the real issue could be dehydration, lack of food or fatigue.

Certain prodromal symptoms (early warning symptoms that a migraine may be about to start) may also be confused with triggers. This is very common. For example, craving sweet things can be a warning sign of an impending migraine attack. However, if you eat some chocolate to satisfy this craving and a migraine ensues, it would be easy to conclude incorrectly that the chocolate had triggered the attack.

It's often not the food itself, but one or more substances in the food that are triggers to your headache. And to make it even harder, the substances that might trigger your headache are present in varying amounts in a wide range of foods and drinks.

Cheese is a good example of this. It's considered to be a headache trigger, however the real trigger is most likely to be tyramine, a vasoconstrictor. Tyramine occurs naturally in cheese. It also occurs in salami, red wine, chicken liver pate, soy sauce and sauerkraut.

The tyramine content of cheese is extremely variable. It differs widely from one type of cheese to the next, between the same type of cheese produced by different manufacturers, and between different batches of the same cheese. It even varies between servings cut from the middle versus near the outside of the same cheese sample.

So, will you get a headache if you finish your meal with some cheese? That depends on lots of factors, such as:

- The average tyramine content of the cheese you eat (which is extremely variable)
- How much cheese you eat
- The amount of tyramine (and other vasoactive substances) in all the other foods and drinks you will consume during the meal – the total dose matters
- Your usual daily diet – if you are consuming cheese and other sources of tyramine faster than it can be cleared from the body, it will accumulate
- Your headache threshold at the time, which can be lowered by factors such as stress, menstruation and muscle tension
- The other non-dietary headache triggers you were exposed to.

When you factor in the time delay between consuming a potential 'problem food' and the appearance of a headache, it's not surprising that food triggers are often misidentified. To add to all of that, exposure to one of your triggers does not always lead to a headache. Whether you get a headache or not depends on how many of your other triggers you are exposed to simultaneously. The effect of triggers is cumulative.

In the following scenario, headache triggers stack up until eventually a headache occurs.

Kathy is running late for work and skips breakfast, so on her way to work she buys a donut to have mid-morning. At work, she spends two hours without a break typing out a report on her computer, and eats the donut sitting at her desk. The donut causes her blood sugar levels to surge and then drop. Two hours later Kathy has a bad headache.

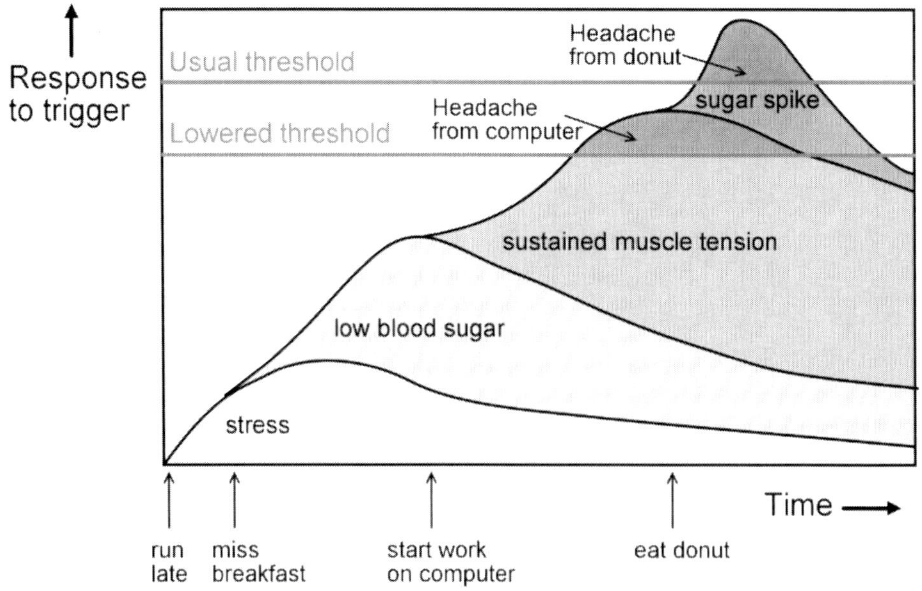

Figure 4.1 – Kathy's Headache – How Headache Triggers Add Together

It would be fair to conclude there's something about donuts that provokes Kathy's headaches. In this instance, it was certainly her response to the donut that triggered her attack, but, if one or more of her other triggers had been absent, her total 'trigger load' would not have been significant enough to cause an attack. Kathy is tired, she's missed a meal, stressed at work, not moving enough and probably sitting in an awkward posture – it seems unfair to blame the donut for all that!

Triggers are a part of headache management – but it pays to remember that identifying and managing your triggers can be a tricky business with variable success.

Key Points

- There's no such thing as a universal headache trigger.
- Dehydration, missing meals, alcohol and caffeinated drinks are the most important dietary triggers to consider.
- The significance of avoiding food triggers is over-rated for most headache sufferers
- Being overzealous in the search for triggers can be counter-productive. Fear that a trigger will provoke an attack can become a self-fulfilling prophecy, or the so-called 'nocebo effect', where your fears create the symptoms.
- Identifying and managing your triggers can be a tricky business with variable success.

5

The Headache Threshold

What is the Headache Threshold?

We often think of a headache as a switch that gets flicked; we eat something, do something or skip something and the headache begins, but headaches are more like buckets than switches.

The bucket gradually fills until it finally overflows. We don't feel any pain as the bucket is filling, only when it overflows. Unfortunately, people who get headaches regularly have smaller buckets than other people, which is why it overflows more often. Your aim is to keep as far below the edge of the bucket as you can.

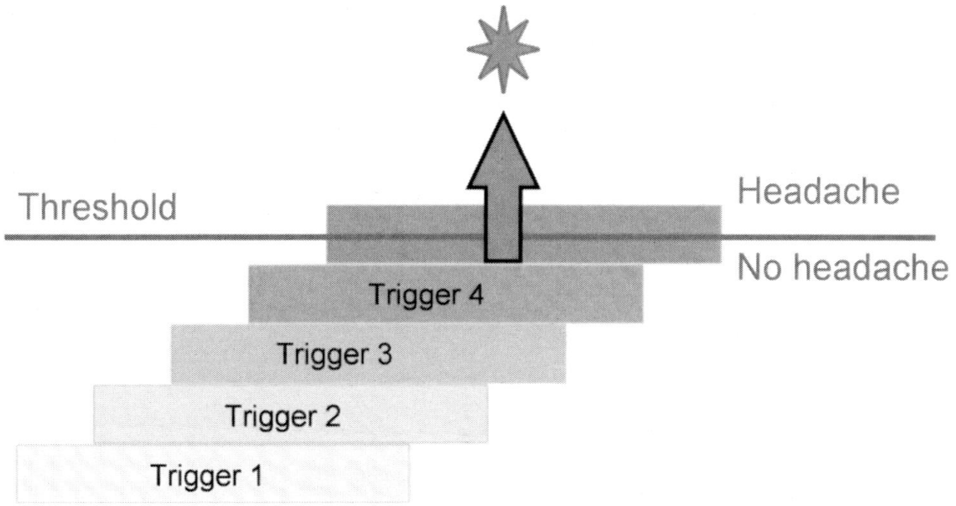

Figure 5.1 – How headache triggers add up to push you over your headache threshold

Some people have a high enough headache threshold that they only get headaches on rare occasions, such as when they're sleep deprived and under severe stress. If you have a low headache threshold, the impact of contributing factors is much more significant than it would be to someone less prone to headaches.

Understanding how the headache threshold works is crucial to managing your headaches. The fundamental aim of a headache management strategy is to keep you as far from your threshold as possible. And the good news is that reducing the impact of just one or two factors can keep you under the threshold a lot more often.

Can You Raise Your Threshold?

Your headache threshold is largely inherited, but you can modify it to a certain extent.

Raising your headache threshold is really just common sense. The better your health and mood, the higher your headache threshold will be. Improving your diet and sleep patterns and reducing your general background level of stress will all help raise your threshold. Of course, it's easier said than done, and I have some strategies on how to help with that in the following chapters.

Keeping Below the Threshold

As well as raising your threshold, you can also work to keep below your threshold. This mostly involves being aware of your triggers and avoiding as many of them as possible. The crucial thing to remember about triggers is that their effect is cumulative. We often think of a trigger as the one thing that initiates a headache, but it's more complex than that.

Returning to our bucket analogy, everyone's headache bucket is filled from lots of different taps. Stress, lack of sleep, diet, muscle tightness and dehydration all contribute to raising the level in your bucket. And these taps all run at different speeds and at different times. Some gush, some drip, some only turn on every second Tuesday. No one tap is responsible for your headache – your bucket could be holding a lot of water from stress, and then it's the drip of a muscular trigger point that causes an overflow. It's the combination of all the taps, or triggers, together that causes the headache, not one individual trigger.

The impact of a trigger depends on your headache threshold at the time, and also on how many of your other triggers you are exposed to simultaneously. For example, some women report that chocolate triggers a migraine, but only if it is eaten just before a menstrual period and not at other times.

Latency or Delayed Response

The latency period, or the gap between when a trigger impacts the body and when the symptoms are felt, varies from one trigger to the next. It can range from several hours to days but is usually less than 24 hours. The latency period for chocolate and red wine, two of the most commonly reported migraine triggers, is 3 hours for red wine and 22 hours for chocolate.[14] An emotionally stressful episode can trigger a migraine after a delay as long as three to four days and there may be an additional delay if your total exposure to triggers is initially below your headache threshold.

Blurred Boundaries between Trigger and Threshold

In practice, the boundary between factors that can raise or lower your headache threshold and factors that can trigger an attack is often blurred.

For example, dehydration will cause a headache even in people with a high headache threshold. But what happens when a regular headache sufferer is mildly dehydrated most of the time? (This is more common than you might expect.) Is dehydration lowering their headache threshold or acting as a headache trigger? In this case, the answer matters less than the message, which is to drink more water, and avoid even mild dehydration.

The same is true for MSG, which occurs naturally in food and is also added as a flavour enhancer. MSG may sometimes cause a headache when eaten in sufficient quantities by those who are sensitive to it, or it could lower your threshold, making it much more likely that you'll experience a headache not long after consuming MSG. Like dehydration, the answer doesn't alter the necessary action, which is to avoid eating large quantities of foods with significant amounts of MSG.

Both migraine and tension headache sufferers list emotional stress, and feelings such as anxiety, worry, fear, anger, and frustration that accompany stress, as one of their most important triggers. But emotional stress is more than a trigger. It is part of the mechanism that produces a headache.

On-going stress can lower your headache threshold, making it more likely that exposure to your other triggers will provoke a headache attack. Specific short-term stressful episodes may trigger a headache attack.

Few headache sufferers are aware that the sustained and excessive amounts of muscle tension that accompany emotional stress may play an equally important role in starting a headache.

Sustained tension in the muscles of our jaw, neck and shoulders is a common response to emotional stress. Muscle tension lowers your headache threshold, making a headache attack more likely. Muscle tension can also act as a headache trigger. On-going tension in your neck, jaw and shoulders acts as a continual low-level source of pain, which can reduce your headache threshold. If you also have trigger points, the tension may irritate them enough to start a headache.

For many women, changing levels of female hormones are a powerful factor in provoking headaches. About half of all women who suffer either migraine or tension headache regularly experience headaches around the time of menstruation. Some women have headaches only at this time. Like emotional stress and muscle tension, changing hormone levels lower your headache threshold and may also trigger a headache attack. A sudden drop in estrogen levels after several days of sustained high levels is the most common hormonal headache trigger.

Regardless of blurred boundaries, the key message is that whatever you can do to raise your headache threshold or lessen your total exposure to headache triggers will reduce the frequency of your headache attacks. This is one of the main principles behind headache prevention, because, regardless of muscular triggers, trigger points and genetics, if you can stay below your headache threshold, you won't have a headache.

Key Points

- The higher your headache threshold, the less likely you are to experience regular headaches.
- Crossing the headache pain threshold is like a bucket finally overflowing due to lots of different taps (triggers) being turned on, rather than a main switch that gets turned on.
- Headache triggers have a cumulative effect on your headache threshold.
- Staying below your headache threshold is the basis of a successful headache management strategy. If you stay below your threshold, you won't experience headache pain.
- The good news is that reducing the impact of just one or two factors can keep you under the headache threshold.

6

Triggers Worth Considering

If you look online for headache triggers, you'll find long, conflicting lists. To help make a pathway through this important, complicated and controversial area, I've summarised the most common triggers under four broad categories:

1. Body-related factors
2. Food, beverages and medications
3. Lifestyle
4. Environment.

1. Body-related Factors

- Shallow breathing (high in the chest)
- Hyperventilation (over-breathing – breathing faster or deeper than normal, especially high in the chest)
- Problems breathing while asleep
- Musculoskeletal triggers
- Eyestrain and vision problems
- Changes to your glasses prescription
- Vitamin and mineral deficiencies
- Obesity
- Allergies and/or allergic reactions
- Minor head or neck trauma, e.g. being hit on the head with a ball, including heading the ball in soccer
- Local pain from teeth, ears, eyes
- Minor illness such as a cold or flu
- Injuries
- Female hormones.

2. Food, Beverages and Medications

- Dehydration
- Alcoholic beverages
- Sugary snacks and drinks
- Caffeine (excessive use and sudden reduction)
- Naturally occurring components of foods such as histamine, tyramine and MSG
- Food additives such as MSG and nitrites
- Fatty foods
- Medications for other conditions.

3. Lifestyle

- Not eating regular meals, skipping meals, delaying meals, dieting
- Changes in sleep patterns
- Lack of sleep, excessive sleep, disturbed sleep
- Fatigue
- Relief from stress, such as the start of the week-end or holiday. (I have doubts about this one. It seems to me that it's more likely to be a delayed effect of the earlier episode of stress. Other factors such as a change of sleeping pattern and caffeine withdrawal may also be important.)
- Physical over-exertion, excessive exercise, sexual activity. Note that a sudden onset headache that starts during exercise or sex is a red flag headache. It is not necessarily serious but it needs to be investigated. Make an immediate appointment with your doctor.
- Tight hairstyle, head gear or goggles
- Lack of movement, insufficient exercise, sedentary lifestyle
- Smoking
- Taking illicit drugs.

4. Environment

- Sun glare
- Bright, glaring, flashing or flickering lights and screens
- Unpleasant odours, perfume, second-hand cigarette smoke, chemical solvent odours
- Traffic fumes, air pollution and smog
- Loud noise
- Lack of fresh air
- Exposure to carbon monoxide
- Weather and weather changes (temperature, barometric pressure, humidity), also constant wind and dust
- High altitude or changes in altitude
- Extended travel
- Aeroplane travel

Some Key Triggers in More Depth

Musculoskeletal Triggers

Musculoskeletal triggers don't get very much attention, but I think they're one of the most important triggers to consider – and one of the easiest to fix. Musculoskeletal triggers are not the same as muscular trigger points (although a musculoskeletal trigger can trigger a muscular trigger point!). Musculoskeletal triggers are postures, movements or activities, such as sleeping on your stomach, grinding your teeth or holding a bad posture. If you wake up with a headache, it's very likely due to a musculoskeletal trigger, as are headaches that follow long, uninterrupted periods of sitting, especially if you were using a computer or behind the wheel of a car.

Just as the musculoskeletal contribution to headache pain is often ignored, musculoskeletal headache triggers are generally not recognised. The exception is teeth clenching and grinding during sleep, which has been recognised as a headache trigger by the dental profession. Unfortunately, most people who clench or grind their teeth are unaware of it. A sleeping partner may be able to tell you, or a dentist may notice wear and tear on your teeth. The only other indication is that your jaw muscles are likely to feel tired and sore in the mornings.

The sort of postures or actions that can act as musculoskeletal headache triggers include:

- Sitting or standing with your neck craned forwards, especially if your head is tilted upwards at the same time
- Sleeping with a pillow that is too high or too low
- Prolonged typing or driving long distances, especially if your back and shoulders are rounded
- Turning your head sharply
- Clenching or grinding your teeth
- Chewing gum
- Half lying down on a couch with your head and neck pushed forwards
- Excessive frowning, wrinkling the forehead or squinting
- Sitting in a slumped posture with your legs out in front of you.

Women of all ages are more likely to suffer from headaches related to head and neck posture than men. Women's necks are thinner and less muscular and their shoulder and neck muscles support the weight of breasts. They tend to have a larger curve in their lower back so their head and neck is held further forward in compensation.

Stress

Both migraine and tension headache sufferers list emotional stress, and feelings such as anxiety, worry, fear, anger and frustration as one of their most significant triggers. But emotional stress is more than a trigger. As part of the integrated model, it's also one of the mechanisms that produces a headache.

Emotional stress can cause and intensify a headache by interfering with natural pain suppression mechanisms, increasing the excitability of the brain, altering blood flow to and within the brain and causing the release of histamine, a vasodilator and inflammatory substance.

The role of emotional stress in provoking headaches is generally accepted, but fewer headache sufferers are aware that the sustained and excessive amounts of muscle tension that results from stress may play an equally important role in triggering a headache. Tension in the jaw, neck and shoulders is a common response to emotional stress and the muscle tension that comes from emotional stress may also act as a musculoskeletal trigger.

Breathing Problems

A lack of oxygen is one of the most common, and most hidden, causes of headache. Low oxygen levels initiate the widening of blood vessels, which can bring on migraines.

If you are not getting enough air into your lungs, it may be because of shallow breathing or a restriction of the airways. Shallow breathing is often due to emotional stress as already discussed, but it can also become a habit even when you are not stressed.

Two other common causes of breathing problems are a hunched restrictive posture and a stiff rib cage. Both stop your lungs from expanding fully when you breathe. Hunched posture is almost inevitable if you use a laptop on your couch at home, whether you lean forward towards a low table, or lean back against the couch.

Except for conditions like asthma, restriction of the airways is most often experienced during sleep. It may be relatively minor, due to nasal congestion from an allergy or a cold, or sleeping on your stomach with your mouth and nose partly buried in the pillow or mattress.

Obstructive sleep apnoea occurs when the tongue and the soft tissue in the back of the throat relaxes, blocking off the upper airway. It can also reduce the amount of oxygen you receive when you're asleep. Shorter pauses have less effect on blood oxygen levels, but they still lead to fragmented sleep, which is itself a headache trigger.

Obstructive sleep apnoea is relatively common. It is estimated to affect about 5% of the population in Australia, including 1 in 4 men over the age of 30.[15] It causes daytime sleepiness and morning headaches but many people who have the condition are unaware of it.

Rhinitis

Rhinitis is the irritation, inflammation and swelling of the tissues inside the nose. Symptoms include a runny nose, itching, sneezing, watering eyes, blocked or congested nasal passages and post-nasal drip down the back of the throat. There are three different types of rhinitis that I think may have an impact as a headache trigger.

However, you need to be careful not to jump to the wrong conclusion. Nasal symptoms, including a stuffy nose and facial pain, are very common during migraine attacks. They are so common that approximately 90% of self-diagnosed sinus headaches are actually migraines.[16] Even doctors are sometimes fooled.

Allergic Rhinitis

Allergic rhinitis, commonly known as hay fever, significantly increases the body's total histamine load. It worsens food intolerance symptoms and is also a risk factor for migraine.

In allergic rhinitis, the immune system mistakes harmless substances, like pollen, for a dangerous micro-organism. This triggers the release of a large amount of histamine and other inflammatory substances, so it's not surprising that a nasal allergy can provoke a migraine attack.

Allergic rhinitis is seasonal, occurring mainly in the warmer months, especially spring. This is usually caused by reactions to pollen grains from grasses, trees and weeds, or to airborne mould spores.

Allergic rhinitis can also occur throughout the year, known as perennial allergic rhinitis. This is usually caused by reactions to allergens around the home, such as dust mites, moulds or animal dander.

Non-allergic Rhinitis

Non-allergic rhinitis, or irritant rhinitis, has very similar symptoms to allergic rhinitis but it's caused by irritation of nerves in the nasal passages by small particles and vapours in the air.

Nasal irritants are everywhere – in the home, in the workplace and in the general outdoor environment. Common examples of irritants include smoke, air pollution, vehicle exhausts, aerosol sprays, perfumes, newspaper ink and paint fumes. We all breath them in, but some people are much more sensitive to them than others.

Food intolerance, in which histamine released in the stomach finds its way into general circulation, can also cause non-allergic rhinitis.

Local Allergic Rhinitis

Local allergic rhinitis is a newly recognised condition, which is thought to affect about 40% of the people previously diagnosed with non-allergic rhinitis. The usual skin prick tests and blood tests are negative but antibodies to specific allergens can be detected in nasal secretions.[17]

Nail polish is a good example. It is actually a refined version of the paint used to spray paint cars. Ethyl acetate, the main solvent used in both products, is known to cause severe irritation of the mucous membranes and the upper respiratory tract. It also causes headaches.

Water

Dehydration is a very common and very powerful headache trigger, even provoking headaches in those who aren't normally prone to them.

The type and amount of fluid you need to drink to stay well hydrated is a controversial area, however the evidence points to many headache patients being mildly dehydrated much of the time.

In one small controlled trial,[18] a group of 18 migraine patients were told to drink an extra 1.5 litres of water a day, on top of their normal fluid intake, for a period of 12 weeks. This corresponds to 6 additional 250ml glasses per day. On average, the study participants managed an additional one litre per day. Monitoring the headaches they experienced during the next two weeks, they found that headache duration was reduced by 21 hours. Headache pain was also less severe.

Caffeine

Excessive caffeine intake and caffeine withdrawal are common headache triggers. Caffeine is a vasoconstrictor and headache sufferers seem to be more sensitive than usual to its effects and to the rebound vasodilation that occurs when caffeine levels fall.

It's easy to underestimate how much caffeine you consume. Caffeine is found in coffee, tea, cocoa, and certain soft drinks, as well as in many over-the-counter and prescription pain-killers. For some people, as little as 100mg of caffeine a day can be sufficient to develop physical dependence and subsequent withdrawal symptoms.[19] This is less than the amount in the typical 240ml cup of brewed coffee.

Alcohol

After caffeine withdrawal, alcoholic beverages are the most potent food trigger for headaches, especially migraine.

Like food, alcoholic beverages contain varying amounts of a wide range of vasoactive substances, such as tyramine and histamine, all of which can trigger a headache.

Some headache sufferers are also highly sensitive to small amounts of alcohol, with these alcohol-related headaches occurring within about three hours of drinking an alcoholic beverage.

Those headaches are quite different from a hangover headache, which is part of a delayed response to excessive alcohol consumption, and begins the next day, when the alcohol has mostly cleared from the bloodstream.

However, a regular headache sufferer is much more likely to experience a hangover headache, which in the words of the International Headache Society (IHS) is due to 'Ingestion of a modest amount of alcoholic beverage by a migraine sufferer or an intoxicating amount by a non-migraine sufferer.'[20]

Wheat and Milk

Most substances in food that act as headache triggers, like tyramine, are only ever present at low levels. However, for a sub-set of migraine sufferers with demonstrated food intolerance, the major proteins in cereals (gluten) and dairy products (casein) may be responsible for their headaches.

For people who are intolerant to cereals and/or milk, significant quantities of histamine are released into the bloodstream when they have these foods, and this may provoke a headache. It's important to distinguish between different types of adverse reactions to cereals and milk, as they each require different dietary changes.

Coeliac disease and (non-coeliac) gluten intolerance both involve adverse reactions to gluten. On the other hand, wheat allergy is an allergic response to any of the many different proteins in wheat (one of which is gluten). Wheat allergy is rare in adults.

Similarly, intolerance to casein, a major protein in milk, is much more common in adults than milk allergy, an allergic reaction to any of the milk proteins.

Both are unrelated to lactose intolerance, the most common cause of adverse reaction to milk and milk products. Lactose intolerance is due to a lack of the enzymes necessary to break down lactose – the naturally occurring sugar in milk. It causes gastrointestinal symptoms but usually not headaches.

MSG

MSG has a serious reputation as a headache trigger, but I think the accusations may often be unjust.

Glutamic acid is part of most food proteins and foods rich in naturally occurring free glutamic acid have long been used to give flavour to cooking around the world.

A few examples include tomatoes, Parmesan cheese, mushrooms, soy sauce, slow simmered meat stocks and certain types of seaweed. A range of other additives, such as hydrolysed vegetable protein and yeast extract, which contain free glutamic acid, are also used by the food industry.

What's interesting is that both artificially added MSG and naturally present free glutamic acid exist in exactly the same chemical form in body fluids, but naturally occurring glutamates have not been implicated as headache triggers.

People vary in their sensitivity to MSG. For some, MSG can cause a collection of symptoms that were first dubbed 'Chinese restaurant syndrome' in 1968[21] and have been automatically associated with added MSG ever since. (It's surprising to me that there is no 'Italian restaurant syndrome', given how widely glutamate-rich tomato paste and Parmesan cheese are used in Italian cooking.)

Symptoms include headaches, facial flushing, tightness in the face and jaw muscles, sweating, nausea and palpitations. However, they only occur when MSG is consumed in high doses on an empty stomach and especially when it is in liquid form like a clear soup.

A meal high in rapidly absorbed MSG will cause blood glutamate levels to spike, but there is no evidence that glutamate affects blood vessels. Glutamate is, however, the most important excitory neurotransmitter in the brain, which means high levels of glutamate in the blood can interfere with the normal processes that remove glutamate from the brain, causing levels in the brain to temporarily increase. This could potentially trigger a headache attack.

Nevertheless, double blind placebo controlled trials have never consistently demonstrated that MSG in quantities normally consumed during a meal can trigger a headache attack.[22]

This is true even for those headache sufferers who believe MSG is a headache trigger for them. MSG in combination with other trigger factors such as stress or alcohol may be the cause of a headache. Alternatively, other food components often found in high levels in the same foods as MSG, such as tyramine or histamine, or large amounts of fat and salt, may be the real headache trigger.

Biogenic Amines

A biogenic amine is, very basically, an organic compound. Tyramine, a vasoconstrictor, and histamine, a vasodilator and inflammatory substance, are the two biogenic amines you are most likely to encounter as headache triggers.

Significant sources of tyramine and / or histamine include:

- Aged (ripened) cheeses, such as English Stilton, Danish blue and Parmesan
- Processed meats produced by traditional fermentation methods, such as fermented ham and dry sausages like salami and pepperoni
- Salted, dried or pickled fish, such as anchovies
- Fermented vegetables including sauerkraut (from cabbage) and tofu (from soya beans)
- Certain alcoholic beverages, such as wine and beer
- Reclaimed yeast extracts used as spreads, e.g. Marmite® and Vegemite® or stock cubes
- Improperly stored fresh meat. Chicken livers and the pâté made from them are common offenders. It's worth noting, histamine has no smell and is not destroyed by cooking, so it can be hard to detect in improperly stored food.
- Improperly stored fresh fish – this can develop particularly high levels of histamine
- Asian condiments produced by fermentation, e.g. fish sauce, soy sauce, miso (from soya beans and rice), shrimp sauce.

Other biogenic amines include:

- Phenylethylamine, found in cocoa beans and hence chocolate products. (Phenylethylamine unlike other biogenic amines, is able to cross the blood-brain barrier)
- Octopamine and synephrine which occur in citrus fruits
- Serotonin found in bananas, pineapples, plums and avocados (especially if they are over-ripe).

The levels of biogenic amines in different samples of the same type of food vary widely. If you have shown to be intolerant of biogenic amines, one of the easiest ways to reduce your intake is to make sure the food you buy, cook and eat is fresh. The longer foods are stored and the higher the storage temperature, the higher the levels of biogenic amines.

More on Histamines

With histamines, it's more effective to think in terms of the total histamine load on your body rather than any one food that will affect your histamine levels. Any factors that increase this load beyond a certain critical value will worsen your headaches and other symptoms.

Food is commonly associated with raising histamine levels. It can also be raised by injury, infections, emotional stress and reactions to air-borne substances. Physical stress associated with vigorous exercise causes a short-term increase in histamine levels.

Activity in your colon (large bowel) can also be significant. Some histamine is produced here by classes of micro-organisms acting on undigested protein, so changes to your gut flora from taking antibiotics can cause your tolerance to alter. So can the treatment of heartburn with antacids or prescription medications, which reduces stomach acid, which will in turn reduce the efficiency of protein digestion in the stomach.

Alcohol acts as an irritant, causing cells in the gut to release histamine. Various food additives, certain drugs and a range of minor natural food components can similarly act as histamine releasers, although the mechanism may be much more complex.

In a few sensitive people, the histamine produced can enter the bloodstream in sufficient quantities to provoke a headache. It may also cause a range of other allergy-like symptoms of histamine excess, like a runny nose, sneezing or itching, which may not appear to be food related.

Aspartame

Aspartame (NutraSweet®, Equal®, E951) is used as an artificial sweetener in place of sugar. Diet soft drinks contribute most to aspartame intake, with smaller amounts coming from a wide variety of products, such as fruit drinks, desserts, chewing gum and pharmaceutical drugs.

Ever since aspartame was first approved by the US Food and Drug Administration in 1981, its safety has been the subject of political and medical controversy. Headache is the most frequent consumer complaint about aspartame.

Studies investigating aspartame as a headache trigger have produced conflicting results. Like other dietary triggers, aspartame is only likely to be important for a small sub-set of headache sufferers.

The current consensus[23,24,25] is that aspartame should be considered as a potential headache trigger, especially for people who consume it in large amounts. For most people, it's probably not worth worrying about minor sources of aspartame but it's best to avoid the main source – artificially sweetened drinks. This is a good idea even if aspartame is not a headache trigger for you. Water is always the best way to quench your thirst.

Nitrites and Nitrates

Nitrites and nitrates are used as preservatives in processed meats such as corn beef, ham, luncheon loaf, bacon, hot dogs and traditional fermented meat products like salami. Nitrites prevent the growth of bacteria and give cured meats their characteristic pink colour.

Processed meats are thought to be responsible for triggering headache attacks, often referred to as 'hot dog headaches'. The actual trigger is thought to be nitric oxide, the most powerful vasodilator known. However, producing nitric oxide from nitrite is one of the body's normal protective mechanisms. It occurs when levels of oxygen in the blood are low, and causes blood vessels to dilate.[26] So, it's unclear why some people are more sensitive to dietary nitrites and nitrates than others.

It's also unclear why leafy green vegetables, like lettuce and spinach, which accumulate nitrates from water and soil, are not reported to act as headache triggers. They actually contribute a larger amount of nitrates and nitrites to the diet than processed meats. I don't want to disregard processed meat as a potential headache trigger, but I would question whether nitrites and nitrates are the culprit.

A Note on Testing for Allergies and Intolerance

Most of us tend to use the word food allergy to describe any sort of adverse reaction to food, but this is not how the medical profession uses it.

Medically the term allergy is reserved for an immune system malfunction, such as the peanut allergy, which in extreme cases (known as anaphylaxis) can be fatal. An allergic reaction to a problem food is rapid and occurs on each and every exposure to the food. Only tiny amounts of the food are needed to produce the response.

Headaches that appear several hours after consuming food and drinks are usually the result of food intolerance, not food allergy. Food intolerance does not involve an immune reaction. It is a delayed adverse reaction to a normal serving of food that doesn't bother most people.

Blood tests or skin prick tests are designed to assist with the diagnosis of allergies. They're good for identifying inhaled allergens, like grass pollen and house dust mites, and for injected allergens like bee venom. They are far less reliable for diagnosing food allergies and are no use for diagnosing food intolerance that doesn't occur by the same mechanism.

You are likely to see advertisements online for tests which claim to be able to diagnose both food allergy and food intolerance for a range of 100 or so foods. These tests measure levels of an antibody known as IgG in your blood. The trouble is that raised IgG levels are a normal finding in healthy people. They're a marker for prior exposure to a food, not intolerance to it.[27,28] IgG tests do not determine food intolerance.

The only way to test for food intolerance is to go on a supervised elimination diet, followed by a food challenge, or even better, a double-blind placebo controlled food challenge. It's not a good idea to make significant changes to your diet based solely on your conclusions from your own observations.

If you believe you have food-based headache triggers you should seek professional help. Look for an allergist or a dietician with an interest in food allergy and intolerance, or a hospital allergy clinic to help you verify suspected headache food triggers. They may also find others that you are not aware of. Once the problem food components have been determined, a dietician will prepare a list of foods you need to reduce or avoid. They will also help you work out what foods you can use as substitutes so you maintain a balanced diet.

Light and Movement

Environmental headache triggers come under the category of intense stimuli of vision and hearing, like flashing lights or glare and loud noise.

These stimuli may initiate the headache process by provoking an excessively large response from the headache sufferer's excitable brain. The sorts of movement that cause motion sickness often also trigger migraine attacks, such as virtual movement, as in IMAX or 3D movies.

Those who suffer from migraine with aura are normally thought to be the most susceptible to sensory triggers – bright light is the second most commonly reported trigger after stress – although some scientists now think that sensitivity to light and other sensory stimuli may instead be an indication that the migraine process has already begun.[29]

Smoking

It isn't surprising that tobacco smoke is an important headache trigger, even for non-smokers. It's an irritant on mucous membranes in the mouth, nose, airways and lungs. Nicotine constricts blood vessels, lessening blood flow to and within the brain. Finally, the carbon monoxide in cigarette smoke preferentially attaches to the red blood cells, displacing oxygen which reduces the amount of oxygen the blood can carry.

In smokers, lungs, airways and arteries are damaged. Less air can get into the lungs and less oxygen is transferred into the blood stream, further reducing the brain's oxygen supply and increasing the chance of a headache.

Air Travel

Sitting in a pressurised cabin is equivalent to being at an altitude of around 2400m (8000 feet). At this altitude, air pressure is only three quarters of its value at sea level and maximum blood oxygen levels are about 93% of normal.

In addition to the reduced supply of oxygen, several other factors associated with air travel combine to make it a powerful headache trigger for many people.

There's the stress of negotiating check-in, security inspection and various possible delays in the airport. Then there's the design of the seats, which makes it almost impossible to maintain good head and neck posture. Cramped seats and narrow aisles don't make it easy to get out of your seat to move around the plane.

The dry, reduced pressure atmosphere of the cabin causes extra fluid loss, so it's easy to become dehydrated without noticing it. You typically lose about 1.5 litres of fluid over a three-hour flight. And lastly, broken sleep and fatigue is a problem, especially on long flights.

Key Points

- Headache triggers fall into four broad categories: Body-related, Food, Beverages and medication, Lifestyle, and Environment.
- Food allergies and food intolerance are two different things and should be confirmed by a professional before you eliminate anything from your diet.
- Musculoskeletal triggers are different to musculoskeletal trigger points. Musculoskeletal triggers are postures, movements or activities that can cause a headache. They are often overlooked and are usually easy to fix.
- Key triggers are musculoskeletal, stress, breathing problems, rhinitis (sinus), dehydration, caffeine, alcohol, wheat and milk, MSG, histamine, aspartame, nitrates and nitrites, smoking and air travel.

7

Female Hormones

Female hormones are significant headache triggers. Under the age of eleven, there's not much gender difference in the prevalence of headaches in children. It's only after puberty that migraine prevalence increases much more sharply among girls than boys, with up to 20% of female migraine sufferers reporting their first attack in the same year as their first period. Onset of migraine with aura tends to occur up to two years earlier. Girls also start to have more tension headaches than boys after puberty although the gender difference is more balanced by the time they reach adulthood.

A significant, sudden change in levels of female hormones, an increase or decrease, can precipitate a new headache or worsen an existing one and sustained low or high levels of hormones act as threshold setters, lowering your headache threshold and increasing the likelihood that exposure to your personal headache triggers will provoke an attack.

Times of hormonal change include:

- Onset of puberty
- Menstruation
- Ovulation
- Use of hormonal contraceptives
- Pregnancy
- Giving birth
- Peri-menopause (the lead-up to menopause)
- Menopause,
- Use of hormone replacement therapy (HRT).

Please note, if you start to experience a persistent new headache, or changes in your headaches, such as the development of a migraine aura for the first time, you should consult your doctor.

Menstrual Headaches

Menstrual headaches are very common. They're usually more severe and last longer than headaches at other times. They are essentially estrogen withdrawal headaches, occurring when estrogen levels drop immediately before the start of a period.[30] Some women experience headaches at mid-cycle when estrogen levels drop following ovulation.

To be considered as a menstrual headache, attacks must occur between two days before to three days after the start of menstrual bleeding in two out of every three menstrual cycles. If you think you are having menstrual headaches, add a calendar to your headache diary and record the date of your headaches and the date your period starts for at least three menstrual cycles.

Over half of all women migraine sufferers experience menstrually related migraines.[31] These are migraines without aura which occur regularly around the time of menstruation, in the time window from 2 days before to 3 days after the start of menstrual bleeding.[32]

Compared with migraines that they experience at other times, women usually say that their menstrual migraines:

- Last longer
- Are more severe
- Occur more often
- Are more likely to lead to nausea and vomiting
- Are less responsive to medication.

About 14% of women migraine sufferers only experience migraines during the menstrual time window above and at no other time. These migraines are called pure menstrual migraines.

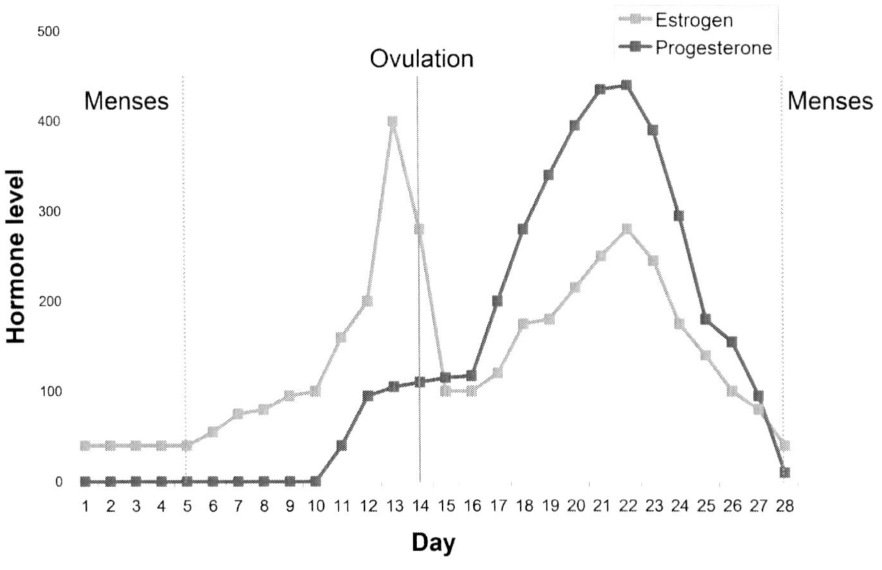

Figure 7.1: The menstrual cycle – typical estrogen and progesterone levels

Figure 7.1 shows the way the important female reproductive hormones, estrogen (also called oestrogen) and progesterone, vary during the menstrual cycle. For convenience, the cycle in Figure 7.1 is 28 days long. The start of menstrual bleeding is day 1 of the menstrual cycle, day 27 will be the last day before the next menstrual period.

During the first half of the cycle, estrogen levels rise and bleeding slows and then stops. The lining of the uterus thickens and several follicles in the ovary start to develop. One follicle becomes dominant and the non-dominant follicles die. Around mid-cycle, the dominant follicle releases an egg during ovulation.

In the second half of the cycle, the remains of the dominant follicle in the ovary start to produce large amounts of progesterone. This prepares the lining of the uterus to accept the implantation of an embryo and sustain a pregnancy. If pregnancy does not occur, progesterone and estrogen levels drop sharply. Withdrawal of progesterone causes the uterus to shed its lining and menstrual bleeding begins again.

There are two peaks in the estrogen levels – one just before ovulation and one about a week before menstruation. Estrogen and progesterone levels reach their lowest values during menstruation.

The major precipitating factor for menstrual migraines is the decline in estrogen levels that occur immediately before the start of a period.[33] The fall in progesterone just before menstruation has been demonstrated not to trigger migraine.[34] It has also been suggested that the prostaglandins which are released into the circulation at the time of menstruation may contribute to the triggering of a headache. Prostaglandins increase pain sensitivity throughout the body. Some women are much more sensitive to small decreases in estrogen than others, but, in general, the larger and more rapid the fall, the worse the migraine.

Several studies indicate that estrogen decline will only trigger a migraine if two conditions are met:

- The decline follows an interval of several days of sustained high levels of estrogen, and Estrogen levels fall below a threshold value.
- The existence of an estrogen threshold is the reason why low doses of an external estrogen are often prescribed to help prevent menstrual migraine. Estrogen supplied by a skin patch or a gel supplements the body's natural estrogen levels and stops them dropping so low. It is normally started 1 or 2 days before a period is expected and continued for 5 to 7 days.[35]

Some women also regularly experience migraines at mid-cycle after ovulation occurs. These migraines are likely due to the rapid drop in estrogen levels that follows the estrogen surge just prior to ovulation. High levels of estrogen mid-cycle are not sustained as long before they drop, as in the second half of the menstrual cycle. This lesser 'priming' of the system may explain why mid-cycle migraines are less common than menstrual migraines.

The pre-menstrual and mid-cycle decline in estrogen is just as important a trigger for tension headache as it is for migraine, affecting approximately half of all female tension headache sufferers,[36] especially those in their thirties and forties. However, the relationship between the menstrual cycle and tension headache has not received much attention until recently.[37]

Headaches During Pregnancy and After Giving Birth

During the first trimester, headaches may worsen as hormone levels fluctuate. After the third month, as levels of estrogen and other hormones stabilise, headaches improve for approximately 70% of women who suffer from migraine without aura, but only about 25% of tension headache sufferers. Migraine with aura may get worse.

Blood volume and resting heart rate increase with pregnancy, putting extra stress on the cardio-vascular system. Women with the common risk factors for cardiovascular disease, including diabetes, high blood pressure and cigarette smoking, are more likely to suffer migraines during pregnancy.[38]

Although the absolute risks are small, it's important to see your doctor to rule out any serious underlying causes if you suffer your first ever migraine, or a migraine with aura, during pregnancy. Aura is hard to distinguish from a transient ischemic attack (a mini stroke) in pregnant women.

If you develop a headache that is more severe than usual, especially in the later stages of pregnancy, consult your doctor immediately. It could indicate pre-eclampsia, a serious disorder characterised by high blood pressure, protein in the urine and severe fluid retention, which affects 5–10% of pregnancies. Pre-eclampsia usually arises in the second half of pregnancy after 20 weeks gestation and can harm both the mother and the unborn child. It can also occur some days after delivery.

After labour and delivery, there is a dramatic drop in the levels of estrogen and progesterone in the first one to two days, with estrogen reaching its lowest level a week after birth. After two weeks, hormone levels have usually returned to levels prior to pregnancy. No surprise then that hormonal headaches often re-start during the first week after giving birth and return to their usual pattern after a few weeks.

Any severe, constant or recurring headaches in the week following delivery should be investigated. Possible serious causes include complications of epidural anaesthesia, stroke or post-natal depression.

Headaches During Peri-Menopause and Menopause

Some women develop a new headache during peri-menopause. New onset tension headaches are moderately common over the age 50, but it is not common for new migraines or cluster headaches to develop at this time. All new headaches at this age should be investigated, as they are more likely to have a serious underlying cause than at a younger age.

Both migraines and tension headaches tend to worsen during peri-menopause as hormone levels fluctuate. Once past menopause, migraines tend to become less frequent and some women stop having them completely. There is less improvement in the case of tension headaches.

During peri-menopause, ovulation becomes more erratic, periods become increasingly irregular, and estrogen and progesterone levels can fluctuate wildly. Estrogen levels may temporarily rise higher than those typical of women in their twenties only to fall again abruptly. It's only during the last year of the peri-menopause, after periods have ceased, that estrogen levels begin to decrease consistently.

Levels of estrogen and progesterone stabilise over the following year so that by two years after the last period, they are low and constant, typical of the post-menopausal state. Many women find that they get more frequent migraines with the fluctuations in estrogen levels that accompany peri-menopause. Other women, who were not previously aware of any connection to their menstrual cycle, may start to suffer repeated menstrual migraines. Tension headaches also tend to worsen at this time.

Migraine frequency tends to decrease with age. For women who go through a natural menopause, by the time hormone levels stabilise a year or two after the last period, approximately two thirds of women migraine sufferers are having less frequent attacks, and some women have stopped having migraines altogether.

There is less improvement in the case of tension headaches, with only one third improving and two thirds suffering more frequent attacks than they did before the onset of peri-menopause.

Women who have a hysterectomy but retain their ovaries will experience similar changes to their headache patterns as women who have not had a hysterectomy. Women whose ovaries are removed as part of the hysterectomy procedure will experience more frequent and severe migraines with a worse long-term outlook. There is very little data available on the effect of a full hysterectomy on tension headaches.

Hormonal Contraceptives and Headaches

Hormonal contraceptives contain a combination of artificial forms of estrogen and progesterone, or progesterone alone. Headache is a common side effect when starting hormonal contraceptives, but tends to improve over the first few months. Some women experience migraines for the first time and a few may develop aura without headache.

Pre-existing migraines with aura may become more frequent and severe, whereas migraines without aura commonly improve. Tension headaches appear to be little affected by hormonal contraceptive use, but not much data is available on this.

For some women who experience new or more frequent migraines and stop taking hormonal contraceptives, the improvement is immediate. For other women, there may be a 6–12 month delay before any improvement is noticed, and some women continue to suffer from migraines in the longer term.

The most commonly used types of hormonal contraceptives include:

- The combined oral contraceptive pill, or 'the pill' for short, which is the most popular hormonal contraceptive.
- A contraceptive patch which is applied to the skin and worn continuously.
- A flexible vaginal ring which is worn for 3 weeks then removed.

All combined hormonal contraceptives provide 3 weeks of active treatment followed by a 1 week break during which progesterone withdrawal bleeding occurs. This replicates what happens during the natural menstrual cycle as progesterone drops.

With the combined oral contraceptive pill, progesterone withdrawal bleeding occurs during the dummy pill week in the last week of the 4-week treatment cycle. It also occurs with the ring and the patch after 3 weeks, when treatment is discontinued for 1 week. The last week of the 4-week cycle can provoke an estrogen withdrawal headache in women who have previously suffered menstrual headaches. In the case of the combined pill, headaches occur most commonly around the third day of the 7-day dummy pill series (shown outlined in Figure 7.2). However, headaches are becoming less frequent with more modern, lower dose pills.

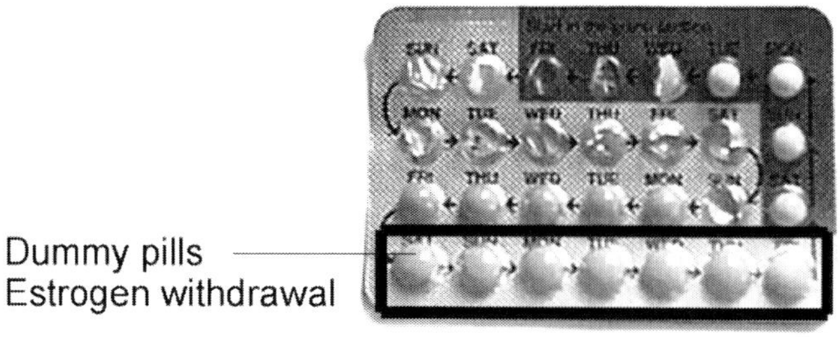

Figure 7.2: The combined pill showing estrogen free days

My recommendation is if you have suffered severe menstrual migraines in the past, you would be well advised to avoid 'the pill' and other types of cyclic hormonal contraceptives. Estrogen withdrawal during the week when estrogen is stopped can trigger a severe form of migraine known as status migrainosus. This headache lasts longer than 72 hours, is usually accompanied by extreme nausea and vomiting and by pain which does not respond to the usual medications. It requires emergency medical treatment.

The other main types of hormonal contraceptives contain progesterone only. Unlike the combination contraceptives, they are used continuously without a break.

Progesterone only contraceptives include:

- The 'mini pill' which relies on thickening the cervical mucus. It only prevents ovulation about 50% of the time so menstrual bleeding tends to be irregular.
- An intrauterine device that releases progesterone over 5 years.
- An intramuscular injection of progesterone every 3 months.
- An implant beneath the skin of a flexible rod that releases progesterone over 3 years.

Progesterone only contraceptives overcome the problem of estrogen withdrawal headache. However unfortunately the forms of progesterone used are more likely to cause headaches than the progesterone produced during the natural menstrual cycle. Higher doses increase headache risk.

HRT Medications and Headaches

Hormone replacement therapy (HRT) medications contain estrogen, either alone, or in combination with progesterone. Many women choose to start HRT in the later years of peri-menopause to combat the effects caused by changes in natural hormone levels.

HRT medications may improve headaches indirectly, by relieving night sweats that disturb sleep. It also seems reasonable to expect HRT to improve headaches directly by stabilising estrogen levels, especially during peri-menopause when hormones fluctuate wildly.

Studies have shown that HRT may indeed improve headaches, but it may also make them worse or it may cause no apparent change. Results depend strongly on the characteristics of the particular HRT formulations tested. There has been very little systematic investigation of the effect of some of the newer HRT medications on headaches.

Overall, HRT appears to have little effect on the frequency or severity of tension headaches.[39] It has a variable effect on migraines, with approximately 20% of sufferers experiencing more frequent and longer-lasting attacks. HRT often worsens migraine with aura and may provoke aura for the first time. Reducing the dose usually prevents this. In contrast, HRT has been shown to be protective for migraine without aura, provided the dose is sufficient to prevent total estrogen levels dropping below the threshold at which a migraine is triggered.

Headache sufferers who have experienced menstrual headaches in the past should avoid cyclic HRT regimens in which there are gaps in estrogen therapy. This type of regimen is likely to provoke an estrogen withdrawal headache during the 3–6 days when no estrogen is taken. Hot flushes are also likely to return at this time.

With any hormonal medication you are taking, I recommend reading the fine print to check that the estrogen dose is constant throughout the entire treatment cycle. If you are in doubt, ask your pharmacist. Some women in consultation with their doctor may choose to obtain separate prescriptions for estrogen and progesterone medications, which allows greater flexibility in the dose and method of delivery.

Key Points

- Female hormones can affect the frequency and severity of headache pain and should be considered, if applicable, as part of your headache management program.
- Fluctuations in estrogen are the main cause of menstrual headaches.
- Migraine frequency tends to decrease with age.
- Hormonal changes can't be avoided, only managed.

8

Painkillers

Painkillers are marketed and used as a quick, convenient fix for headache pain, but I believe they cause more problems than they solve. Not only do they have unwelcome and sometimes damaging side effects, the long term use of painkillers can actually cause a type of headache, known as a rebound, or medication overuse, headache.

Headaches are the most common reason for taking OTC pain-killers, accounting for 30-40% of their total use.[40] People who suffer from headaches use OTC pain-killers on average 3 times per week,[41] which means headache sufferers as a group are at a significant risk of damaging their health from overuse of OTC pain-killers.

They may get you feeling better in the moment, but long-term use can increase the frequency and intensity of your headaches and start a cycle of dependence that can lead to addiction and detrimental side effects, without ever tackling the source of the problem.

Before we start, a cautionary reminder – if you are already taking headache medication, please consult your doctor before you stop taking your medication, or alter your dose.

Over-the-Counter (OTC) Painkillers

All medications designed to relieve pain contain an analgesic – a substance that reduces the sensation of pain registered by the brain. The word comes from the Greek an = without and algos = pain. There are three different types of analgesics used in OTC painkillers.

Paracetamol

No one really knows how paracetamol (known as acetaminophen in North America) works, but it's thought to act on the parts of the brain that receive pain messages and control body temperature. It can ease pain and lower a fever, but it won't reduce any swelling or inflammation.

NSAIDS

NSAID stands for non-steroidal anti-inflammatory drug and includes drugs like aspirin and ibuprofen. NSAIDs reduce fever, pain, and inflammation. Not all NSAIDs are the same – some work in slightly different ways from others.

Codeine

Codeine is a weak opioid (substances obtained from opium as starting material, and which include morphine and heroin) available as an OTC painkiller in some countries.

Choosing an OTC painkiller

Contrary to the impression drug company advertising tries to create, analgesics do not target a specific part of the body. All the drugs above are absorbed into the bloodstream and travel to most tissues, not just the site of pain.

Nor is there nearly as much choice between OTC painkillers as there appears to be from the vast array of products with different brand names on the shelves of supermarkets or pharmacies.

It's important to look beyond brand names, appearance and packaging of OTC painkillers and get into the habit of checking the labels to find out the active ingredients and the dose of each one. When you start reading the labels, you'll discover that many of these products have the same active ingredients, often in the same amounts.

And there is the reverse issue. There are lots of products with very similar brand names and packaging, but different active ingredients. For example, the time of writing, packets of Lemsip Max Cold & Flu sachets and Lemsip Flu 12 hour capsules looked very similar. But Lemsip Max Cold & Flu contained 1000 mg of paracetamol, the maximum recommended dose to be taken at any one time. On the other hand, Lemsip Flu 12 hour capsules didn't contain paracetamol – instead they contained 300 mg of ibuprofen.

Becoming familiar with the different types of active ingredients in OTC painkillers will make choosing the right painkiller a lot easier to do. If in doubt, ask for advice from your pharmacist.

Prescription Drugs

This very brief overview covers some examples of the multitude of prescription-only medications used to treat headaches. It includes medications used for acute and preventative treatment. All these medications have significant side effects and there are many precautions associated with their use.

If you are already taking one of these medications, consult your doctor before altering the dose in any way.

Acute Treatment

Acute, or abortive, treatments are short-term treatments designed to relieve or stop the symptoms of a headache once it has begun. These include prescription NSAIDs, opiates, muscle relaxants, anti-nausea drugs, Butabil, ergots, Triptan and Midrin.

Some of these drugs, such as Butabil and opiates, are highly addictive and should be taken with great caution.

Preventative Treatment

Many different medications are used as preventatives against migraine, tension headaches and cluster headaches. Many were initially introduced for another medical condition but were observed to reduce headache. Some of the most commonly used classes are medications used to treat high blood pressure (beta-blockers), antidepressants, anti-seizure medications and some anti-allergy drugs.

Why are Painkillers so Popular?

They Offer a Quick Fix

Painkillers offer an instant, inexpensive, easy solution to an immediate problem. When time is money and we're expected to keep 'soldiering on', it can be very tempting, and understandable, to reach for a solution that promises so much return for very little effort.

We Overestimate the Success of Drugs

A preventive medication is considered successful if it reaches or exceeds a 50% responder rate, which is an arbitrary measure defined as a 50% reduction in headaches in 50% of patients receiving medication.[42]

The placebo response in testing medication is usually quite high in both acute migraine and preventive studies (approximately 20% to 30%, or higher).

Even prescription pain relievers or migraine abortives may not work much more than half the time. When they do work, it can take up to four hours to get the full effect,[43] and that's still considered a successful time frame.

When set against their unpleasant and sometimes dangerous side-effects, the success rates of migraine medications starts to look less impressive.

Marketing

Aggressive marketing targeted at both doctors and consumers is by far the most powerful force in promoting the use of medications. The problem is pharmaceutical marketing is often promotion disguised as information.

In Australia, as in most countries except for the USA and New Zealand, drug companies cannot market prescription-only drugs to patients directly. However, promotional information still reaches patients via the media, self-help groups for patients suffering various illnesses and the internet.

We Live in a Culture of Treating Rather than Preventing

Thomas Edison believed 'the doctor of the future will give no medicine, but will interest his patients in the care of the human body, in diet, and in the cause and prevention of disease.

Although there have been many medical advances since Edison's time, the doctor is unfortunately still 'giving medicine'. The traditional approach in Western medicine has always been to diagnose a disease or condition from known symptoms and then treat it with medication, surgery or various procedures.

This focus on diagnosis and treatment works well for infectious diseases, but has not been very useful for multi-factorial chronic diseases like cardiovascular disease and headache, which benefit from preventative measures and long-term changes to lifestyle and diet.

Especially when a patient is in pain, many doctors feel helpless if they can't provide some form of immediate pain relief.

Acute, Abortive and Preventative Treatment

There are three main categories of prescription headache medications which are designed to provide different types of treatment. These are:

- Acute treatment – medication taken to relieve pain or other symptoms like nausea after the headache has already begun.
- Abortive treatment – medication used to stop (abort) the migraine process after an attack has already begun. It is important not to wait too long to take it or it won't be properly absorbed. Stopping the migraine process relieves pain and nausea. The medications used are meant to be specific for migraine but they are sometimes also used to stop tension headaches which have some migraine-like characteristics.
- Preventative treatment, also known as prophylactic treatment, are medications which must be taken daily, irrespective of whether or not you have a headache. These medications reduce the frequency, duration and severity of future headache attacks but certainly don't completely prevent them. All have very significant side effects.

Prescription-only pain-killers used for acute treatment of headaches are similar to their OTC counterparts, except they are more effective and their side-effects are more pronounced.

The main active ingredient is an analgesic. Sometimes the analgesic is combined with other active ingredients which have different functions. These can include a sedative (a substance with a calming effect which allows sleep), a muscle relaxant and caffeine, which aids absorption.

For treating the nausea and vomiting that often accompanies migraine, anti-nausea drugs are available on prescription, sometimes combined with an analgesic.

The usual protocol for treating headaches with medication is to start with an OTC pain-killer. If this proves ineffective you will normally progress to a more powerful prescription pain-killer and/or to an abortive treatment.

Doctors will usually recommend preventative medications if acute or abortive treatments are required more often than twice a week, as these treatments almost certainly lead to rebound headaches. So you can be in a situation where the medication you are taking is causing more headaches, which you take more medication to manage.

If you are facing this possibility, I believe it is time to start looking for non-drug alternatives to headache prevention and treatment. Many headache researchers are starting to agree.

Some of the many disadvantages of preventative medications include:

- In spite of their name they do not completely prevent headaches – in fact a reduction of 50% in frequency, severity and duration of attacks is considered a good result for any particular medication in this group. Hence abortive / pain relieving medication will also be needed to treat those headache attacks that do occur.
- Even though any particular medication has only an approximately 50% chance of working, to see if it is effective, it generally needs to be trialled for several weeks at a time, each time with a staged increase in dose. A total time of at least 2 to 3 months is needed for this.
- All have very significant side effects.
- You tend to focus narrowly on monitoring of your pain levels and other symptoms to decide whether or not this medication and dose work for you. This can actually make the pain worse.
- You will need to take the medication for a minimum of 6 months to 1 year. After that the dose is gradually reduced to see whether the headaches return.
- You surrender a lot more control. Once you take the decision to start preventative headache medications, it tends to close off the search for non-drug alternatives, such as having treatment for trigger points in your neck muscles.

A Lack of Awareness of Alternatives

Many headache sufferers are not aware there are non-pharmacological methods of treating headache pain.

Comprehensive and unbiased information about non-drug methods of headache prevention and treatment is hard to find, either in books or online. In contrast, a vast amount of detailed information on headache medication is readily available online from sources such as medical information sites, various national headache and pain foundations, self-help groups and consumer organisations.

Such sites are likely to spend some time discussing how to identify and avoid headache triggers, including stress. However, alternative treatments are generally only mentioned in passing. In the end, there's not much money to be made in advising people about the importance of drinking enough water, or the need to seek treatment from a manual therapist for tight jaw, neck and shoulder muscles.

Why Painkillers Should be Less Popular

Tolerance and Dependence

Tolerance occurs when your response to a drug decreases, and you need to take larger doses of the drug to achieve the same effect. Without carefully managing your intake of painkillers, it's easy to become trapped in a vicious cycle of worsening headache attacks and increasing reliance on painkillers to get through a week.

As drug use continues, tolerance can progress to physical dependence, which is characterised by withdrawal symptoms if you stop taking the drug. People who fear a headache attack and start taking pain relievers just in case they develop a headache are the most at risk of developing tolerance and physical dependence. Physical dependence is different to addiction, which is a compulsion to seek out the drug.

One of the main withdrawal symptoms from OTC and prescription painkillers is a rebound headache. If you take non-opiate painkillers or abortive medications for headaches for more than 10-15 days a month, for over three months, and then stop taking them, you will suffer rebound headaches.

For painkillers containing opiates like codeine, or barbiturates like butalbital, tolerance and physical dependence develops much more quickly and withdrawal is much more severe. This is partly because psychological dependence is quick to develop for these opiates, with cravings for the pleasurable emotional effects that the drugs induce.

My advice would be to avoid any headache medications containing opiates or butalbital because of their dependent and addictive potential. I also believe these medications are unsuitable for migraines. They can increase nausea in a migraine attack and increase the likelihood that an episodic migraine will progress to a chronic migraine.[44]

There are Other Ingredients in There Too

It's worth checking to see what else is in your painkillers – some of the extra substances might not be helping you in the long run.

Caffeine

Caffeine acts as an enhancer in painkillers, added to accelerate the absorption of analgesic ingredients into the bloodstream and to enhance the pain relieving effect. Caffeine seems to have little pain relieving effect of its own, although, if dilated blood vessels are contributing to headache pain, caffeine acts to constrict the blood vessels. In fact, some people report that the caffeine in a cup of coffee assists with managing migraine if taken at the first signs of an attack.

However, caffeine is a double-edged sword and products containing caffeine are among those more likely to lead to withdrawal headaches.

Doxylamine

Doxylamine succinate is a sedating antihistamine (anti-allergy agent) with anti-nausea properties. Apart from drowsiness, side effects include dry mouth, lack of coordination (ataxia) and urinary retention. Combination drugs containing paracetamol and codeine with doxylamine succinate are marketed for treatment of tension headache, migraine and other types of pain, e.g. Mersyndol, Dolased, and Syndol.

They All Have Side Effects

You should make sure you're aware of the side effects of every drug you take, but here is an overview of the side effects that make me wary of painkillers.

One of the most common side effects, which I am especially interested in, is the rebound headache. It's one of the main reasons I encourage people to avoid taking painkillers in the first place.

Rebound Headaches

Rebound headaches are a vicious cycle of worsening headaches, triggered and driven by taking painkillers, especially if you overuse or misuse your medication, which, for most OTC painkillers, means taking the prescribed dose for longer than three days – easy to do when your head hurts! You are also very likely to develop a rebound headache if you take migraine abortives more often than twice a week for 10–15 weeks.

A rebound headache is a response to withdrawing from your medication, especially if your medication contains caffeine[45], which is included in lots of medications to speed up the reaction of the other ingredients. Caffeine in medications, combined with consuming caffeine in coffee, tea, soft drinks or chocolate, makes you more vulnerable to a rebound headache.

A rebound headache happens as the effect of the medication wears off. You experience a withdrawal headache, prompting you to take more medication, which eventually wears off and leads to another headache and the desire to take more medication. And so the cycle continues until you can start to suffer from chronic daily headaches.

You might have a rebound headache if:

- Your headache occurs every day or almost every day
- The pain is present on waking and generally worst then
- The pain gets worse if you stop taking painkillers
- The pain is a dull pressure on both sides of the head
- The pain is not made worse by routine activities
- There is no nausea, vomiting, sensitivity to light or to noise.

Reducing the amount of medication you are using will initially increase the intensity of your headaches, so it's very important you consult with your doctor if you think you are suffering from rebound headaches, so you can plan and monitor your treatment or strategy. The headaches get worse for a while, making it much harder to remain convinced that it's the pain-killers that are the cause of the headaches, and not the solution. It's so important to remember that painkillers are not the solution, but in fact the reason for headache.

When first reducing the amount of painkillers they are taking, many people sleep badly, and feel restless, anxious and nauseous. After 7-10 days, headaches usually return to their 'normal' frequency. However, some people can take several weeks or even months to get the medications out of their system.

Symptoms of codeine withdrawal include:

- weakness
- yawning
- runny nose
- sweating
- headaches
- muscle pain and twitches
- irregular heartbeat
- nausea
- vomiting
- fever
- insomnia.

For barbiturates, such as butalbital, withdrawal symptoms include:

- nausea
- weakness
- anxiety
- tremors
- elevated blood pressure and pulse
- sweating
- possibly seizures, which may be life-threatening.

It can be helpful to know what to expect and understand the symptoms you might experience when reducing your painkiller dosage is normal and part of the healing process. All of these symptoms are superimposed on those of rebound headache, due to withdrawal of the non-opiate analgesic.

Ideally, you should avoid becoming physically dependent on pain-killers in the first place. They should only ever be taken very occasionally, as it is easy to become trapped in a vicious cycle of ever worsening headache attacks and increasing reliance on painkillers to get through your week.

Addiction

Addiction is more likely with opiate based painkillers, in particular codeine[46], because its use is usually less closely supervised. In countries where codeine is freely available in OTC painkillers, the potential for addiction is increased.

Many cases of overuse and addiction start with the pain of an injury or a severe headache. I recommend avoiding all painkillers containing any type of opiate because they are so likely to be addictive.

If you believe you are addicted to your painkillers, I recommend talking with your doctor.

Gastro-intestinal Bleeding

Gastro-intestinal bleeding is the most common side effect of treatment with NSAIDs. Damage to the stomach lining occurs within the first three days of use of NSAIDs and approximately 5% of people experience blood loss of greater than 5ml per day.[47] Up to half develop gastro-intestinal lesions that can readily be seen with an endoscope.[48] Unfortunately, because they are taking painkillers, people usually have no stomach pain to act as an early warning sign that something is wrong. By the time they seek medical attention, they are often seriously ill.

Kidney Failure

Kidney failure is another risk of prolonged use of NSAIDs, especially at high doses. Approximately 10% of all cases of end-stage kidney disease are attributed to overuse of NSAIDs.

Liver Damage

Liver damage is a common side effect of high doses of paracetamol. Although paracetamol is normally thought to be safe, a recent study showed that two weeks of use at the recommended dose led to abnormal liver function tests, indicating minor, reversible liver damage[49] and paracetamol is responsible for over 50% of all cases of acute liver failure.

Safe Use of Painkillers

Taking a painkiller shouldn't be your first response every time you get a headache, but there are some occasions where a painkiller can temporarily relieve your headache symptoms, break the pain cycle and give you chance to get yourself together.

The warning here is that the more you use them, the greater your risk of experiencing serious side effects and developing rebound headaches. You can also get trapped in a cycle of taking ever more medications, all with their own side effects, where each medication is meant to treat the side effects of the one that went before.

See Your Doctor

If you do decide to use an OTC painkiller for headache pain, don't just grab something on the way past in the supermarket or convenience store. Check first to make sure it will be suitable for you. You should check with your doctor, but at the very least, you should check with your pharmacist.

Take the medication in accordance with the directions given on the packet or by your doctor, and do not exceed the specified dose. It is important that you read and fully understand the label on the packet, especially any important warnings and possible side effects.

To protect your own health, it's important to know what the active ingredients are in all drugs you are taking. Many OTC medicinal products for different purposes contain the same active ingredients and you want to be sure you don't accidentally take an overdose. Accidental overdoses are surprisingly common.

Be Aware of Side Effects

Most side effects are minor and don't affect most people taking painkillers. However, people with certain medical conditions, the elderly, and women who are pregnant or breast-feeding need to be especially careful.

Make sure you read the packet for listed side effects before you start taking painkillers and contact your doctor if you think you are experiencing any side effects.

Some Painkillers to Avoid

The table below lists a few well-known brand names of OTC and prescription painkillers which contain butalbital, codeine or other opiates.

I strongly advise against taking them because of their addictive potential and because they cause rebound headaches to develop more rapidly than alternative painkillers.

Some Painkillers to Avoid	
Active Ingredients	**Well-known Brand Names**
Over-the Counter (Pharmacy)	
Aspirin with codeine	Codis, Aspalgin, Disprin Forte
Paracetamol with codeine	Panadeine, Solpadeine
Ibuprofen with codeine	Nurofen Plus, Panafen Plus
Paracetamol, codeine & doxylamine succinate	Mersyndol, Dolased, Syndol
By Prescription	
Paracetamol, butalbital & caffeine	Fioricet, Esgic
Paracetamol, butalbital, codeine & caffeine	Fioricet #3 with Codeine
Aspirin, butalbital & caffeine	Fiorinal
Aspirin, butalbital, codeine & caffeine	Fiorinal #3 with Codeine
Paracetamol and hydrocodone	Vicodin

For More Information

The book *Pain and Profits: The History of the Headache and Its Remedies in America* by Janice Rae McTavish is a fascinating look at the pivotal role played by headache remedies in development of the US OTC pharmaceutical industry.

There are many useful and reliable sources of information about medications online that can help you find out more about side effects and precautions, dosage instructions etc.

Useful sites include:

- MedlinePlus at http://www.nlm.nih.gov/medlineplus/druginformation.html. This is a service of the US National Library of Medicine (NLM) and National Institutes of Health (NIH). You can browse lists of drugs, supplements, and herbal products alphabetically according the first letter of the generic (scientific) name of the active ingredient, e.g. ibuprofen, or the brand names under which it is sold in the United States, e.g. Advil, Motrin IB.
- RXMed at http://www.rxmed.com/ under the drug and illness section (detailed information on many prescription medications listed under US brand names).

Key Points

- Painkillers are not a good long term solution for managing head ache pain because they produce side effects and can make your headaches worse in the longer term.
- Both prescription and over-the-counter pain killers can cause rebound headaches.
- Rebound headaches are caused by withdrawing from pain medication, which can establish a cycle of dependence on pain killers to keep the rebound headaches under control.
- If you suspect you are suffering from rebound headaches, you should consult your doctor before stopping your pain medication so you can plan and monitor your treatment or strategy.
- Withdrawing from pain medication will initially make rebound headaches worse.

Part C

Managing Headaches:

Diagnosis

9

Taking Charge

Recurring headaches can make you feel powerless, especially if you're relying on medication that sometimes works and crossing your fingers to get through a week.

Knowledge is power and now it's time to put that knowledge into action. Successful strategies to manage your pain can turn frustration into hope. With some effort and persistence, I know you will be able to stop walking on egg shells, constantly worrying about when the next attack will strike, and instead, implement tested strategies for prevention and relief that you can rely on.

The following chapters are all about helping you manage and prevent headaches without drugs. The main benefit is, obviously, a reduction in the frequency and severity of your headaches, but working to find successful non-drug therapies will bring other, profound benefits to your life.

With some investigation and exploration, you will be able to start managing your headaches instead of letting them manage you.

It's time to take charge.

Diagnosis

First things first, you need to know what you're dealing with, which isn't always easy. The broad diagnosis of a headache is simple – your head hurts, you have a headache – but it's much harder to be accurate about what type of headache you have.

Many people who believe they suffer from migraines have tension headaches. On the other hand, approximately half of all migraine sufferers have never been diagnosed,[50],[51] especially those whose headaches are less severe. Getting an accurate diagnosis is crucial – once you know what you're dealing with, you can develop a targeted strategy to manage it.

Where does it hurt?

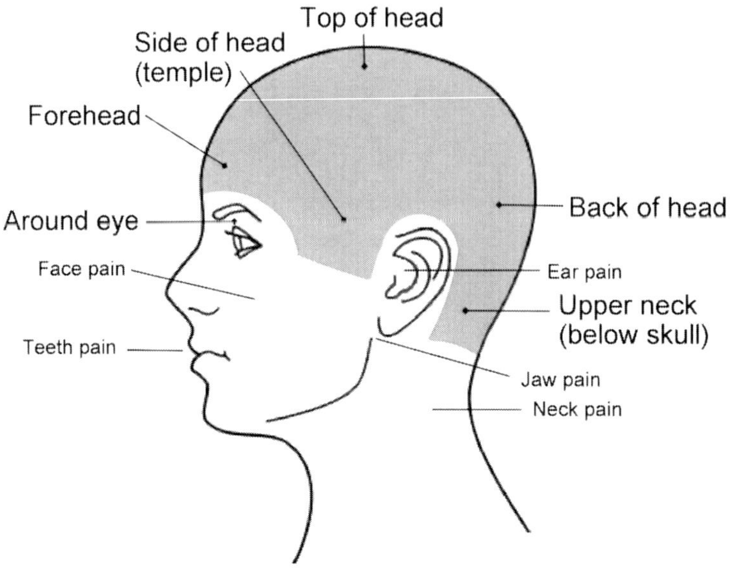

Figure 9.1 – Areas where we feel pain which we would call headache (shaded area) (Other areas that may hurt during a headache attack are also included)

Primary and Secondary Headaches

Medically, headaches are divided into two broad categories – primary and secondary. Essentially, a primary headache, such as a tension headache or migraine, is a medical condition in itself, whereas a secondary headache is a symptom of another medical condition, such as depression or an injury.

Doctors use this classification, so it is worthwhile being aware of it, but the distinction between primary and secondary headaches isn't always obvious or helpful.

Many secondary headaches cause pain that is hard to differentiate from the pain caused by tension headaches or migraine. To add to this difficulty, it's possible to have both a primary headache and a secondary headache at the same time.

My process of treating headaches is the same, whether they are secondary or primary, so I will discuss 'headaches' without using this classification.

I'm going to concentrate on the six main categories of headache:

- Tension
- Migraine
- Rebound
- Sinus
- Neck and jaw
- Cluster.

The three most common are tension, migraine and rebound.

Tension Headache

Tension headaches often occur near the start or end of the day, during or after periods of stress, and may last 30 minutes to 7 days, although most last less than 24 hours.

The onset of pain is usually gradual and intensifies progressively. The pain is steady and non-pulsating. It's often described as a dull, aching, pressing or squeezing sensation, like a band tightening around the head.

Most sufferers experience pain in the temples, across the forehead, especially above the eyes, at the back of the head and neck, and sometimes in the shoulders. The pain usually starts at the base of the skull and spreads around to the forehead.

Tension headache is not accompanied by nausea or vomiting, but there may be loss of appetite. Sometimes sensitivity to light or sound occurs. The intensity of pain varies from person to person and from one episode to the next, but is normally mild to moderate. A tension headache isn't aggravated by routine physical activity such as walking or climbing stairs.

Migraine Headache

Migraine attacks often develop at night or in the early morning. The headache phase of the attack can last from 4–72 hours, although most last from 6–12 hours.

The onset of migraine pain intensifies progressively and gradually abates. The pain is usually pulsating in character, often described as throbbing or pounding, and tends to throb at the same rate as the heartbeat and the pain is aggravated by movement. Sometimes the pain is in the forehead, around the eye or at the back of the head. It mainly affects one side of the head around the temple region and stays there for the entire attack.

A migraine attack is frequently accompanied by nausea and vomiting. Other symptoms can include diarrhoea, a pale face, cold hands and feet, a runny or blocked nose, extreme scalp tenderness, muscle or neck pain and a sensitivity to light, sound and odours.

Migraine Early Warning Signs

For up to 70% of migraine sufferers, an impending attack is preceded by one or more early warning signs, often more than 24 hours beforehand.

This phase, called a prodrome, is the first stage of the migraine process. Symptoms include:

- Neck stiffness
- Constant yawning
- Fatigue
- Mood swings
- Intense food cravings (especially for sweets and chocolate)
- Irritability and restlessness
- Slowed thinking, difficulty concentrating and memory problems
- Increased urination or fluid retention
- Constipation or diarrhoea
- Cold hands and feet
- Extreme sensitivity to light or sounds
- Aura.

Aura with Migraine

About 20% of migraine sufferers experience a highly characteristic warning sign called an aura. This is a temporary visual disturbance lasting from 5–60 minutes. The most common aura symptoms include bright zigzag lines, flashing lights, difficulty in focusing and blind spots. These symptoms are sometimes accompanied by pins and needles, numbness and speech difficulties.

There is very little written information about prodrome for tension headache, but this may simply be because tension headache has received so much less study than migraine.

A recent paper[52] reported that sufferers of episodic tension headache experienced similar prodromal symptoms to those listed for migraine, but that they were less pronounced. So if you suffer from tension headache, it is still well worth checking to see if you can notice any potential prodromal symptoms.

Rebound Headache

Rebound headache (or medication overuse headache) is a well-known effect of regular, long-term use of OTC and/or prescription painkillers for headache pain. If you become physically dependent on pain-killing medication, the rebound headache you experience is actually a withdrawal symptom which appears near the time that the next dose is due, most frequently in the morning.

Overuse of painkillers is responsible for approximately one third of chronic daily headaches. You are very likely to develop rebound headache if you take painkillers or migraine abortives, such as triptans, more than twice a week for between 10–15 weeks.

Rebound headaches usually occur every day. The pain is present on waking and generally gets worse during the day. The pain also intensifies if you stop taking the painkillers.

The pain is similar to a tension headache. There is often a dull pressure on both sides of the head. The symptoms aren't aggravated by movement, and there isn't any nausea, vomiting, sensitivity to light or to noise.

Comparison of Tension, Migraine and Rebound Headache Symptoms

Feature	Headache Symptoms		
	Tension	Migraine	Rebound
Onset	gradual	gradual	gradual
Aura	no	sometimes	no
Duration	30 min–7 days	4 hours–3 days	Remains until a painkiller is used
Pain intensity	mild/moderate	moderate/severe	mild/moderate
Pain character	ache/pressure	throbbing	ache/pressure
Pain on one or both sides	both (mostly)	one (mostly)	both
Aggravated by movement	no	yes	no
Normal activities possible	yes	no (rest needed)	yes
Nausea	no	yes	no
Vomiting	no	yes	no
Sensitivity to light	sometimes	yes	no
Sensitivity to noise	sometimes	yes	no
Sinus (eye / nose)	no	sometimes	no

Three Less Common Headaches

These next three headache types are less common, but worth being aware of:

Sinus

A sinus headache usually occurs after either an infection following a head cold, or an allergy attack, when you would have typical hay fever symptoms such as sneezing. They are quite rare and symptoms disappear when the infection is successfully treated. There is a perception that sinus headaches are quite common, but often, what is perceived as a sinus headache is a migraine with very similar symptoms.

Migraine is often misdiagnosed as sinus headache, especially by headache sufferers themselves, but also by their doctors.[53] Migraines are commonly accompanied by sinus symptoms, including stuffy or running nose, sinus pressure, sinus pain and watering eyes.

Unlike migraines, sinus headache pain is localised to a specific area of the cheekbones, forehead or bridge of the nose, depending on which sinus is affected. The headache is also accompanied by a stuffy or running nose, sinus pressure, sinus pain and watering eyes. The area often feels tender when pressed.

Neck and Jaw Headaches

Neck and jaw-related headaches caused by musculoskeletal problems are two of the most common types of headache.[54,55,56,57,58]

Both types of headache have variable symptoms and are often misdiagnosed[59,60] as tension headache or migraine. When nausea is present in addition to pain, they may be indistinguishable from migraine.[61] To complicate matters further, neck and jaw related headaches can occur on their own, or they may co-exist with tension headache or migraine.

Cluster Headaches

Cluster headaches are a chronic disease. They mostly affect young men and tend to run in families. They often recur at the same time each year. However, in about 10-15% of sufferers, attacks occur daily without remission.

The onset of pain is very rapid, and the pain, which is non-pulsating, is always on one side of the head, especially behind one eye. It may spread to the forehead, temple, cheek and upper gum on same side of face. The pain is described as sharp, penetrating or burning.

Red Flag Headaches

Just a reminder that some headaches are symptoms of serious conditions and several of these are immediately life-threatening. Of course, having headaches with these characteristics doesn't mean you have a serious brain disorder – most people don't. However, you should have the headaches assessed.

Important symptoms to watch out for:

- A new headache, especially after age 50
- A change in your old pattern of headaches
- A headache that is unusually severe or has a very rapid onset
- A headache that starts after a head injury (even several weeks later)
- A headache associated with severe pain in the eye or ear
- A persistent headache that progressively worsens over days or weeks
- A sudden-onset headache that starts during exercise or sex
- A headache triggered by coughing, bending over or lying down.

Additional danger signs include:

- A stiff neck and fever
- Severe nausea or vomiting and neurological symptoms such as weakness, difficulty speaking or walking, vision changes
- A very rapid onset where pain reaches peak intensity in seconds or minutes
- Pain so severe you would describe it as your 'worst ever headache'.

If you ever experience a headache with these features you should either phone your doctor or call for an ambulance.

Getting an Accurate Diagnosis

Self-diagnosis for headache is very common and, most of the time, for a one-off, mild headache, it's all you need. But if your headaches are frequent and debilitating, or you are taking OTC painkillers regularly, you should seek professional advice. The Internet is not your friend here, and there is also a chance your headache might be a symptom of something serious. Instead of avoiding the issue or scaring yourself, you should seek professional advice to help you identify exactly what you have.

When you are seeking professional advice for your headaches, there are two different assessments you should get – one from a medical doctor and one from a manual therapist.

Medical diagnosis of headaches is primarily based on your headache history and symptoms. If your doctor is unable to find any obvious cause for your headaches, it's likely they will decide they are either tension headaches or migraines based on their characteristics and often prescribe medication.

A manual therapist will assess your headaches from your medical history, by observing and testing your posture and movement and especially by feeling your muscles and joints. Most medical doctors are not trained to recognise untreated musculoskeletal problems as a cause or a contributing factor in headaches.

Manual therapy is one of the most successful strategies for reducing the frequency and severity of your headache attacks, but it's vital to check there are no undiagnosed medical conditions which could be perpetuating your headaches or aggravating your musculoskeletal problems.

The only way to be sure you're getting a thorough diagnosis is to see both a medical practitioner and a manual therapist.

Even for medical professionals and experienced manual therapists, an accurate diagnosis can be a challenge. There is a significant overlap of symptoms between each category of headache. A migraine without aura can feel a lot like a tension headache. Migraines are often misdiagnosed as sinus headaches because they share so many symptoms.

This overlap is compounded further because not every person with a particular type of headache will exhibit all of the symptoms, and the symptoms may change from one attack to the next. It is also quite possible to have more than one type of headache simultaneously. Variations can occur between each attack for the one person, especially in symptoms such as severity and location of pain. Some attacks are milder than others and there may even be variation within the one attack, as when pain moves from one side of the head to the other.

To add to the confusion, there is the temptation to call all severe headaches migraines. A diagnosis of tension headache can seem like a liability. This is partly due to the different meanings of the word tension. Although tension headaches were thought to result from muscular tension, the underlying cause was said to be emotional stress and tension. So they were, and sometimes still are, referred to as stress headaches or muscle contraction headaches. Migraine has been called a neurovascular headache and even a neurological disease – both labels that are far more likely to be taken seriously than tension headache.

Your Role in Diagnosis

The greatest resource you have in correctly diagnosing and treating your headaches is you.

You need to know your headaches, inside and out, so you can work with medical professionals and manual therapists to correctly treat and manage your headaches. You may not rid yourself of headaches completely, but if you take charge, you will, at the very least, significantly reduce the frequency and severity of your headaches.

One of the most important tools in your kit will be a headache diary. Keeping a close, ongoing record of what is happening, when and why, will give you an insight in to potential triggers, identify treatments that work and give your medical health professionals an invaluable insight into your condition.

Key Points

- It's difficult to accurately diagnose the type of headache you have, even for medical professionals.
- You should get your regular headaches assessed by both a medical professional and a manual therapist.
- You need to play an active role in diagnosing and monitoring your headaches.
- A headache diary is an invaluable tool for you and your medical practitioners in diagnosing and treating your headaches.

10

Headache Diary

Why?

A detailed headache diary is a crucial step to getting a clear and accurate understanding of what's happening with your headaches and gaining control over them, and it's an invaluable resource for the medical professionals you choose to work with.

Keeping a diary can feel like an overwhelming task. It takes time and effort, and it requires you to think about pain and other unpleasant symptoms, probably when you feel least like doing it, but the benefits of keeping a diary far outweigh the time and effort required.

A diary:

- will help you accurately record your use of headache medications, which is important, because we routinely underestimate our medication use
- can help you identify personal headache triggers, which helps you minimise or avoid those triggers, and so reduce the number and severity of headaches
- can also help you identify possible early warning signs and any actions that worked to reduce the severity of headaches. This means that when you feel a headache starting you can quickly start effective actions which may reduce the effects of the headache. Started early enough, therapies such as self-treatment of muscular trigger points or relaxation may prevent your headache from developing, or at the very least, reduce its severity.

Motivation is one of the big benefits of a diary. Treating your headaches successfully without drugs can take time and patience. Manual therapy should deliver some improvement in your headaches after one or two treatments, but most of the methods of headache prevention are likely to show more gradual improvements. For example, relaxation techniques take time to learn and changes in diet and sleep patterns tend to take a while to show an effect.

A diary helps remind you of the improvements you've made. Signs that your headaches are improving include less frequent severe pain, pain not lasting as long, more headache-free days, a generally lower pain rating and a decrease in the use of headache medications. These are indicators that are easy to miss if you're not keeping a diary. All of this can help you stay the course, not get discouraged and remember you are engaged in a long-term solution.

Downloadable Headache Diary

I developed a downloadable, printable Headache Diary. You can use the diary to record information about your headaches, and enable you to better review and analyse them.

Information on where to download the Headache Diary is in the Conclusion section at the end of this book.

The diary contains instructions and worksheets to record headaches, symptoms and your actions. You can then review and analyse your experience over a number of headaches – the diary provides for details of eight headaches. This means you will be able to see any patterns and trends occurring with your headaches.

What the Headache Diary Sheets Do

It can be hard enough to concentrate on writing anything during or after a headache attack, let alone deciding on what to write or thinking about what it means.

The pre-formatted question and answer sheets are intended to make the process as easy as possible, while still gathering vital information. The diary sheets guide you on what to record, with very short answers required, usually just a yes or no. After you've recorded information about your headaches, there are sheets to guide you through interpreting your information.

There are:

- Data sheets, to record symptoms and triggers for about 8 headaches. You need to fill in these sheets as soon as you feel able to after the pain and other symptoms have eased off so you can record as many details as accurately as possible
- Summary sheets, so that after you've recorded all headaches, you can see any patterns in those headaches
- Interpretation sheets, to help you better understand the effectiveness of treatments, the impact of early warning signs, and possible triggers
- Success sheets, to be used 2-3 months later for highlighting improvements to your headaches.

I suggest repeating the process of recording, summarising and analysing your headache symptoms after a gap of two to three months. This should be enough time for any methods of headache prevention you have been using to start showing an effect.

Here is sample data sheet from the diary, showing how the details for headache symptoms are recorded:

HEADACHE DIARY 6
A New Approach to Headache and Migraine Sample Sheet – Four Headaches – Symptoms

Sample Sheet – Four Headaches – Symptoms

SAMPLE

Early warning signs, symptoms and treatments: Q1 to Q16

Question		Headache _	Headache _	Headache _	Headache _
Q1:	When did the headache start?				
	Date	*21 June*	*15 July*	*24 July*	*10 August*
	Day of week	*Fri*	*Mon*	*Wed*	*Sat*
	Time (to nearest hour)	*5 pm*	*9 am*	*1 pm*	*10 am*
Q2:	Time when the headache ended? (Was it the same day?)	*3 pm Sat*	*10 pm*	*11 am Fri*	*6 pm*
Q3:	How many hours did the headache last? (From Q1 and Q2)	*22 hrs*	*13 hrs*	*about 2 days!*	*8 hrs*
Q4:	Did you notice any **early warning signs** (up to 24 hrs before)?	✓	☐	✓	✓
	Neck stiffness— *2 x yes*	✓	☐	✓	☐
	Incessant yawning	☐	☐	☐	☐
	Fatigue	☐	☐	☐	☐
	Mood swings from elation to depression	☐	☐	☐	☐
	Irritability and restlessness	☐	☐	☐	☐
	Slowed thinking, difficulty concentrating and memory problems	☐	☐	☐	☐
	Intense food cravings (especially for sweets and chocolate)	☐	☐	☐	☐
	Increased urination — *2 x yes*	✓	☐	✓	☐
	Signs of fluid retention (rings tight, ankles swelling)	☐	☐	☐	☐
	Constipation	☐	☐	☐	☐
	Diarrhoea	☐	☐	☐	☐
	Cold hands and feet — *3 x yes*	✓	☐	✓	✓
	Extreme sensitivity to light or sounds	☐	☐	☐	☐
	Other (a difference from normal)				

Key Points

- A detailed headache diary gives you a clear, accurate understanding of your headaches.
- A headache diary is the best way to identify personal headache early warning signs, triggers and actions which are most effective in reducing headache effects.
- A combination of strategies may be best.
- We frequently underestimate the amount of painkillers we take. A headache diary helps you keep an accurate record of how much and what type of pain medication you are taking.
- Staying motivated with long-term, incremental change is challenging. A headache diary gives you reassuring evidence of the improvements you've made.
- You should complete the diary every two to three months, to see changes over time.

11

Choosing Your Team

Who is the Best Doctor for You?

Now you've got your information (and have hopefully sought some interim relief from a manual therapist) it's time to find the right doctor to partner with you on the next stages of your journey.

You should seek out a doctor who is willing to take the time to listen and consider your situation, not just rush you out the door with a recommendation to take painkillers. Good communication is essential. They should encourage you to ask questions and be prepared to work with you.

It's important to take an active role in determining what medical treatments you receive. If you don't know a suitable doctor, perhaps your local pharmacist or the headache sufferers among your friends, family or co-workers may be able to recommend someone.

General practitioners associated with sports medicine or multidisciplinary clinics are likely to be more in tune with the musculoskeletal contributions to headache and work as part of a team with manual therapists.

Getting the Most from Your Doctor

Go through your headache diary before your appointment and summarise your symptoms, your use of headache medications and the success of any treatments.

Make sure you tell your doctor:

- Your medical history, including your existing and past illnesses and medical conditions, e.g. childhood asthma, allergies
- Past falls, accidents or injuries
- Major medical procedures and surgery (these can lead to musculoskeletal problems)
- Major dental procedures
- All prescription medications you are taking
- All OTC medicinal products you are taking. As well as painkillers, don't forget things like cough mixtures, nasal sprays and antacids. These can interact with prescription medications and some, like certain nasal sprays, can cause rebound headaches
- All complementary therapies, such as vitamins, minerals, nutritional supplements, and herbal products, you are taking. These may interact with regular medications and some may have headache as a side effect
- Any family history of headaches – talk to your family, especially some of the older members.

It is often hard to remember the details on the spot – you may find having your information written out helps make the best use of your appointment time.

It's important you're completely honest with your doctor – it's not just medicinal products that can cause headaches as a side effect.

Headache sufferers tend to be more sensitive to the effects of tobacco and alcohol, as well as to drugs like cocaine, amphetamines, ecstasy and cannabis.[62]

All are well-known headache triggers. For example, cocaine can trigger a severe headache which typically begins within one hour of use and can last for up to 72 hours.[63]

You should tell your doctor if you use illegal drugs, even if your doctor doesn't directly ask you about illegal drugs. Only with full disclosure can you hope to get to the bottom of your headaches.

You should also consider different sources of caffeine in your diet. Caffeine is present in several over-the-counter and prescription painkillers as well as in coffee, tea, certain soft drinks and chocolate.

If you think you could be suffering from depression, don't try to hide this from your doctor. The sooner you get treatment, the sooner your mental state and your headaches will improve.

Ask your doctor what additional tests could be useful to verify that your headaches don't have any contribution from some underlying medical cause that could easily be fixed, such as sub-optimal levels, or even actual deficiencies, of certain key vitamins and minerals.

Such tests would not be performed routinely as part of an overall check-up, but would need to be specially ordered. Doctors are the only health professionals able to authorise collection of venous blood for testing and testing a sample of venous blood is the only way of obtaining reliable and meaningful results for large number of parameters. Ask for a copy of your tests and any report that comes with them, so you can take this information with you when you visit another health professional.

If you are committed to using non-drug treatments for your headaches (and I hope you are!), you will need to be clear with your doctor that you are looking for non-pharmaceutical methods of headache treatment and, preferably, prevention.

Ask what other health practitioners may be able to help you, such as a manual therapist for tight neck muscles and stiff joints, a dietician for advice about a proper diet and food triggers or a counsellor for advice on stress management.

Key points

- Choosing the right doctor is an important step.
- Seek a doctor who is willing to take the time to listen and consider your situation, not rush you out the door with a recommendation to take painkillers.
- Your headache diary will be an invaluable source of information for your doctor and a great way for you to monitor the success of different strategies.
- It's important to be open and honest with your doctor.

Part D

Managing Headaches:

Manual Therapy

12

Manual Therapy – Why?

In Chapter One, I introduced the Integrated Headache Model – the idea that headache pain, regardless of what type, is the sum of musculoskeletal and neurovascular factors, after they have been modified by emotional factors. The key to this model is the musculoskeletal system. It causes pain on its own, it affects both the emotional and neurological systems, it's the easiest system to treat – and the key to treating the musculoskeletal system is manual therapy.

Most of us, especially if we suffer from headache pain, have had a massage to release tension and help us relax, and that's a great massage to have. Your emotions and stress levels play a crucial role in keeping you above or below the headache threshold. Your stress levels affect your neurological system by releasing histamine, increasing the excitability of your nervous system and altering blood flow to and within the brain. Stress can also increase musculoskeletal pain by 'lighting up' your muscular trigger points. A massage is one of the best ways to relax and help you reduce the impact of your emotions in intensifying your headache pain.

But I'm not talking about a relaxing deep tissue or Swedish massage. Complete manual therapy for headache management should target specific muscles, the muscular trigger points associated with those muscles and mobilisation of the cervical joints. If you don't treat muscular trigger points, the associated muscles and cervical joints, you will never be free from headache pain.

Knowing which muscles and joints should be targeted for headache relief, understanding how muscular trigger points work and how they can be treated is vital if you are going to manage your headaches successfully. Most doctors, neurologists and migraine specialists do not acknowledge muscular trigger points or musculoskeletal input as a factor in headaches and so they ignore manual therapy as a crucial part of a headache management plan. Often, you will be the one who needs to continue to investigate and search for a better treatment of your pain, as was the case for John.

Case study – John and His SCM (Sternocleidomastoid Muscle)

John had suffered chronic headaches for 25 of his 43 years, but had no history of neck injury. His pain was continuous and moderate to severe in intensity. For several years, it was located above his right eye, but eventually spread to include the right side of the base of his skull and neck.

A range of symptoms accompanied his head pain and varied with its intensity. The right side of his nose was stuffy and running, his right eye swollen, red and watering and he heard rushing, pulsating sounds in his right ear. He was unable to sleep for more than 1 – 2 hours and he had fatigue, decreased appetite and difficulty in concentrating. Over the years, John saw neurosurgeons, neurologists, pain specialists and a chiropractor and underwent five trials of physical therapy.

His headaches were variously diagnosed as occipital neuralgia, hemicrania continua (a rare type of primary headache similar to migraine) and cervicogenic headache combined with medication overuse.

During this time he was subjected to invasive medical interventions, including injections into the facet joints and the use of radio waves to destroy part of the small nerves that carry pain signals from the facet joint to the spinal cord.

On most occasions, these procedures worsened his head pain. At best, they provided 24 hours of pain relief. Not surprisingly, John 'had a medical history of overuse of pain medication'. At the time of documenting his case, his prescribed medications included paracetamol, a NSAID, a synthetic opiate and an anti-epileptic drug used for migraine prevention.

Previous unsuccessful medication trials had included other migraine preventatives (two other anti-epileptic drugs, a blood pressure drug and an anti-psychotic drug), an alternative NSAID (since withdrawn after safety concerns) and two migraine abortives.

John had also spent 16 days in hospital, during which he received intravenous medication in an unsuccessful attempt to control his headache pain.

On his discharge, he was referred for more physical therapy. Fortunately, this time, the therapist examined him for muscular trigger points. Pressure on the middle of the sternal branch of his right SCM (sternocleidomastoid) muscle immediately reproduced the pain over his right eye and at the base of his skull.

Quoting from the case study: 'He volunteered that during previous evaluations by various practitioners, the SCM had not been palpated', which is the only way muscular trigger points can be detected. Treatments included trigger point release, biofeedback to learn how to relax the SCM muscle, stretching and advice on sitting posture, including reduction of forward head posture.[64]

Six months after completing 16 sessions of manual muscular trigger point therapy, John was 'pain free one third to a half of the time and had mild discomfort for the remainder'. He continued with home exercises and being mindful of maintaining correct posture.

John might have avoided years of pain, hours of pointless medical investigation and expense if he had understood the Integrated Headache Model, how muscular trigger points work and which muscles should be targeted in manual therapy.

Manual therapy is beneficial, regardless of the symptoms. Even if your symptoms are migraine-like, musculoskeletal problems are almost certainly playing some part in your headaches. Taking medication to calm your neurological system will never improve your musculoskeletal system, but treating your musculoskeletal system will not only reduce referred pain, it can also improve the function of the neurological system. Neurovascular pain may even be an indirect effect of musculoskeletal problems causing irritation of nerves, blood vessels or dura.

Whether your headache has been diagnosed as tension headache or migraine, or as a secondary neck or jaw-related headache, all relevant muscular trigger points need to be located and properly treated. Manual therapy is the only way to treat muscular trigger points and it is the best way to reduce both direct and indirect musculoskeletal contributions to headache pain, regardless of whether you have a tension headache or a migraine.

Composite Pain Patterns

One of my favourite parts of treatment is explaining composite, or overlapping, pain patterns to my patients. For so many of them, it is an 'a-ha' moment that opens up a world of understanding and a path to the successful, sustainable treatment of their headaches.

When a muscular trigger point becomes active, it's like a light switch being turned on. Each muscular trigger point 'lights up' its own specific area of the shoulders, jaw or head and just one of these 'light switches' turned on would be enough to create pain, stiffness and soreness. But for headache sufferers, it's very common to have numerous light switches turned on, each referring pain to a specific area and these areas overlap each other. This is called a composite pain pattern ... no wonder your head hurts! The painful area may get larger, or, if several muscles refer pain to the same area, the pain may become more intense.

Images of heads below show muscular trigger point pain referral patterns for the labelled muscles that refer pain to the head.

- Crosses X indicate the common sites of muscular trigger points in these muscles, but they are a general guide only – muscular trigger points have to be located with palpation for each individual.
- The solid pattern shows where (almost) everyone with active muscular trigger points in labelled muscle(s) will feel pain.
- Some people will feel additional pain in part or all of the dotted area and this may be just as intense.
- Where several muscles are in the same image dashed lines show the extent of each muscle.

All of these diagrams are based on the pain referral patterns given in Travell and Simons[65].

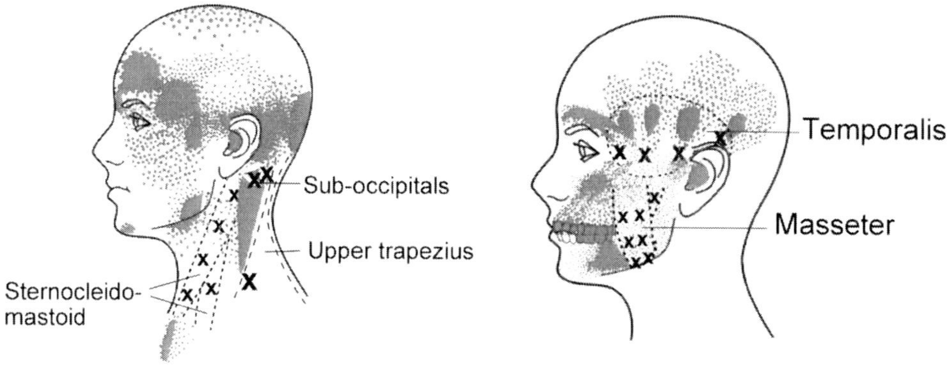

(a) Neck (b) Jaw

Figure 12.1 Composite pain patterns from the neck and jaw

Figure 12.1 shows what the composite pain pattern looks like when all the muscular trigger points in the SCM, upper trapezius and sub-occipital muscles of the neck and the masseter and temporalis muscles of the jaw are active.

Forward head posture can cause all five of the muscles shown in Figure 12.1 to independently develop muscular trigger points.

If you spend a lot of your time in front of a computer which has not been set up properly, or don't take adequate breaks, your headache pain pattern may look like the one in Figure 12.2. If you clench or grind your teeth you will make the muscular trigger points in your jaw muscles much more sensitive.

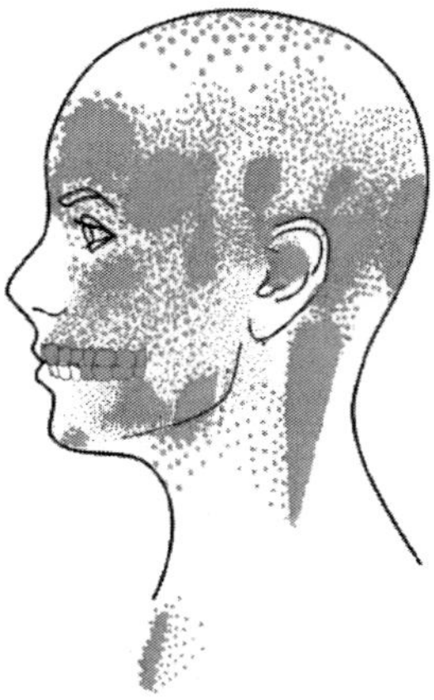

Figure 12.2 – Composite pain pattern from outer neck and jaw muscles

The Big Three

For any headache, the most important muscles to treat are those that control the movement and posture of the head and neck. This will automatically take in the most important direct sources of headache pain, but there are three muscles that are responsible for most of the pain you are feeling.

You've heard of the Magnificent Seven, the Dirty Dozen and the Famous Five, well, now meet the Big Three – the three muscles responsible for producing most of your headache pain. Getting to know them will change your life.

They're all neck muscles and they are called the SCM (sternocleidomastoid), upper trapezius and sub-occipital muscles. When we talk about the musculoskeletal factors of the Integrated Headache Model, we are mostly talking about these three muscles and their muscular trigger points.

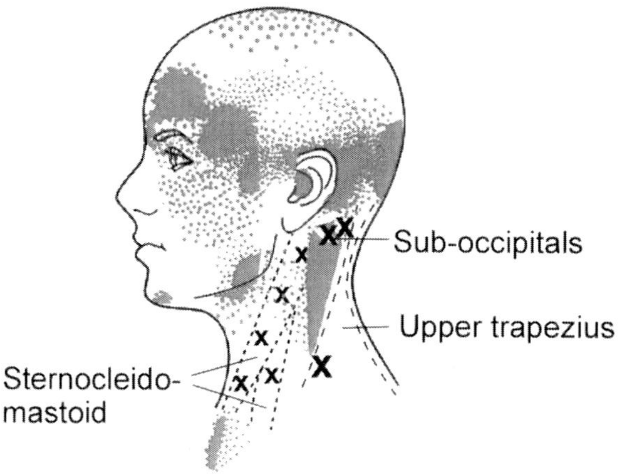

Figure 12.3 – The Big Three muscles, their muscular trigger points and combined pain pattern

SCM

The SCM (sternocleidomastoid muscle or 'neck cord') at the front of the neck attaches to the side of the skull just behind the ear. The muscle splits into two branches. The front branch attaches to the breast bone, the rear branch attaches to the collarbone.

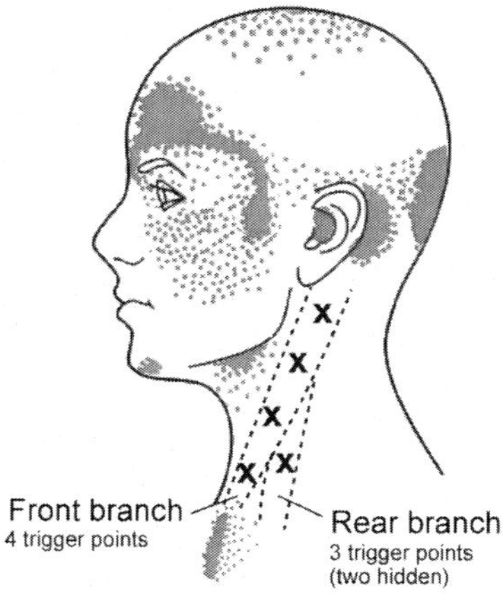

Figure 12.4 – SCM (Sternocleidomastoid), its muscular trigger points and pain pattern

Upper Trapezius

The upper part of the trapezius muscle is at the back of the neck, attached to the back of the skull and to the collarbone. The trapezius acts as a shoulder muscle and a neck muscle, which makes it an important postural muscle. The upper trapezius muscular trigger points are the most frequently identified muscular trigger point in the body. You've probably found it yourself, when you've rubbed your shoulders after a long day and found a sore or tender spot along there. And if you pressed hard enough, you might have even experienced referred pain emanating up into the neck and head – that's a muscular trigger point!, shown below as **X** TrP1

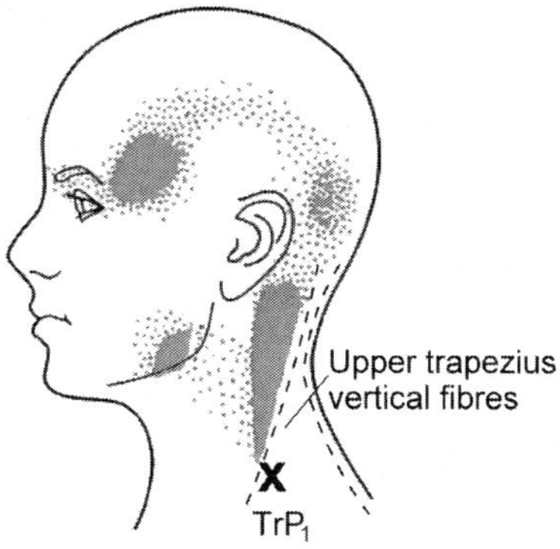

Figure 12.5 – Upper trapezius muscular trigger point and pain pattern

Sub-occipital

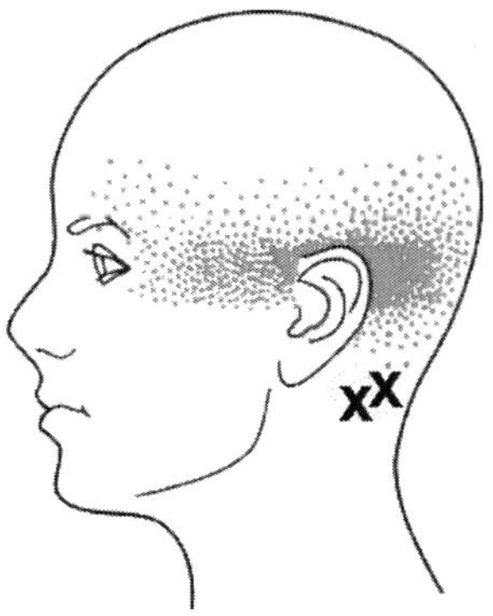

Figure 12.6 – Sub-occipital muscular trigger points and combined pain pattern

The muscles of the sub-occipital group move the head separately from the neck. They consist of eight relatively small muscles – four on each side of the spine that connect the base of the skull to the top two cervical vertebrae. The main functions of the sub-occipital muscles are to tilt the head backwards, rotate it from side to side and restrain it from moving too far forward. They are our 'yes/no' muscles. They also act as position and movement sensors for the head and the top of the neck.

Working Together

These three muscles are among the most common and powerful sources of headache pain, so treating them almost always leads to a very rapid and dramatic improvement. It can even stop a full-blown migraine in its tracks.

Overlap of the composite pain patterns from muscular trigger points in the SCM, upper trapezius and sub-occipital muscles can account for pain in all the different locations considered to be characteristic of tension headaches and migraine, such as the top and back of the head, the forehead, the temple area (at the side of the head), above the eyebrow and behind the eye socket. Muscles on one or both sides of the head may be affected.

The longer you have had your headaches and the more severe and the more frequent they are, the more muscles will be affected and the more active muscular trigger points they will have, which means, left untreated, the area affected by pain can increase and the pain can become more intense.

SCM and Upper Trapezius Trigger Points

Active muscular trigger points in the SCM and upper trapezius muscles tend to spread to nearby muscles along nerve pathways within their pain referral zone. They produce satellite trigger points, which act as additional sources of headache pain. Examples include muscular trigger points in the muscles of the jaw, which are often SCM and/or upper trapezius satellites, the muscles in the deeper layers at the back of the neck, which can be upper trapezius satellites, and the smaller muscles of the face and scalp, which are commonly satellites of long-standing SCM muscular trigger points.

All these muscles refer pain to the head and, as when composite pain referral patterns overlap, the headache pain grows. Where several patterns coincide, the pain is more intense. The area just above the eyebrow is a good example of this. It's a site where SCM and its satellites all refer pain, so the pain will progressively increase as more muscles develop muscular trigger points.

Fortunately, treating the original muscular point, called the key trigger point, will also inactivate its satellites, which is one of the main reasons treating muscular trigger points in the upper trapezius and SCM muscles is so effective in reducing headache pain.

SCM and Autonomic Pain

Not content with just causing you pain, active muscular trigger points in the SCM muscle can also produce a whole raft of bizarre and unpleasant autonomic symptoms, many of which will be familiar to migraine sufferers. They include:

- Dizziness, balance problems, even fainting
- Nausea and loss of appetite
- Partial hearing loss, strange sounds in the ear
- Cold, pale, sweaty forehead
- Sinus congestion and runny nose
- Red and watering eyes, twitching or drooping eyelid
- Visual disturbances including dimmed, blurred or double vision, print moving
- Sore throat, persistent dry tickling cough.

Active muscular trigger points can produce autonomic symptoms spontaneously once they are sufficiently irritated. However, because the symptoms occur some distance away from the muscle housing the muscular trigger points, and are not always accompanied by pain, the connection between the two may be missed.

Episodes tend to follow certain movements which require the affected muscle to be strongly contracted or stretched, such as staying in a position which keeps the muscle in a shortened or a lengthened state for a prolonged period.

Two common examples of a movement that can cause a reaction in the SCM muscle include looking back over your shoulder while reversing the car, or typing on a keyboard with your head to one side to read poorly placed documents or books.

If you have active muscular trigger points in the upper third of the rear SCM branch, moving your head too quickly can provoke bouts of dizziness that may last anywhere from seconds to hours.

Nobody knows how these muscular trigger points cause autonomic symptoms. Fortunately, you can treat the autonomic symptoms caused by SCM trigger points with manual therapy. Many symptoms, including dizziness and nausea greatly improve as muscular trigger points are made less sensitive.

Sub-occipital Trigger Points

Muscular trigger points in the sub-occipital muscles produce a migraine-like pain that feels like it's inside the skull, extending from the back of the head to the eye and forehead. The sub-occipital muscles also provide a good illustration of how sustained awkward postures or repetitive movements which overuse the normal functions of a muscle will cause muscular trigger points to develop. For example:

- Forward head posture – the sub-occipital muscles will automatically contract to tilt the chin upwards and level the eyes with the horizon
- Bending the head and neck forward to read, or to use a laptop or mobile phone – the sub-occipital muscles are strained by preventing the head from pivoting forward onto the chest
- Looking upwards to read or watch television with the head propped up on the elbows – the muscles are held in a shortened position
- Looking sideways to view a movie, to look at documents to one side of the keyboard or sleeping on your stomach with your head turned to one side – again the muscles are held in a shortened position.

Muscular trigger points in the sub-occipital muscles and tightness in the top three neck joints tend to coexist and perpetuate each other. Their headache pain referral patterns partially overlap. Severe headaches due to irritation of some of the many important pain-sensitive structures between the skull and the second vertebra are more likely to occur when the sub-occipital muscles are tight and upper neck joints are stiff.

One of the muscles of the sub-occipital group is linked to the dura at the base of the brain stem by a band of connective tissue that was only discovered in 1995. In 2011, another of the sub-occipital muscles was found to connect to the dura, this time at the top of the spinal cord. If the sub-occipital muscles are tight because of trigger points, neck movements can put abnormal traction on the dura of the brain stem and spinal cord, causing severe headaches.

Treatment of muscular trigger points in the sub-occipital muscles and treatment of tightness in the top three neck joints will help prevent these headaches.

The Big Three and Migraine Symptoms

After years of treating people with migraine, I believe that muscular trigger points in the big three muscles play a significant role in starting and intensifying migraine headache. Sometimes this is because the symptoms induced by muscular trigger points mimic classic migraine symptoms, but it's also because muscular trigger points and tight muscles can have a direct impact on our neurological system, increasing the input of both musculoskeletal and neurological factors in the integrated headache model.

Muscles containing muscular trigger points are tighter than normal and may compress nearby blood vessels, especially when they are contracted. The irritation of blood vessels can alter blood flow to or from the brain. This is very likely to provoke a migraine attack in someone who is susceptible to migraine.

This type of irritation may occur intermittently because of particular movements or sustained postures of the head and neck. Forward head posture and tilting the head back are likely to be major culprits of triggering this type of headache.

Damaged tissues, such as muscular trigger points, release a complex mixture of chemicals that stimulate our pain receptors and increase our pain in order to trigger the body's natural pain suppression mechanism. This 'inflammatory soup' present in muscular trigger points may irritate the fine network of nerves that surrounds blood vessels, causing the blood vessels to dilate, which is another example of how the musculoskeletal system and the neurological system are integrated in causing headache pain.

The 'inflammatory soup' present in muscular trigger points in the temporalis muscle is the likely cause of tenderness in the scalp arteries, which persists between attacks in many migraine sufferers. Actions such as clenching your teeth, which contracts the temporalis muscle, make muscular trigger points more irritable and compresses the arteries, which may be enough to provoke a migraine attack.

A similar mechanism is likely to be involved with the muscles of facial expression. Prolonged frowning or squinting may also trigger a migraine attack. SCM trigger points may also provoke a migraine attack by irritating the nerves surrounding the occipital artery and by increasing compression on the internal jugular vein when the head is rotated.

Treating muscular trigger points is the most beneficial strategy you can employ for reducing the frequency and severity of your headache, whatever type of headache you have. Not only do you reduce the impact of the musculoskeletal system in the Integrated Headache Model, you also potentially lessen the impact of the neurological system.

Now you have a better understanding of why manual therapy is so important, let's look at different types of manual therapy and the best types of manual therapy for eliminating muscular trigger points.

Key Points

- Manual therapy for headache treatment is more than just a relaxing massage.
- Manual therapy can help reduce the frequency and severity of both migraine and tension headaches but for it to be effective it needs to target specific muscles, the muscular trigger points associated with those muscles and mobilisation of the cervical joints.
- When a muscular trigger point becomes active, it's like a light switch being turned on.
- Composite pain patterns, or overlapping pain from multiple muscular trigger points (numerous 'light switches' turned on), will intensify your headache pain.
- The three most important muscles to treat for headache pain are the SCM, the upper trapezius and the sub occipital muscles.
- These three muscles and their composite pain patterns play a significant role in migraine and tension headaches.

13

Manual Therapy – What?

The greatest and most rapid relief of headache pain is almost always obtained by treating muscular trigger points in the SCM, upper trapezius and sub-occipital muscles. So, let's start by looking at the best manual therapy for treating muscular trigger points.

Dry Needling

The technique of dry needling developed from treating muscular trigger points with injections of local anaesthetic. This was first used for treating myofascial pain by Dr Janet Travell in the early 1940s and gave long-lasting pain relief.[66] As therapists experimented to find the best substance to inject, they discovered it didn't matter what substance they used[67], anaesthetic, saline, or nothing at all, the effect was the same. What mattered was the mechanical effect of the needle[68] producing a local twitch response in the affected muscle.[69,70]

The aim of dry needling is to induce the local twitch response, which increases blood flow to the area and disperses the 'inflammatory soup' that has built up around the muscular trigger point.[71] This is the main reason dry needling relieves the pain from muscular trigger points, and one reason why obtaining the local twitch response is so important. The local twitch response also helps the over-contracted muscular trigger point to relax, which helps the taut band of muscle relax too.

Dry needling treats central muscular trigger points by inserting a fine solid filament needle through the skin into the muscle and cautiously moving the needle around within the muscular trigger point. Nothing is injected – hence the name 'dry' needling. The needles are the same type as those used for acupuncture, however that is where any similarity to acupuncture begins and ends.

Dry needling is often associated and confused with acupuncture but they are different practices. Although both techniques use the same needles, acupuncture is an ancient practice based on the pre-scientific teachings of Chinese traditional medicine. It aims to restore the flow of energy ('chi') along meridians in the body by inserting needles into pre-determined locations shown on charts. Dry needling is founded on modern Western scientific principles and a detailed knowledge of anatomy, physiology and neurochemistry. Muscular trigger point sites are located by specialised palpation techniques and a needle is inserted only when the muscular trigger point has been located.

How It's Done

A muscular trigger point contains a highly variable number of contraction knots, all of which must be treated and all of which vary in size. The therapist manually palpates the muscle to locate the taut band and the suspect muscular trigger point site, which they continue to hold firmly in position.

With a quick tap, they insert the needle through the skin above the muscular trigger point and guide it through the muscle. An increase in resistance indicates to the therapist that the needle is in the taut band.

The therapist then looks for the muscular trigger point with small movements of the needle, going in and out in different directions, attempting to elicit the local twitch response. The local twitch response happens when the needle passes through a contraction knot in the muscular trigger point. A pain signal is transmitted to the spinal cord, causing an involuntary reflex contraction of the muscle fibres in the taut band. The muscle may grasp the needle and the taut band may gradually relax, similar to the reflex muscle contraction you experience when you automatically withdraw your hand if you touch something hot.

The therapist can readily feel the local twitch response. Larger twitches in muscles close to the surface of the skin can also be easily seen, as the taut band momentarily tenses and bulges outwards. You will probably feel the taut band twitch too, although sometimes you may feel a deep ache, a mini-cramp or a burning sensation instead.

You may also experience referred pain in areas other than the part of the muscle being needled. This can provide important diagnostic information for the therapist. Fortunately, any local or referred pain is short-lived.

The therapist will normally continue to explore the same muscular trigger point area with small needle movements until no local twitch response or further relaxation of the taut band occurs for between three to five passes of the needle.

When several muscular trigger points are close together, more than 20 local twitch responses can sometimes be produced from the one small area.

The same procedure is used to treat other muscular trigger points in the muscle and then the muscle must be stretched. Stretching helps equalise the length of the affected muscle fibres and restores the muscle to its normal resting length. The therapist may also perform some general remedial massage strokes to relax the muscle, improve circulation and reduce treatment soreness.

Several muscles may be treated within the one dry needling session and it's important that you continue to stretch all treated muscles after you get home to maintain their new length. While it is not a good idea to do strenuous activities or vigorous exercise immediately after dry needling treatment, you should make sure you keep moving to keep blood flowing through your muscles and keep putting them through their newly increased range of motion so the body can adjust.

How Many Sessions Will Be Needed?

A number of muscular trigger points can be dry needled in the same session, however, each muscular trigger point will usually need to be treated on several separate occasions to eliminate all the contraction knots. The tighter the taut band, the more difficult it is to distinguish the muscular trigger point area. It becomes easier after the first treatment as the taut band progressively releases. The second and any subsequent treatments also produce much less soreness.

The effectiveness of dry needling and hence the number of treatments needed also depends on the skills of the therapist. These include:

- Good manual palpation skills to identify trigger points for treatment
- The ability to form a three-dimensional mental image of the location and depth of the trigger point within the muscle
- The ability to translate changes in firmness of the tissues into a picture of where the tip of the needle is and the path it is taking.

These are all learned skills which develop with experience.

It is not really possible to answer how many dry needling treatments are typically required in total. Each muscle may contain several trigger points and each of these in turn is likely to require several treatments.

A published case study in which a patient had been diagnosed with a combination of migraine, chronic tension headache and jaw problems can serve as an illustration of a worst-case scenario.[72] Trigger points in the following muscles were treated by dry needling:

- Upper trapezius (5 right, 8 left)
- Sternocleidomastoid (5 each side)
- Masseter (5 each side)
- Temporalis (5 each side)
- Lower trapezius (3 left).

The number of times each muscle was needled is given in brackets, but how many trigger points were present in each muscle was not stated. Not all these trigger points contributed to the patient's headache pain, however the aim was not just to reduce pain but also to improve head and neck posture and range of motion.

Trigger point dry needling was one part of a comprehensive treatment program designed to correct a collection of musculoskeletal problems. This included manual compression and stretch based techniques, remedial massage, joint mobilisation and manipulation, exercises and postural advice.

How Effective is It?

When done correctly, dry needling has been found to be a very effective technique for eliminating muscular trigger points.[73] It is especially useful for muscular trigger points that have existed for a long time and may be extensively adhered.[74]

In my experience, one dry needling session produces the same benefits as three concentrated treatments with manual compression and remedial massage techniques. Likely reasons for this include:

- A local twitch response is a lot easier to provoke with dry needling, confirming that the muscular trigger point was accurately located
- The pain referral pattern can also be produced more easily.75 Whether or not you recognise the pain as familiar allows the therapist to determine if the muscular trigger point is active or latent and hence how important it is in producing your headache
- Muscular trigger points in taut bands or in areas that feel tender can be located more precisely and small ones are less likely to be missed when a needle is used as a diagnostic tool to supplement manual palpation
- Muscular trigger points can be treated more completely as the individual contraction knots within a trigger point complex can be separately located and treated
- Muscular trigger points can be treated in deeper muscles that are not readily accessible to manual pressure
- Dry needling helps loosen tight adhered fascia that is often found within and around long-standing muscular trigger points. It also helps to loosen tight, thickened or adhered fascia that surrounds muscles and separates them into layers. This is particularly useful when treating areas such as the upper back and shoulders.

The beneficial effects of dry needling on fascia are something I regularly observe but have not seen anything written about. I use this analogy to explain it to my patients: imagine a bowl covered with plastic cling wrap stretched tight. If you make a few small holes in the wrap with a pin then the plastic wrap becomes looser. Fascia is much like that plastic cling wrap, stretched too tight around the affected muscle.

The local twitch response, which is most easily produced by dry needling, also makes the myofascia surrounding the muscle looser and easier to treat. As the taut band releases, the muscle becomes less tense and puts less stretch on the fascia which covers it.

Why Dry Needling Works

It is most likely that the main way dry needling gets rid of trigger points is by mechanically disrupting the collection of contraction knots within the bundle of muscle fibres that make up a muscular trigger point.

When the needle is passed through a contraction knot, it makes a very tiny hole in the muscle. This stimulates muscle fibre repair and regeneration by muscle stem cells (satellite cells) which takes place over the next few days.[76,77,78]

The needle is a little larger than a single contraction knot. Figure 13.1 shows a magnified view of how their sizes compare. Notice that the contraction knot in one muscle fibre also affects adjacent fibres, so these need treatment too.

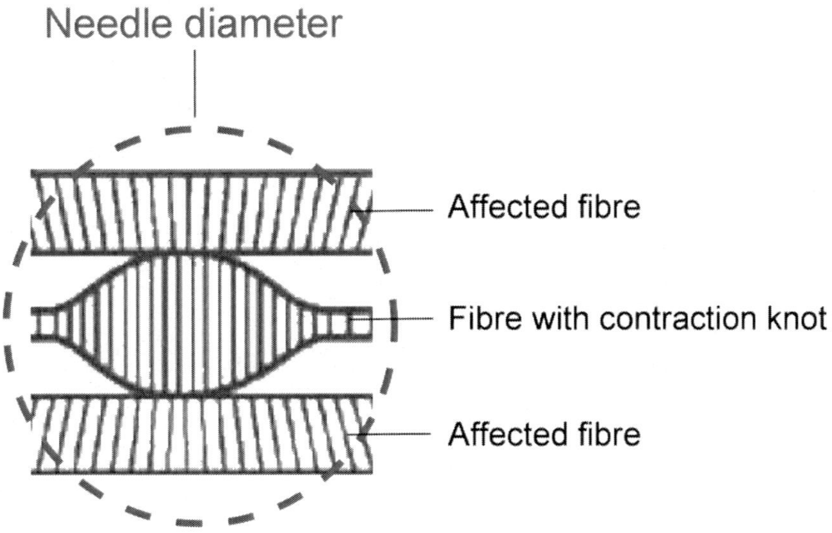

Figure 13.1 – Relative sizes of the needle and a single contraction knot within a muscular trigger point complex

The real size of a single contraction knot in one muscle fibre is a little smaller than a full stop (period) on a printed page. An entire trigger point complex will contain many muscle fibres with contraction knots spread amongst normal fibres.

The more irritable the trigger point, the more contraction knots it contains and the more treatments it will take to 'get them all'. In addition to disrupting the contraction knots, other ways dry needling may help to mechanically release trigger points include:

- The local twitch response, including small less obvious twitches, may stretch muscle fibres deep within the muscle. This may help unstick other contraction knots and may relieve pain by decreasing the pull of tight muscle fibres on tiny pain sensitive nerves and blood vessels[79]
- Movement of the needle – this may provide a localised stretch to the over-contracted sarcomeres within contraction knots.

Does It Hurt?

Although most people don't look forward to being treated with a needle, dry needling is different to getting an injection.

The needles used for dry needling are very fine and they are solid (unlike hypodermic needles, which are thicker and hollow) so they normally cause very little pain when they are inserted through the skin and move through healthy muscle.

You may feel some tenderness when the needle enters the taut band if it's very tight, and probably some twitching, aching or a burning sensation when the needle encounters a contraction knot. If the contraction knot is part of a highly active muscular trigger point, the local twitch response can be quite painful.

However, the pain is short-lived and it's a good sign. It means you've found something that is almost certainly making a large contribution to your headache pain and it's being treated.

You can expect some soreness in the muscles that are needled, but it generally only lasts one to two days. Stretching and movement is the most effective way of alleviating it. A heat pack may also be helpful.

Medical Trigger Point Injections

Some doctors treat muscular trigger points, but mostly they do so by injection rather than dry needling. The procedure is identical, except that local anaesthetic is injected in stages, first as the needle approaches the taut band and then every time a local twitch response occurs (up to one ml in total).

Unfortunately, not all doctors performing trigger point injections are very good at palpating for them. Some inject areas of referred pain and tenderness rather than actual muscular trigger points and others inject in pre-determined locations. In neither case are they trying to elicit a local twitch response, which is vital for treating muscular trigger points.

A good dry needling therapist will palpate your muscles to find the muscular trigger points and will always be seeking the local twitch response.

Muscular Trigger Point Massage

What It's Not

Muscular trigger points are not the same as acupressure points, pressure points or reflexology points. Some clinics may offer acupressure in the form of traditional Chinese or Japanese massage (Tuina or Shiatsu). However, acupressure does not treat muscular trigger points.

Muscular trigger point massage techniques may look superficially similar to acupressure, but they're completely unrelated. Acupressure is sometimes referred to as acupuncture without needles. It is a pre-scientific method of treatment, developed in Asia more than

5000 years ago. Acupressure uses the same fixed pre-determined locations as acupuncture, which are read from a chart. Pressure is applied to these points to unblock the flow of energy ('chi') along the meridians in the body.

In contrast, muscular trigger points are detected by modern scientific methods and the location of each muscular trigger point must be determined individually by specific palpation techniques.

Muscular trigger points are also sometimes incorrectly referred to as pressure points. One type of pressure point is the area above an artery to which pressure is applied to stop blood loss. The other is a vulnerable point on the body that's attacked in martial arts. Neither have anything to do with muscular trigger points.

Finally, muscular trigger points have nothing to do with the reflex points to which pressure is applied in reflexology. This is a non-scientific system with similarities to acupressure in which practitioners believe every part of the body maps onto a particular area on the feet or hands.

What It Is

The three massage techniques used to treat muscular trigger points are ischemic compression, transverse friction and longitudinal friction.

Ischemic compression is sustained, deep static pressure applied perpendicular to the skin directly above the trigger point. Pressure temporarily reduces blood flow to the muscular trigger point area making the skin go pale. When the pressure is released, blood rushes back in, reddening the skin.

Transverse friction involves repeated short, deep, slow massage strokes to the muscular trigger point across the muscle fibres of the taut band. Very little or no lubricant is used so that the therapist's hands do not slide over the surface of the skin. Instead the skin is moved relative to the underlying fascia and muscle, exerting a slowly moving sideways pressure on the muscular trigger point. It's also known as strumming.

Longitudinal friction is similar to transverse friction except the short massage strokes to the muscular trigger point are directed along the muscle fibres of the taut band, rather than across. It's also known as deep stroking massage or stripping massage.

How It's Done

A therapist may use their fingertips, thumbs, knuckles, hand, elbow or forearm to apply pressure in any of these three techniques. The amount of pressure used depends on the muscle being treated and the size of the area they wish to concentrate on at the time.

By repeatedly applying and releasing pressure, muscular trigger point massage has a pumping effect on the local circulation. It brings in fresh, fully oxygenated blood to the muscular trigger point area, renewing depleted energy supplies and helping each contraction knot to release.

Other variations include putting the muscle to be treated in a neutral position or under a gentle stretch. Alternatively, rather than being held stationary, the muscle may be moved through its entire range of motion several times by either therapist or patient during the treatment. Muscular trigger point diagnosis and massage treatment are normally combined.

When a likely muscular trigger point is located within the taut band, it's usually treated straight away, along with any adhesions felt while examining the taut band.

During ischemic massage, the use of sufficient pressure to produce referred pain both confirms and treats the muscular trigger point. The therapist gradually increases the pressure on the muscular trigger point until they feel a definite increase in resistance in the muscle, or you report you are starting to feel some referred pain away from the site being treated. The pressure is maintained at this level until the therapist senses some softening of the muscular trigger point area. This usually takes about 20 seconds or so, and you should feel some lessening of pain when it happens. The same procedure is then repeated three or four times during the one treatment session.

Longitudinal friction stretches the taut band using very slow movement from one muscle attachment to the other. This treats any remaining adhesions, helps equalise the tension along the affected muscle fibres and increases the overall length of the muscle fibres.

In transverse and longitudinal friction, the therapist also uses firm sustained pressure, sufficient to cause a feeling of resistance, as they move slowly across or along the taut band. When they encounter the hard, muscular trigger point area they slow the movement down even further, waiting for the muscular trigger point to give a little. With successive strokes, the muscular trigger point will gradually soften, the taut band will start to relax and pain will lessen.

These same three techniques used to treat muscular trigger points are also used to break up adhesions that occur within and around the central muscular trigger point and elsewhere in the taut band. Once the muscular trigger point and taut band have been treated, the fascia and entire muscle are targeted by more broad-based remedial massage techniques. Finally, the whole muscle is lengthened by therapist-assisted stretching.

How Many Sessions Will Be Needed?

The number of sessions depends on how many muscles are affected, the number of muscular trigger points in each and how long they have been present. A study measuring the effectiveness of muscular trigger point treatment for tension headache, showed that an average of ten treatments is usually enough to produce lasting results.[80]

It's likely that every muscular trigger point will require several treatments to progressively eliminate all the contraction knots. Long-standing muscular trigger points tend to have extensive adhesions as well as more contraction knots and take more time to treat.

One important factor to note is that muscular trigger points become less sensitive with repeated massage, which makes them increasingly difficult to locate and more pressure can be required to produce the initial referred pain patterns. This is a good sign, but it does mean subsequent treatments can be longer, to allow for locating the muscular trigger points.

How Effective Is It?

The combination of ischemic compression, transverse friction and longitudinal friction used in muscular trigger point massage is an effective treatment for muscular trigger points. However, it takes longer to produce results compared to dry needling.

This is not surprising when we consider that the needle is only a little larger than a single contraction knot. It can precisely locate and treat each contraction knot within the muscular trigger point complex. In contrast, even the tip of a therapist's thumb is a lot larger than most muscular trigger points. It can only apply pressure indirectly to the entire collection of contraction knots through the intervening tissue.

All three techniques provide a combination of localised stretch and pressure to the muscular trigger point area and the taut band.

It seems likely that this combination mechanically disrupts some of the contraction knots within the muscular trigger point. Mechanically disrupting the contraction knots is the most efficient way of getting rid of muscular trigger points and gives the longest lasting results. It is also the most effective way of dispersing the inflammatory soup within muscular trigger points and hence reducing the amount of pain generated.

Does It Hurt?

The techniques used in muscular trigger point massage can be painful, however the pain is short-lived and should be always be within your pain tolerance, say a maximum of seven out of ten on a scale where zero is no pain, one is slight discomfort and ten is extreme pain.

The advantage of a pain scale is it gives you a point of reference. This makes it easier to tell whether pain is lessening during the treatment, and on subsequent treatments. If the pain level is less than last time but the therapist is exerting the same pressure, you are making progress.

Communication with your therapist about pain levels and referred pain is vital to the success of trigger point massage. The therapist needs to work with you and your body. There is no place for the adage 'no pain, no gain'. Too much pain is counterproductive, causing the muscle to tense up. Breathing slowly and deeply helps relax the muscle and decreases your pain sensitivity.

As with dry needling, you are likely to experience some treatment soreness but it generally only lasts one to two days. Stretching and movement, but not vigorous exercise, is the most effective way of alleviating muscle soreness after treatment. A heat pack or a hot bath with Epsom salts usually helps.

Beyond Muscular Trigger Points – Other Types of Massage

Targeting muscular trigger points is one of the main benefits of manual therapy, but to maintain long-lasting relief from headache pain, you need to also correct poor shoulder posture, improve overall spinal posture and increase mobility in the thoracic spine and rib cage. Muscles must be also lengthened to restore normal function after thickened fascia and muscular trigger points have been treated, otherwise muscular trigger points will recur. Soft tissues need to be loosened in preparation for joint mobilisation, and, especially for manipulation, surrounding soft tissues should be loosened.

This is where massage comes into play.

The Minefield of Massage Options

Massage therapy is one of the oldest forms of medical treatment and has been practiced across the world since prehistory. Taking the simplest view, a massage therapist manipulates the soft tissues of the body with pressure, stretch and movement. And, in the end, there aren't very many distinctly different ways this can be done. In other words, the number of basic massage techniques is relatively limited.

One of the problems with prescribing massage therapy is the inconsistency of names for the same technique, which causes confusion for practitioners and patients alike, and the number of names for what is often the same technique. What does vary, depending on the overall purpose of the massage treatment, is the combination of techniques chosen, the detailed way they are carried out and the areas of the body they are used to treat and why. This is what defines a massage style.

Each massage style uses a specific set of basic techniques with an aim in mind. The three most commonly practiced massage styles, with shared techniques but clearly different aims are:

- Swedish massage (also called relaxation, traditional and classical massage) relaxes the muscles and moves tissue fluids. It normally provides an overall treatment of the entire body within the one session.
- Sports massage for improved sports performance, prevention of athletic injury and speedier recovery after training and competition. It is similar to Swedish massage but is adapted to the needs of athletes.
- Remedial massage for treatment of acute and long-standing musculoskeletal problems in specific regions of the body. It includes several additional specialised techniques that are not part of the two previous styles.

Deep tissue massage uses strong focused pressure to reach deeper muscle layers. I don't think of it as a style of massage, more a description of the depth of treatment, which can apply to several different massage styles. Most commonly, deep tissue means Swedish massage performed using heavier pressure.

The term deep tissue massage is also used to mean remedial massage. I feel this is misleading because both superficial and deep tissues need to be treated to remedy musculoskeletal problems. Just to add to the confusion, deep tissue massage is also used as a simpler name for neuromuscular therapy, which includes muscular trigger point therapy.

If someone is offering deep tissue massage, it's important to ask some questions to find out exactly what you are getting.

Remedial Massage

By treating muscle structure, remedial massage leads to sustained improvement in muscle health and function and relief from pain. Its effects on the circulatory, lymphatic and nervous systems produce additional, shorter-term benefits. It's the massage I recommend to complement muscular trigger point treatment.

Aims of Remedial Massage Treatment

The overall aim of remedial massage is to improve muscle health and functioning and to reduce pain. In the previous section we focused on techniques used to treat trigger points and the taut band. In this section, we look at a range of techniques which can be used to treat the entire muscle and its fascia which are shown in Figure 13.2. Before we examine the techniques, let's take a moment to get better acquainted with your fascia.

What is Fascia?

Fascia (pronounced 'fash-aa') is a type of connective tissue which contains strong fibres embedded in a moist gel-like material. It forms membranous sheets or bands throughout the body. (The name comes from Latin and means band or bandage.)

Although most people haven't heard of fascia, anyone who has ever skinned a chicken breast will have noticed the thin white filmy membrane located between the skin and the muscles of the meat. This is an example of fascia.

Fascia extends throughout the entire body, from head to feet, covering and interconnecting muscles, bones, organs, nerves and blood vessels with an uninterrupted three-dimensional fibrous web. It varies in how dense, fibrous and flexible it is depending on its location and its function.

This continuity means that tension created in one part of the body can be transmitted much further afield. Just as in a wet suit, if you stretch your arms above your head you will feel a pull on other parts of the suit. Hence the stretch produced by moving a tight muscle, or holding an awkward posture, may be transmitted through the fascial network, causing irritation of distant pain sensitive structures.

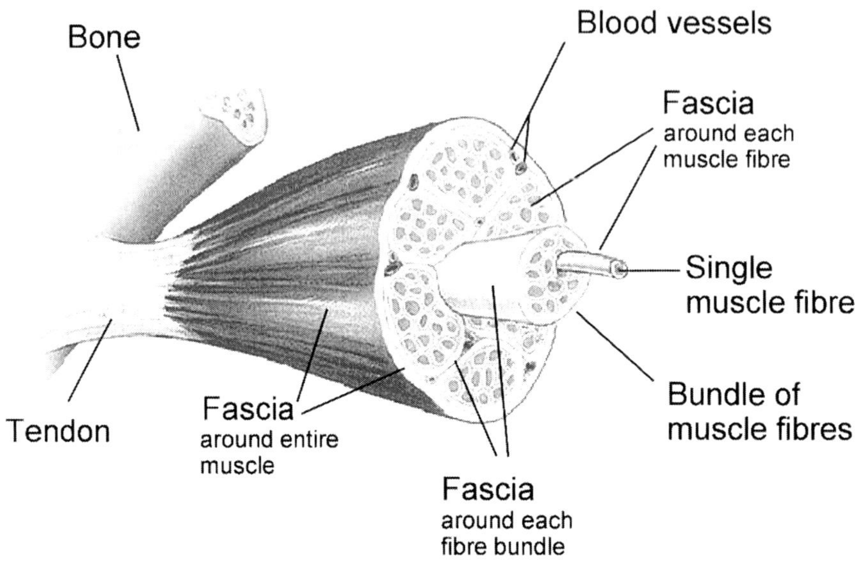

Figure 13.2 – Muscle structure showing the muscle fibres and fascia

This effect is the most likely explanation of why patients undergoing manual therapy sometimes experience pain a long way from the treatment site which does not follow any known pain referral pattern. It may even occur on the opposite side of the body.

When this happens in everyday life, rather than on the treatment table, the pain produced will appear unrelated to the activity that caused it. Fascia itself is well supplied with pain receptors and may act as a source of pain in its own right, however this subject has not received much study.

How Does Fascia Become Restricted?

For fascia to stay healthy, it needs the intermittent stretching that ordinary movement supplies to keep it moist and pliable.

When fascia remains immobile, its gel component loses water and becomes stickier and more viscous. This makes the fibres less able to slide past each other and reduces their separation.

When it is unhealthy, fascia becomes drier and more fibrous. Abnormal cross-links start to form between the fibres and these restrict how much the fascia can stretch. Fascia shortens and loses its elasticity. Instead of being moist, slippery and stretchable, it starts to resemble a hard sheet of plastic.

If the strong myofascial sheath covering the muscle becomes too short and tight, it will limit how much the muscle can expand outwards as it contracts and it will compress the nerves and blood vessels which supply the muscle. The tiny capillaries which take blood to the individual muscle fibres and return it to the general circulation are particularly vulnerable to compression.

Treatment of a fascial layer involves breaking apart abnormal cross-links which have formed between the fibres. Reducing the amount of cross-linking improves flexibility and increases the distance between the fibres, allowing more water to be absorbed. Abnormal cross-links also cause fibrous adhesions to develop between adjacent fascial layers. These adhesions, which prevent fascial layers gliding smoothly past one another, must be disrupted to restore normal muscle movement. Each muscle must be able to move freely and independently as it contracts and relaxes.

The remedial massage techniques discussed in this section aim to:

- Disrupt any adhesions which are causing the muscle to stick to nearby structures. Adhesions sometimes cause separate muscle layers to stick together and individual muscles to stick to their neighbours within the same layer. Muscles may also stick to tendons, ligaments and bones
- Disrupt adhesions between the multiple layers of myofascia which cover the whole muscle, the various bundles of muscle fibres and each individual muscle fibre (see Figure 13.2)
- Soften and stretch the myofascial layers covering the muscle, making them moister and more extensible
- Disrupt local adhesions and areas of thickening within the muscle which prevent it from contracting and relaxing evenly. Groups of muscle or myofascial fibres can mat together, forming hard and often painful knots and ropy bands. These are poorly supplied with blood and tend to accumulate waste products from muscle metabolism
- Stretch specific localised areas of tight muscle – this may not be possible with ordinary stretching
- Lengthen shortened muscle fibres and myofascia and hence the whole muscle. This produces similar but longer-lasting effects to stretching the muscle yourself
- Reduce excessive muscle tension maintained by the central nervous system. This may be a result of on-going emotional stress, muscle spasm, fear of pain, muscle overuse or consistently holding the muscle in a shortened state. After a while the nervous system comes to regard this increased level of tension as normal
- Massage techniques in which pressure is applied to the outside of the muscle across the muscle fibres exert a rotational drag on the tissues. This helps break up adhesions between the separate myofascial layers. The effects extend deep into the centre of the muscle
- Applying pressure along the muscle fibres helps lengthen the individual sarcomeres and so lengthen the entire muscle.

Some Additional Benefits of Remedial Massage

By treating muscle structure, remedial massage leads to sustained improvement in muscle health and functioning and relief from pain. Its effects on the circulatory, lymphatic and nervous systems produce additional, shorter term benefits.

Remedial massage, like all forms of massage, reduces the perception of pain by blocking transmission of pain signals to the upper regions of the brain. It does this by:

- Reducing emotional stress through the calming effect of touch and warmth. This lessens pain by allowing the body's natural pain suppression mechanisms to work more effectively and by helping tense muscles to relax
- Closing the pain gate. Massage activates receptors for the sensations of touch and pressure. Rapidly transmitted nerve signals from these receptors close the gate on slower moving nerve signals from pain receptors in muscles. This can be sufficient to break the 'pain-muscle tightening-pain' cycle
- Certain remedial massage techniques, such as ischemic compression, provide additional pain relief through the pain gate mechanism. Faster moving pain signals from receptors in the skin close the gate on muscle pain. They also stimulate the release of pain-killing endorphins, providing more effective and longer-lasting pain relief.

Remedial massage also improves the circulation of blood[81,82] and lymph within the muscle. Improved circulation reduces pain in two main ways:

- It supplies muscle fibres with additional fresh arterial blood, rich in oxygen and nutrients, to speed up the normal processes of repair and regeneration
- It speeds up the removal of tissue fluid from the spaces between muscle fibres into the venous blood and lymph. This lowers the concentration of pain producing metabolic wastes and irritants like substance P within the muscle.

Remedial massage improves blood and lymph flow within the muscle because external pressure forces blood out of the veins through a series of one-way valves towards the heart. When pressure is released, arterial blood floods in to take its place.

Pressure also triggers histamine release. This causes the capillaries surrounding each muscle fibre to dilate and their walls to become more permeable. Blood flow to and from the muscle fibres increases and nutrients and wastes are transferred more rapidly between the blood and the tissue fluid.

In the case of lymph, relatively light external pressure is sufficient to increase flow. Circulation of the lymph normally relies on the increase in fluid pressure that occurs when muscles contract.

Key Remedial Massage Techniques

Remedial Massage Techniques – Gliding

Gliding is the most frequently used remedial massage technique for assessing and treating the muscle and its fascia. It involves repeated long, slow strokes to the area being worked on. The action is one of applying pressure and pushing down and away. At the end of the forward part of the stroke, the pressure is reduced and a dragging action is used to return to the starting position. This back-and-forth sequence is repeated many times over. Some lubricant is used, but not too much – good contact with the skin should be maintained throughout the procedure.

Gliding can be carried out either along the muscle fibres (longitudinal gliding) or across the muscle fibres near the fleshy central part of the muscle (transverse gliding). The pressure ranges from light to heavy and hence the depth of treatment varies from superficial (near the surface of the body) to deep. The area of contact with the skin may be broad, e.g. the palm or forearm, or specific and focused, e.g. thumb, fingertip or elbow. The deeper the pressure, the shorter and slower the movement.

Superficial longitudinal gliding is a basic but effective technique in which light to moderate pressure is applied to the muscle from one attachment to the other. More pressure is exerted when moving in the direction in which the veins return blood to the heart. Superficial longitudinal gliding is used to:

- Reduce emotional tension and relax and warm tense muscles. This enables the muscles to be more easily palpated and prepares them for treatment. It also provides a soothing effect after deeper work
- Identify general areas in the muscle that feel harder or tighter than others and which need deeper and more focused treatment
- Broaden and stretch the muscle and its fascia and increase muscle length
- Move tissue fluid out of the muscle bring in fresh arterial blood.

Superficial longitudinal gliding is the technique typically chosen to start and end a remedial massage session and as a transition between other techniques. It's also used to clear the tissue fluid of metabolic wastes, inflammatory substances and small particles of tissue debris released by treatment of muscular trigger points and adhesions.

Superficial transverse gliding has less effect on the circulation but it is very useful for locating areas of tension in the muscle. These tend to occur in bands running lengthwise through the muscle and so can be easily felt with transverse strokes. Transverse strokes also help loosen adhesions between separate muscles and muscle layers and between the many myofascial layers that cover the muscle and lie within it.

Deep gliding focuses more closely on the hard, tight areas previously identified. It locates and treats areas of thickening, ropy bands and knots that may lie deep within the muscle.

Deep transverse strokes separate adhered muscle and myofascial fibres. Deep longitudinal strokes stretch these fibres and realign them and stimulate local circulation. The two techniques are commonly used in combination.

Remedial Techniques – Kneading

When kneading, both the therapist's hands work together, moving along the muscle, lifting it away from the bone or underlying tissues. The action of rhythmically lifting and squeezing the muscle is like kneading bread dough. The pressure ranges from superficial to deep.

Kneading is used to warm, loosen and soften the muscle and its fascia and to stimulate the circulation. It also helps separate groups of muscles that have become stuck together. Kneading is often done as a prelude to deeper techniques such as muscular trigger point treatment.

Remedial Techniques – Ischemic Compression and Friction

We've examined how the techniques of ischemic compression, transverse friction and longitudinal friction are used to treat muscular trigger points. All three techniques are used in the same way to treat localised adhesions, which may involve muscle fibres, myofascial fibres or both. These techniques provide deeper treatment and focus on smaller areas compared to deep gliding techniques. Ischemic compression is also often applied along the muscle from one attachment to the other to provide temporary pain relief and help the muscle relax.

Remedial Techniques – Sustained Myofascial Tension (Myofascial Release)

Sustained myofascial tension is used to treat restrictions in broad areas of deep fascia. It focuses on reducing tightness in particular 'fascial trains/lines' (a term made popular by Thomas Myers, a cartographer and integrative manual therapist) of the body, such as the front, back or lateral lines, rather than in an individual muscle. The aims are to soften and stretch tight, thickened myofascia of the muscles in the region, and disrupt fascial adhesions between muscles and nearby structures. These include other muscles in the same or adjoining layers, tendons, ligaments and bones. The therapist will work on one layer at a time, starting with the superficial fascia, moving on to deeper layers. This is often described as 'peeling the layers from an onion'.

When the deep fascia is healthy, the skin and superficial fascia can be comfortably stretched in all directions by a surprisingly large amount; however, when the deep fascia is restricted, not much stretch is possible. Having located a tight area, the therapist presses deeper into the tissues until they encounter resistance. Then, keeping the pressure and hence the depth of treatment the same, they slowly push or drag the fascia in the direction which feels tightest.

Not much lubricant is used so the therapist can keep a good grip on the skin surface. Applying sustained myofascial tension has an effect rather like ironing out the wrinkles out of a sheet. Its effect is to move the skin and superficial fascia ahead of the layers of deep fascia and muscle beneath. This creates an overall traction or drag on these underlying layers which is thought to stretch the deep fascia and disrupt adhesions.

The therapist will sense an increase in resistance where the deep fascia is restricted. They maintain the same pressure until they feel a definite change as the tissues relax. Only then do they move slowly through the previously restricted area. At the end of stroke, they release the pressure before starting the next stroke. To affect the fascia in the deeper muscle layers, more traction must be created.

The name 'sustained myofascial tension' emphasises the need for the technique to be performed slowly to be effective. If the fascia is only stretched for a short time it behaves like elastic – returning to its original position when the stretch is released. A sustained stretch causes it to deform like heated plastic, leading to longer term lengthening.

Alternative names for sustained myofascial tension include myofascial release and a range of trademarked names. These are often marketed as an entire treatment system, rather than as minor variants on a remedial massage technique.

Massage for Immediate, Short Term Relief

If you already have a headache and need treatment straight away, but you can't find a remedial massage therapist, myotherapist, or your usual practitioner is not available, I would recommend a Swedish massage. It's the best known and most popular type of therapeutic massage practiced in the West and the most readily available. It's also the oldest and the one on which more recent massage styles, including remedial massage, are based.

Although it doesn't treat muscular trigger points, or aim to affect muscle structure, Swedish massage will provide short-term pain relief. This is often sufficient to stop a headache attack or at least reduce its severity.

Now you know more about what you need and why you need it – the next step is to find the right manual therapist to work with!

Key Points

- Dry needling is one of the most effective ways to treat muscular trigger points.
- The aim of dry needling is to induce the local twitch response.
- Dry needling is not the same as acupuncture.
- A muscular trigger point is not the same as a pressure point.
- Muscular trigger point massage is also an effective way to treat muscular trigger points.
- Both dry needling and manual therapy are founded on the scientific study of the body and involve palpating the muscle to locate the trigger point before treatment.

14

Manual Therapy – Who?

In this chapter, I discuss some of the key skills you want your therapist to have, what type of therapists you should consider and the therapists to be wary of when looking to treat muscular trigger points and headaches.

How Do You Find a Manual Therapist?

You do not need a referral from a medical doctor to see a manual therapist for headache treatment (although you may require a referral to claim from your medical insurance).

Like so many services, word of mouth is generally the best way to find a good therapist. I get more than three quarters of my headache patients through recommendations from existing clients. Ask around among people you know – you may discover at least one headache sufferer who has experienced real benefits from specific manual therapy treatment for their headaches and who can give you the name of a practitioner you can contact.

If you don't have any luck with this, another useful starting point is to compile a short list of practitioners in your area by searching the internet, including the websites of the various professional societies.

When you call the offices of the practitioners on your list, ask what techniques they use and how long the appointments are. You are now armed with enough information to help you decide whether it is worthwhile proceeding further.

You may have to try out several different practitioners before you find one who suits you. Some people tend to opt for the therapist who is closest to them but it is definitely worth travelling a bit further to discover someone who is right for you.

Qualified or Not?

The massage profession is currently unregulated by the Australian government, although it is self-regulating through membership of a professional body.

There are several of these – Massage and Myotherapy Australia (MMA) and the Association of Massage Therapists (AMT) are two of the largest.

To be entitled to join these organisations, a therapist must have been awarded a massage qualification from a government-accredited training organisation. Registered therapists must complete ongoing professional development, abide by the association's code of ethics and have a current first aid certificate. There are different levels of membership for those with diplomas versus certificates. Each professional body maintains a register of qualified massage practitioners and can also provide advice to the public.

There is no legal compulsion for a therapist to be on a register. This means that anyone can practice massage, even without any formal training or experience.

When you make an appointment, it's important to check the qualifications and experience of the person treating you. If you suffer from headaches, the muscles at the front and side of your neck will need to be palpated. This is not an area that someone without sufficient qualifications should be working on.

Fundamentals of a Good Manual Therapist

Regardless of who you choose, there are some basic standards your therapist should meet.

A manual therapist treating your headaches should base their assessment on information from:

- Your medical history
- Examination of your posture, general mobility and gait
- Range of motion testing
- Palpation of your muscles, joints and fascia. Note – if you want to get your muscular trigger points treated, palpation of muscles is essential – not all manual therapists do this
- Reproduction of pain that you recognise as your familiar headache pain by palpation and/or movement

As with any field, knowledge, skill and experience are paramount. A good manual therapist needs to have a 'good pair of hands' because the success of diagnosis and treatment is heavily dependent on sensitive and accurate palpation. A good manual therapist will listen carefully to you. They will explain what musculoskeletal problems they identified in their assessment and how their treatment plan will help, using terms you understand.

They should offer to educate you about prevention of musculoskeletal problems and advise you about correcting your posture, stretching and the need for movement. They may also ask questions about your daily activities, stress levels, diet and sleep patterns to help you identify any factors which may be making your headaches worse.

During the session, they will respond to your requests for variation, such as more or less pressure or a change in position, and show concern for your comfort and well-being. During or after the session they will take some time to answer your questions. Rather than focusing exclusively on the joints or the muscles, or restricting attention to just the one area, a good manual therapist will take a holistic view of the body. Muscles, joints and fascia work together and can't be considered in isolation.

They will also allow sufficient time for appointments, which they should spend entirely with you. Anything less than 30 minutes is not good treatment. For remedial massage, one hour appointments provide optimal progress.

Some Key Skills

Palpation

Palpation is the use of touch to examine the tissues of the body, which includes the skin and body surface, muscles and their tendons, fascia, joints and ligaments. Palpation is a highly specialised skill, which is learnt and improved with experience. A good manual therapist should demonstrate a thorough knowledge of anatomy and be able to palpate the deeper tissues of the body accurately and safely.

Palpation is done slowly and carefully. The therapist applies increasing pressure as they palpate more deeply, moving from the skin and superficial fascia to the myofascia and muscles, and then along the muscles in the direction of the muscle fibres. Tendons, ligaments and joint capsules may also be examined.

A healthy muscle feels firm yet elastic – it has 'give'. It is not painful when pressed and has an even consistency throughout. The therapist will be looking for muscles which are too tight. These feel hard and rigid. They may be painful when pressed and are difficult to stretch. The job of the therapist is to work out why they are too tight, to determine the best type of treatment.

In palpating the spine, the therapist will attempt to reproduce your headache to determine whether your upper neck joints are contributing to the pain. They will also locate any stiff joints which are restricting the range of motion of your head and neck and reducing the overall flexibility of your spine.

Range of Motion Testing

The neck is the most mobile region of the spine. Its range of motion is assessed in six different directions – bending forward and back, bending sideways to the left and right (ear to shoulder), and rotating to the left and right. The head moves with the neck.

For the assessment, you will usually be asked to move as smoothly and as far as you can, keeping your head and neck in the neutral position (head very slightly retracted). This procedure is called 'active range of motion testing'.

The therapist may provide a little light guidance with their hands on how to perform the movement but that is all. It's your neck muscles that do the work. How far you are able to move your neck is compared with the normal range. For example, you should be able to bend your neck forward until your chin touches your chest.

A number of additional tests are often performed, particularly by practitioners whose major focus is on treating the joints. They are used to assess whether your neck joints are making an important contribution to your headaches.

These additional tests include:

- Active range of motion testing with the therapist adding overpressure at the end of the range. This is often done if no pain was previously observed
- Active range of motion of the head independently of the neck. This provides more information about restrictions in the top two neck joints and the muscles that move the head. Your head and neck will be specially positioned by the therapist so that your lower cervical spine is kept relatively fixed. You will then be asked to move your head in the same six directions as before
- Passive range of motion testing in which the therapist moves your head and neck. This allows them to better assess the limits to your range of motion, especially if your active range was very restricted
- Various passive combined movements of the head and neck and compression tests if earlier tests have not yet reproduced your symptoms.

In passive range of motion testing the feel of the movement, especially at the end of the range, provides the therapist with direct feedback on the nature of the restriction in range. Range of motion testing may also be done on the thoracic spine, lumbar spine and the jaw.

Neural Tension Tests

Some manual therapists with a focus on joints might perform a range of what are called neural tension tests, which asses the mobility of nervous tissue of the spinal cord and peripheral nerves. A positive test means that your headaches have a dural component.

Neural tension tests require you to adopt various combinations of body positions that are known to stretch the nervous tissue and its dural covering. An example is bending your head and neck forwards while keeping one leg straight out in front of you, which mimics the movement you do when you get into a car.

The Best Manual Therapists for Treating Headache

The main health care professionals who provide manual therapy are remedial massage therapists, myotherapists, osteopaths, physiotherapists and chiropractors.

The following provides general information about what each different type of manual therapist does. This information is necessarily subjective. The variations between different countries, states, and even cities, in training and licencing requirements, titles and scope of practice are so large that it is next to impossible to make general statements that will hold true everywhere.

It's impossible to say with certainty what techniques any manual therapist will use. One problem is terminology. Some terms, like deep tissue massage and neuromuscular therapy, can be interpreted in different ways. The same technique may also be known under different names, as in the case of spinal manipulation.

Each practitioner also develops their own working style. They will choose techniques they are comfortable with and that suit their physical strength and the height and weight of the patient. Individual practitioners will add new skills and some will adopt ideas or methods from other disciplines. A few may even alter their whole way of approaching treatment from what they were originally taught. And of course, like members of any professional group, manual therapists vary in their abilities and what parts of their training they make use of in their practice.

So, with those caveats in mind, here is an overview of different manual therapists, what they offer and the most successful therapies for treating headaches.

Remedial Massage Therapists

The most important consideration for people looking to manage their headache pain is to find a therapist who treats muscular trigger points. And for that, a remedial massage therapist or a myotherapist is the best choice. Rather than being bound to one massage style, they will select techniques and styles to treat muscular trigger points, the fascia and entire muscle. Most myotherapists and some remedial massage therapists are trained to carry out muscular trigger point dry needling. Both are also able to treat joint stiffness by targeting the muscles, with indirect methods such as contract and stretch and, depending on the regulations in the area they work, using joint play mobilisation.

Remedial massage therapists and myotherapists spend a large part of their standard training learning how to palpate muscles for muscular trigger points and myofascial restrictions and how to treat them. They also routinely assess stiffness in the spinal joints, which they treat with massage, passive stretching and with contract and stretch for the major muscles and the various basic movements.

Their expertise is in treating the pain and restricted mobility caused by muscular trigger points and by myofascial thickening and adhesions. They will also treat stiff spinal joints with methods that lie within their scope of practice. Depending on their training and the regulations in their area, they may use joint play mobilisation to treat joint stiffness. In many cases, this is all that's required to restore joint mobility. However, massage therapists and myotherapists are not allowed to perform spinal manipulation (or manipulation of any joint for that matter). If your spinal joints remain stiff, they can refer you to an osteopath, physiotherapist or chiropractor for additional mobilisation and / or manipulation.

Remedial massage therapists have a thorough knowledge of anatomy and physiology. They are also trained in physical examination, assessment of musculoskeletal problems, clinical reasoning and advanced massage techniques. They will identify the musculoskeletal sources of your headache pain. They will then devise a comprehensive treatment plan. This should do more than just relieve your pain. To truly fix the musculoskeletal problems that are contributing to your headaches, a good remedial massage therapist will determine why these problems have occurred and how to prevent them recurring in the future.

Treatment will focus on a limited number of muscles during each session. Repeated treatment will be required to get rid of long-standing muscular trigger points. Commonly used and effective remedial massage techniques include:

- Ischemic compression
- Friction (longitudinal and transverse)
- Superficial gliding (longitudinal and transverse)
- Deep gliding (longitudinal and transverse)
- Kneading
- Sustained myofascial tension (myofascial release)
- Passive stretching
- Contract and stretch (MET – Muscle Energy Technique)
- Mobilisation of spinal joints using joint play assessment techniques.

Some remedial massage therapists will also have studied muscular trigger point dry needling. Dry needling gives results in fewer sessions than manual methods. It is very effective for treating large thick muscles like the upper trapezius and for easily reaching muscles, such as the levator scapulae, that lie further beneath the surface of the skin.

A remedial massage therapist will give you stretches to do to help prevent treated muscles from shortening and to increase overall flexibility. They will discuss how to improve posture and carry out your daily activities so that your musculoskeletal problems don't recur and may also talk generally about the effects of factors like stress, sleep, diet, and exercise on the musculoskeletal system and headaches.

Myotherapists

A myotherapist (myo means muscle) occupies a position somewhere between a remedial massage therapist and a physiotherapist. They have training in remedial massage techniques, muscular trigger point dry needling and certain methods of treatment from physiotherapy, including the prescription of stretching and strengthening exercises and the use of equipment, such as ultrasound, TENS (Transcutaneous Electrical Nerve Stimulation), heat and cold.

In Australia, most myotherapists hold an Advanced Diploma of Remedial Massage (Myotherapy) and are members of the Institute of Myotherapists of Australia (IRMA). Myotherapy grew out of the work of Travell and Simons on muscular trigger point therapy.

The term myotherapy was popularised by American physical fitness and exercise guru Bonnie Prudden in her book *Pain Erasure*. First published in 1980, it has been in print ever since. At the time, Prudden was assisting a medical practitioner to perform muscular trigger point injections. Her role was to locate and mark the muscular trigger points on patients' muscles and to devise individual corrective exercises. She discovered she could often eliminate the pain simply by exerting pressure on the muscular trigger points, in other words, by performing what is now known as ischemic compression.

Bonnie Prudden's form of myotherapy which combines manual muscular trigger point treatment with remedial exercise (range of motion movement and stretching) is still taught at the Institute she established in Arizona and ran until her death at the age of 97. The Institute maintains an online directory of Certified Bonnie Prudden Myotherapists (CBPM) in the USA.

Osteopaths

Osteopathy was developed in 1874 by Andrew Taylor Still, a country doctor on the American frontier. Still had become disillusioned with orthodox medicine ten years earlier, after three of his children died in a meningitis epidemic and a fourth child died of pneumonia not long after.

He wanted to reform existing nineteenth century medical practices. Patent medicines containing opium and morphine were unregulated and freely available over-the-counter and doctors regularly gave morphine for pain relief. Not surprisingly many people became addicted, including Still's older brother, who was also a doctor.

Still was looking for an alternative system of medicine that would help the body resist disease and would only use drugs or surgery sparingly.

He became convinced that the body could heal itself and remain healthy, provided mechanical barriers, such as misalignment of the musculoskeletal system and poor posture, were removed. He believed that by treating the musculoskeletal system with manual therapy, doctors could treat a wide variety of diseases including infections without the need for drugs.

His two main principles were:

- 'Structure governs function' meaning musculoskeletal problems can interfere with the normal functioning of the other main body systems
- 'The rule of the artery is supreme' stressing the need for a healthy blood supply to all parts of the body. (He considered venous return and lymph flow as part of this).

Osteopathy has moved on since Still's time. Osteopaths today are mainly concerned with alleviating musculoskeletal problems, while acknowledging this can have a positive flow-on effect to other body systems. They treat the spine and other bony joints, muscles, tendons, ligaments, and fascia. In developing a treatment plan, an osteopath will regard the entire musculoskeletal system as a single unit. They will also consider how the musculoskeletal system affects and is affected by the other major body systems, especially the circulatory and nervous systems. For example, tight fascia surrounding a muscle can restrict venous return and lymphatic drainage.

Biomechanics, the structure and mechanical functioning of the musculoskeletal system, is central to osteopathy. An osteopath will always check for asymmetry – differences in position or mobility between the two sides of the body.

For example, if one side of your pelvis is higher than the other this will have effects all the way up your spine to the joints and muscles in your neck. It will also make one leg appear and function as if it is shorter than the other. Restoring symmetry is one the aims of treatment. So is correcting muscle imbalance, which leads to poor posture, such as rounded shoulders or excessive curvature of the lumbar spine.

Osteopaths diagnose musculoskeletal problems by palpation and testing range of motion. They will also examine posture and gait. All osteopathic treatments are hands-on and use a range of different methods to treat joint and soft tissue problems. Treatment sessions generally last for at least 30 minutes and are spaced well apart.

An osteopath will perform massage with deep pressure to loosen tense muscles and stretch tight fascial structures. Frequently used techniques include longitudinal and transverse friction, ischemic compression and sustained myofascial tension. The amount of massage is typically a lot less than a remedial massage therapist would do because osteotherapy is usually targeted at a specific area, with the aim of correcting biomechanics.

Osteopaths may also do passive stretching, move joints through their range of motion and perform regional MET to help correct muscle imbalance. Most, but not all, will perform spinal manipulation – a HVLA (High-Velocity, Low-Amplitude) thrust[83,84] – to treat stiff spinal joints.

The technique of counterstrain (positional release) is also commonly used to treat tight painful muscles, including muscles in spasm. The practitioner first locates what they refer to as a tender point in the muscle by firm palpation. They then place the patient in a position of ease (least pain). In this position the tight muscle is in a shortened state so stretch on it is minimised. They continue to apply firm pressure to the tender point for 90 seconds before returning the patient very slowly to a neutral position.

On re-testing, pain should have decreased. The mechanism is meant to involve interruption of the pain cycle and allowing enough time for resting muscle tension to be re-set, although I wonder if they're not simply treating muscular trigger points under another name. The locations of tender points in the body have been mapped.

In addition to the types of manual therapy treatments discussed above, osteopaths are likely to offer advice about exercise, posture, diet, stress reduction and other aspects of daily life.

Manual Therapists to be Mindful Of

Physiotherapists

Physiotherapists, known as physical therapists in the USA, are movement specialists. They are much better known for prescribing stretching and strengthening exercises rather than providing manual therapy.

Exercise works well when teaching stroke victims how to walk again, getting people up and moving after hip replacement surgery or treating and preventing sporting injuries. What physiotherapy doesn't work as well for are conditions in which muscle pain is often due to long-standing muscular trigger points, such as 'frozen shoulder', chronic neck pain or headaches.

It is not possible to strengthen a muscle containing muscular trigger points and stretching it will cause more pain. Once muscular trigger points and myofascial restrictions have been treated, muscles should be stretched.

Physiotherapists will palpate muscles for increased tone and tenderness but they do not routinely palpate for muscular trigger points and adhesions. These topics are not taught as part of standard physiotherapy training. Nor do they receive much, if any, attention in additional course work done by physiotherapists who intend to specialise in treating musculoskeletal conditions. Even though physiotherapy clinics that offer manual therapy will mention massage or soft tissue work, the focus is still very much on the joints.

If your headaches have a musculoskeletal component, most physiotherapists will see it as a problem of your neck joints. They will treat stiff joints with mobilisation and manipulation, and a combination of other techniques including traction, muscle stretching and strengthening, postural advice and retraining and home exercises.[85,86,87]

Prior to treatment, they will generally do extensive testing. They will identify which joints in the cervical and thoracic spine are causing pain and / or restricting movement and in what way. They may perform some neural tension tests and check that the mobilisation and manipulation of the upper cervical vertebrae, C1 and C2, can be performed with little risk. Physiotherapists appear to have been gradually moving away from cervical manipulation because of concerns about the potential risks of stroke due to damage to the vertebral artery.

In published case reports, physiotherapists sometimes mention the possible contribution to headache pain from trigger points in the neck muscles,[88,89] but they don't report carrying out any specific tests or treatments.

They may not even perform ordinary massage as often we would have expected. For example, in one local study, only 36% of a sample of 202 headache patients treated with multiple sessions of physiotherapy received any massage, and half of this was in the first session.[90]

Your neck joints almost certainly will need treatment, but so too will muscular trigger points and myofascial restrictions. It is always possible (but not very likely) that your upper neck joints may be the dominant source of your headache pain. In that case, you are in the right hands – physiotherapists are good at fixing stiff neck joints and correcting posture.

However, if you aren't careful, you may end up on the medical merry-go-round. Physiotherapists are the only profession that most doctors will refer to for manual therapy treatment of headaches. If physiotherapy is not successful the next steps are usually invasive medical tests and trials of ever more powerful pain-killing drugs.

Make sure you find someone to treat your muscular trigger points. There are physiotherapists who treat muscular trigger points as well as joints, but they are not very common.

Chiropractors

Spinal manipulation – HVLA thrust or 'cracking joints' – is the main method chiropractors use to treat musculoskeletal problems and they have many different ways of carrying it out.

A chiropractor will usually manipulate your neck while you lie on your back, while you're sitting upright on a chair or bench, or sometimes while you are lying face down. Some may manipulate the upper part of the cervical spine while you lie on your side.

In at least some of their treatments, the majority of chiropractors will use an instrument to deliver the thrust to the spine, rather than their hands. The Activator, a spring-loaded mechanical device is the best known example. It delivers a pulse of energy in a chosen direction to the vertebra to be moved. The force is less than in manual manipulation because the movement is more rapid.

Chiropractic treatment was founded in the United States in 1895 by Daniel David Palmer, a self-taught magnetic healer, who was studying spinal manipulation. According to some accounts, he spent six weeks studying with Andrew Taylor Still, the founder of osteopathy. Palmer came to believe that most diseases were a result of interference to nerve signals, caused by 'vertebral subluxation' (misalignment of the spine). This is sometimes called the 'law of the nerve.'

Most chiropractors combine osteopathic, medical, and chiropractic principles of diagnosis and treatment. In addition to manipulation, they may give you exercises and stretches to do, advise on posture and lifestyle, and use modalities such as ultrasound, electrical muscle stimulation, heat and cold. Some will do massage.

If you are intending to see a chiropractor, it's a good idea to get some massage from a remedial massage therapist before your appointment.

A good chiropractor will limit their practice to treating musculoskeletal conditions. They will use joint play and palpation of intervertebral movement to determine which joints need treatment and will use manual treatment methods. They will prepare the muscles with massage and stretching and avoid direct HVLA thrusts, which involve forceful rotation of the neck.

They will also provide you with an indicative time frame for completing treatments.

As far as I can tell, chiropractic students are not taught how to perform muscle palpation, except for the muscles along the spine, which they examine for signs of misaligned vertebrae.

Chiropractors are starting to do short courses in muscular trigger point dry needling. However, to be able to perform dry needling successfully on patients, they need to be able to palpate muscles and to palpate muscular trigger points.[91]

In short, ask questions, be critical of your treatment and work with someone who can treat muscular trigger points. Muscular trigger points aren't the whole answer, but they are a significant and overlooked part of the solution.

Now we've covered the treatments you can seek from professionals to help you reduce the frequency and severity of headaches, it's time to look at what you can do for yourself – including stretches, self-massage and common-sense diet and lifestyle adjustments.

Key Points

- The most important consideration for people looking to manage their headache pain is to find a therapist who treats muscular trigger points.
- Remedial massage therapists and myotherapists provide the best manual therapy for treating muscular trigger points.
- Osteopaths use the technique of counterstrain (positional release) to treat tight and painful muscles.
- Physiotherapists (physical therapists) do not usually treat muscular trigger points during their consultations.
- A good chiropractor will limit their practice to treating musculoskeletal conditions.

Part E

Preventing Headaches:

Stretches

15

Self Massage and Simple Stretches

Most people wanting to reduce the frequency and severity of their headaches will need professional manual therapy to treat the musculoskeletal sources of their headache pain. In between visits, it's great to be able to maintain the benefits of your treatment by being mindful of your posture, avoiding prolonged sitting, stretching regularly and applying self-massage. This set of self-massage techniques and simple stretches are designed to help you maintain the benefits of professional manual therapy and keep you feeling better for longer and if you don't get headaches very often, stretching and self-massage, together with some prevention strategies may be all you need to keep your headaches at bay.

The instructions on self-treatment which follow include detailed instructions with photos. Techniques covered include:

- Simple massage to relax neck and shoulder muscles
- Simple massage to relax face and scalp muscles
- Treatment of muscular trigger points in the muscles responsible for headache pain using compression
- Several important stretches done with deep slow breathing to relax the muscles and mind and to mobilise joints
- Self traction for the neck
- Treatment to relax the muscles attached to the spine.

It is a good idea to practice massage and muscular trigger point treatment when you don't have a headache, so you know what to do when you need it. The descriptions and diagrams of trigger points in Chapter Twelve provide a good background for this chapter.

A note before you start: don't be alarmed if pressing on a muscle causes referred pain in the same area that you normally feel pain during a headache attack. It's a good sign – you have discovered a source of your headaches and one that you can do something about. Maintain the pressure for about 20 seconds. The pain will gradually decrease and you will have made a muscular trigger point less sensitive. Professional muscular trigger point treatment can sometimes stop a migraine attack that is underway and you may be able to learn to do the same thing. And lastly, remember when massaging or stretching, make sure you are breathing slowly and deeply.

Preparing the Shoulders and Neck

The muscles at the back of the neck and the top of the shoulders tend to carry a lot of tension much of the time. However, when a headache attack is on its way, they can feel more tense and stiff than usual.

Breathe slowly and deeply using your diaphragm (belly breathing) while you massage these muscles.

Begin with small circular movements on the back of the neck as in Figure 15.1, using enough pressure to move the underlying muscle a little, not just the surface of the skin.

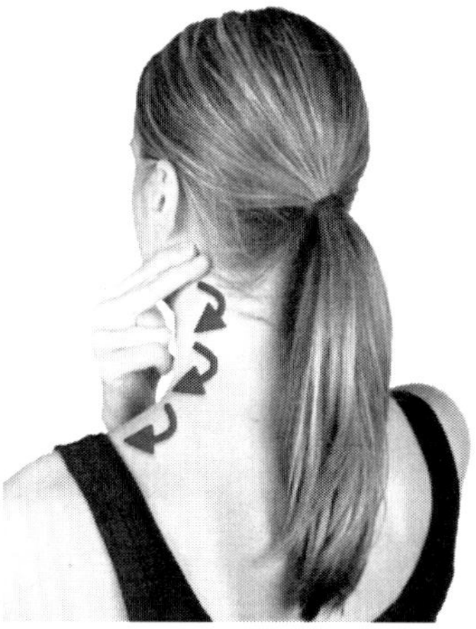

Figure 15.1 – Circular movements on the back of the neck

You can also use one hand to grasp and gently squeeze the muscles along the back of your neck on one side, working upwards from the shoulders towards the head. Then repeat on the other side. The technique you use doesn't matter so much, but it should feel relaxing and make the muscles less tight.

Now, using the opposite hand, squeeze the thick upper trapezius muscles along the top of both of your shoulders. Once some massage and slow breathing have reduced muscle tension, you can move on to treating potential muscular trigger points in a few specific muscles.

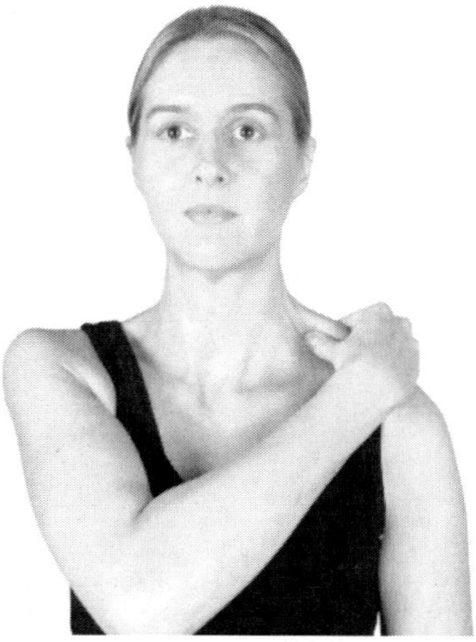

Figure 15.2 – Squeeze the thick upper trapezius muscles along the top of both of your shoulders

Treating Sub-Occipital Muscular Trigger Points

One of the easiest and most effective ways to stop a headache in its tracks is to apply static pressure to muscular trigger points in the sub-occipital muscles.

The eight small muscles of the sub-occipital group are situated at the base of the skull (the occiput), roughly in line with the bottom of your ear lobes. The sub-occipital region is outlined in Figure 15.3. The sub-occipital muscles lie beneath several other muscle layers, which makes taut bands hard to find, so, at home, it's best to apply pressure to the entire sub-occipital region, which tends to be very tense anyway and will respond well to pressure. Areas over muscular trigger points will feel especially tender – spend more time on these.

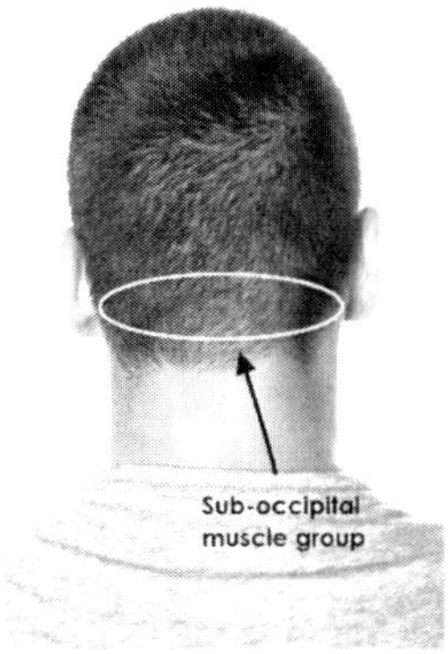

Figure 15.3 – Location of sub-occipital muscular trigger points

The easiest way to apply pressure to the sub-occipital area is to use your thumbs and press upwards as shown in Figure 15.4. You can do this while you are sitting or standing.

When you find a tender spot, maintain the pressure for up to 20 seconds, or until the muscles soften and tenderness decreases. Then move to the next position. If you want to increase the pressure a little, try tilting your head backwards and forwards by a small amount while keeping your thumbs in the same place.

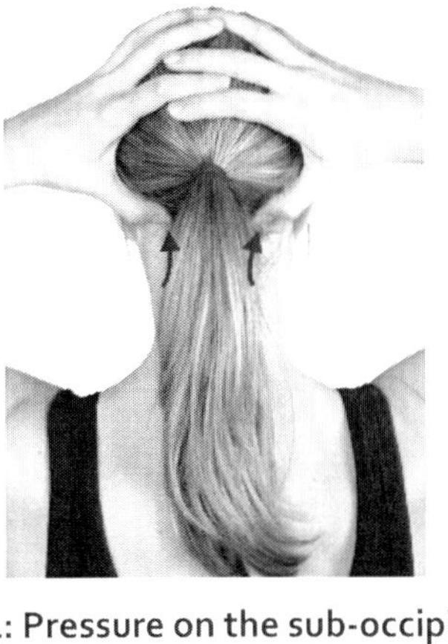

Figure 15.4: Pressure on the sub-occipital region

Tennis Balls Muscular Trigger Point Treatment

If you can lie down, you can use a tennis ball as a massage tool. Lie on your back with your knees bent and both hands behind your head, using one hand to help support your head. Position the ball against the area being treated with your other hand. Release your head onto the tennis ball. The weight of your head applies the pressure.

You could also create a tennis ball massager, by putting two tennis balls next to each other in an old sock as shown in Figure 15.5. Tie the sock to hold the balls firmly in place or fasten the ends with rubber bands.

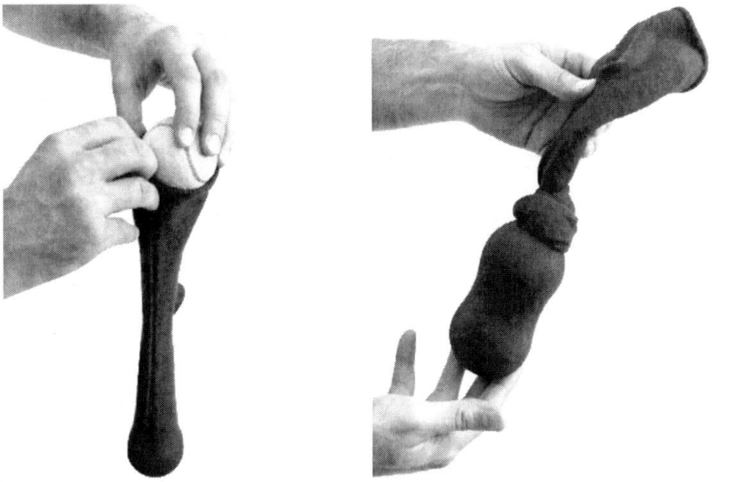

Figure 15.5 – Tennis ball massage

Depending on the size of your head, you may also want to tie a knot between the two balls to space them slightly further apart. Once you have the tennis balls secured, position the tennis ball sock so that the bony ridge on the back of your skull is resting on it. Let the weight of your head settle down onto the tennis ball and your chin dropping towards your chest. Close your eyes and relax for a few minutes.

Lying in this position will gently stretch the muscles at the back of your neck, as well as applying pressure to the sub-occipital region.

Upper Trapezius Massage and Muscular Trigger Point Compression

Massage

The entire upper trapezius muscle along the side of the neck and the top of the shoulder is commonly very tense and hard. Taut bands and muscular trigger points can be palpated relatively easily.

TrP1 is perhaps the most common muscular trigger point and it's a very important muscular trigger point for headache sufferers.

TrP1 is located right in the corner of the neck, not far beneath the surface of the skin. It is marked with an X on the over-developed trapezius muscles of the body builder in Figure 15.6.

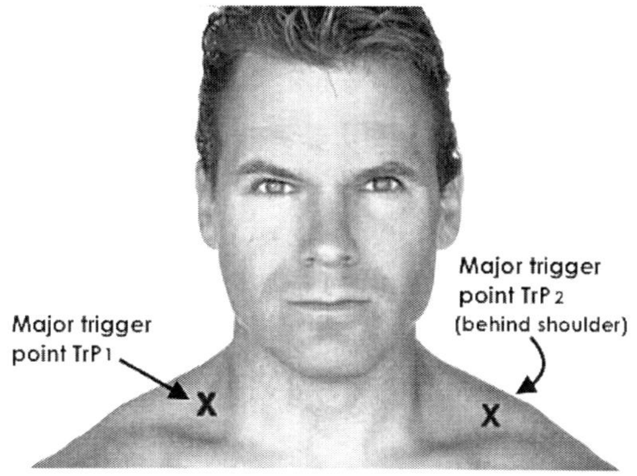

Figure 15.6 – Upper trapezius trigger point locations

A second upper trapezius trigger point, TrP2, lies just behind the top of the shoulder from TrP1 and a little further away from the corner of the neck. A therapist normally treats both muscular trigger points together. TrP2's pain referral pattern extends as far as the base of the skull but not beyond.

Before searching for these two muscular trigger points, it's a good idea to loosen the entire area with some massage. The aim is to relax and lengthen the muscle and to explore the area for muscular trigger points. You may find two locations close together that feel especially painful where TrP1 and TrP2 are located.

If your muscles are very tight, first try squeezing the tops of your shoulders with your hands. Then massage both left and right sides of your neck and shoulders as shown in the Figure 15.7 below. If it's convenient, you may want to use a little lubricant, such as baby oil or hand cream.

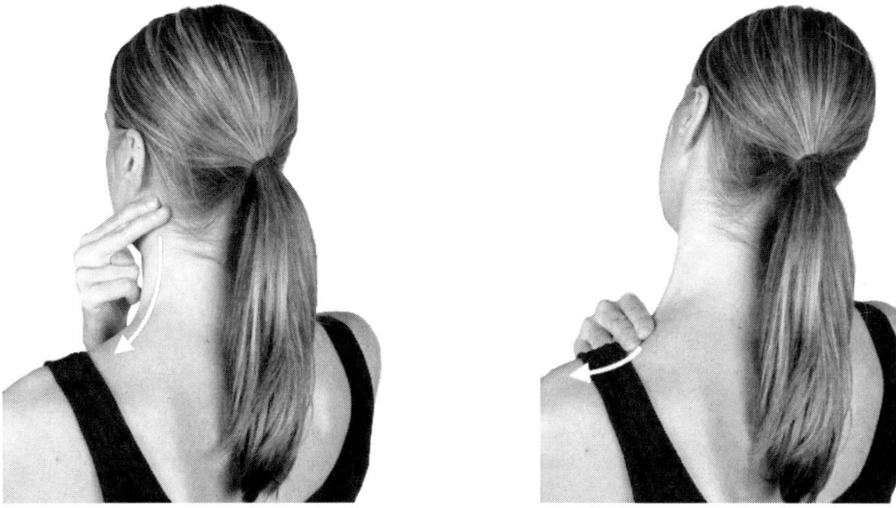

Figure 15.7 – Upper trapezius massage

Use the middle fingers of your opposite hand to apply a firm massage stroke along the muscle fibres (yellow arrows). Start just below your ear. As you move slowly down along the side of your neck and across the top of your shoulder, tilt your head to the opposite side (shown by the arrow) to put the muscle on stretch. Repeat the stroke three or four times, each time tilting your head to the opposite side. Repeat the same process on the other side of the body.

Upper Trapezius Muscular Trigger Point

Figure 15.8 demonstrates the pinch technique you can use to treat yourself. Don't worry if you don't find either of the upper trapezius muscular trigger points. Just performing the treatment procedures described will have a beneficial effect by reducing muscle tension and increasing blood flow.

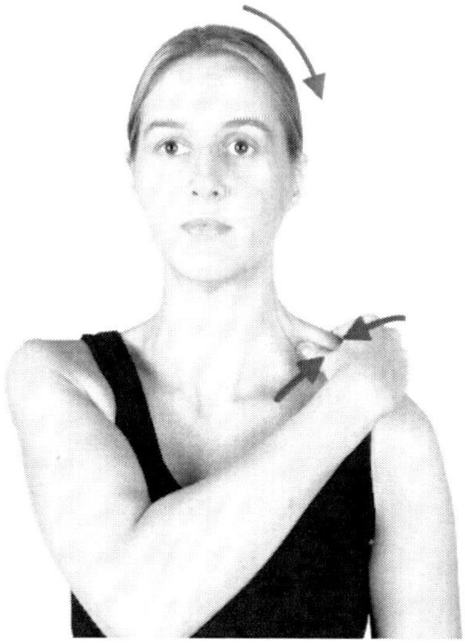

Figure 15.8 – Pinch compression of upper trapezius trigger point TrP1

For TrP1:

- Tilt your head slightly toward the side you are working on. This will relax the thick upper trapezius muscle enough for you to grab hold of it.
- Use your opposite hand to pinch the roll of muscle at the top of your shoulder beside the neck. The muscular trigger point is not far beneath the surface of the skin. Caution – don't stick your thumb in the hollow just above your collar bone.
- Continue to apply pressure with your thumb while you tilt your head a small amount to the opposite side to stretch the muscle and then return to your original position. Repeat this 2 or 3 times.
- You may also like to experiment with rolling this part of the muscle between your thumb and first two fingers.
- If you feel extra tenderness or pain maintain the pressure for up to 20 seconds, or until you feel the muscle soften and become less tender.
- Work your way along the top of your shoulder, maintaining pressure on any tender spots you find.
- Repeat the treatment on the muscle on the other side of your body.

You will need more pressure to find and treat TrP2 as it lies deeper below the skin. Figure 15.9 below shows its approximate location.

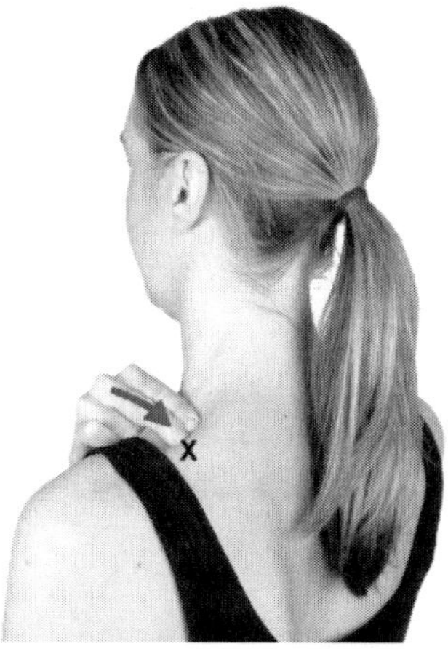

Figure 15.9 – Compression of upper trapezius trigger point TrP2

- Use two fingers of your opposite hand to explore the area shown.
- If you find a tender or painful spot press down on it for up to 20 seconds as shown, waiting for it to soften and become less tender.
- You may also like to try making small circles with your fingers while pressing down.
- Repeat for the opposite side of the body.

Because of its position, it can be hard to exert enough pressure with your fingers to adequately treat TrP2. Some people use a muscular trigger point self-treatment tool to apply pressure to muscular trigger points at the back of the body which are otherwise inaccessible.

SCM Muscle Massage and Muscular Trigger Point Compression

Massage

Muscular trigger points in one or both SCM muscles are very likely to be making an important contribution to your headache pain.

A therapist would normally first loosen tight fascia with remedial massage. They would then separately palpate the full length of the two branches of each SCM muscle, using a pincer grip to apply pressure. This encircles the muscle and moves it away from underlying structures.

In principle, you could do the same thing, however I believe you should only treat the top half of each SCM muscle, where the division into two branches can be easily felt. It requires specific instruction and practical supervision to learn how to treat the lower parts safely.

Figure 15.10 shows how the SCM muscle runs diagonally across the side of your neck. To find it, place the fingertips of your opposite hand just behind your ear where it joins your skull. You should be able to feel the bony base of your skull close by. This is also near where the SCM attaches. Turn your head away from the side you will be working on. As you do this you will feel the SCM muscle get more tense and stand out, as seen in the photo.

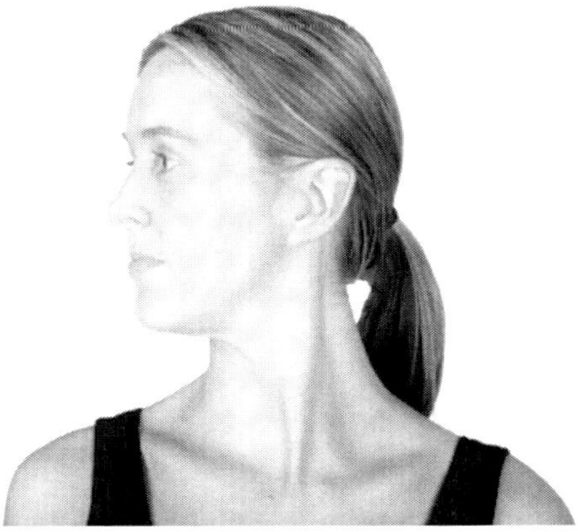

Figure 15.10 – Finding the sternocleidomastoid muscle

Massage the side of your neck to relax and lengthen the top half of the SCM muscle. If it is convenient you may want to use a little lubricant – baby oil or hand cream will do – but it's not essential.

- Keep your fingertips in the same place and apply firm pressure with your fingers as you move slowly down along the muscle fibres as shown in Figure 15.11 below, starting from your ear. Stop about half way down.
- Repeat 3 – 4 times.
- Repeat the entire massage process for the SCM muscle on the other side of your neck.

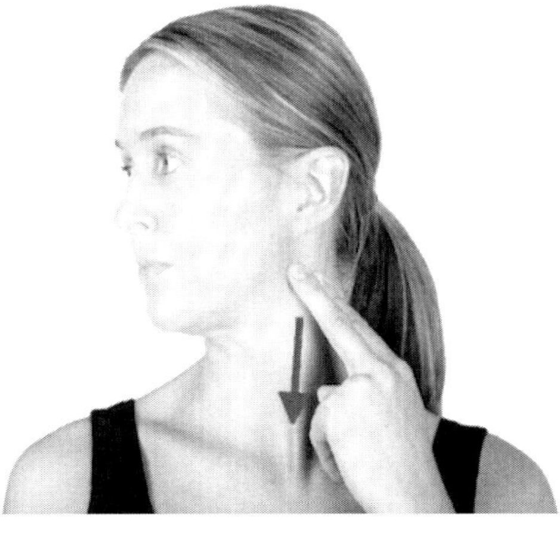

Figure 15.11 – Massage of the sternocleidomastoid muscle

SCM Muscular Trigger Point

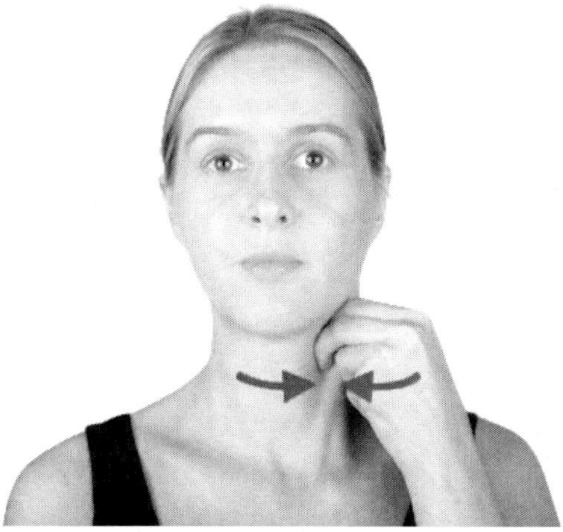

Figure 15.12 – Pincer treatment to the top of the sternocleidomastoid muscle

- Turn your head away from the side you will be working on so that the muscle stands out. Use your opposite hand to locate the SCM muscle as before.
- Gently place your fingers in a pincer grip on the top of the muscle as shown, just below the chin.
- Keep your fingers in the same place while you turn your head to face forward.
- Use the pincer grip to apply pressure to the top part of the muscle and maintain the pressure for about 20 seconds. This will relax this part of the muscle further and treat any muscular trigger points in the area.
- Now move a little further down the SCM muscle and repeat the pinch and hold. Do not go beyond the middle of the muscle.
- Repeat the entire pincer grip process for the SCM muscle on the other side of your neck.

Temporalis Muscles Massage and Muscular Trigger Points

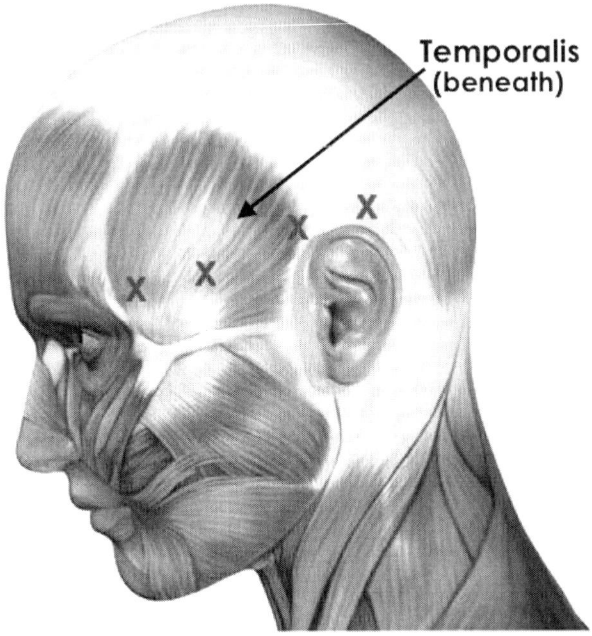

Figure 15.13 – Temporalis trigger points

The temporalis muscle is a large flat thin muscle in the temple region on each side of the head. It is not a face muscle but a jaw muscle, lying beneath the area indicated in Figure 15.13. Temporalis trigger points are extremely common and are a major source of headache pain.

You will almost certainly have temporalis trigger points if you grind your teeth, chew gum or you hold your head too far forward. 'X's in Figure 15.13 shows their approximate position. Temporalis trigger points may also be satellites of untreated key muscular trigger points in the SCM and upper trapezius muscles.

Massaging your temporalis muscles is an instinctive action to relieve pain during a headache attack. If you then treat the muscular trigger points in the temporalis muscles, it can stop the headache occurring in the first place.

Apply firm pressure to the muscle, working slowly backwards, exploring the region above the ears for tender areas. If you find a painful spot, maintain the pressure for 20 seconds, while you open and close your jaw – see Figure 15.14. This will deactivate muscular trigger points and stretch your jaw muscles at the same time.

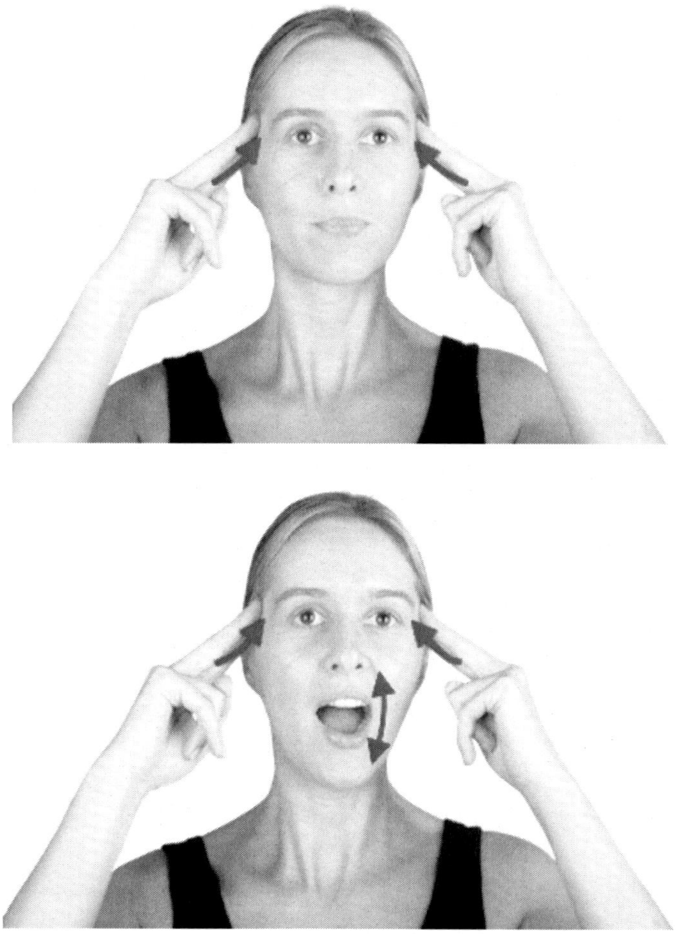

Figure 15.14 – Temporalis trigger point treatment

Scalp and Face Muscles

If you have suffered from frequent, severe headaches for a long time, active muscular trigger points in the muscles of your scalp and face could be a significant source of your headache pain. They are common satellites of long-standing, untreated muscular trigger points in the SCM and trapezius muscles. Other causes of muscular trigger points in the scalp and face can include a blow to the head or brow and muscle overuse – due to habitual frowning, wrinkling the forehead or squinting.

If you are in any of these categories, treating muscular trigger points in your own scalp and face muscles will reduce your overall 'pain load'. This will provide temporary pain relief during a headache attack and may even be sufficient to stop a headache attack that's on its way. It won't be as effective as applying pressure to your neck muscles or the temporalis muscles of your jaw, however the scalp and face muscles are thin and lie just below the surface of the skin which means they're easy to treat.

Figure 15.15 shows two of the more important muscles to treat – the frontalis muscle across the forehead and the occipitalis muscle at the back of the scalp. These are the front and back parts of the large 'worry' muscle on each side of the head. They connect to each other through the white coloured fascia – dense connective tissue – which can be seen covering the top of the head.

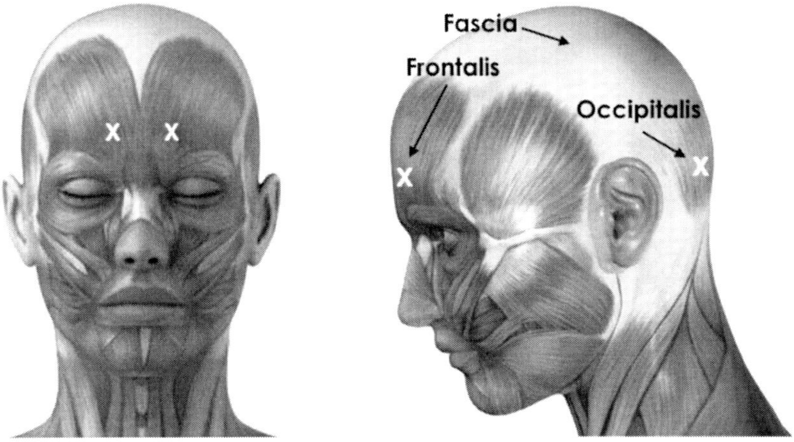

Figure 15.15 – Forehead and scalp trigger point locations

Approximate positions of muscular trigger points are marked with '**X**'s. Before you treat the muscular trigger points, you need to relax the muscles and stretch tight fascia.

The skin of the scalp should move freely on the underlying fascia. It will often feel tight where muscular trigger points are in the muscles beneath, like above the eyebrows. And even if they don't contain muscular trigger points, the scalp and face muscles are often very tense and tender.

A simple massage for the scalp and face muscles can help relieve pain during a headache attack by reducing muscle tension, improving blood flow and aiding overall relaxation.

The procedures described below use much the same sort of actions that people tend to perform instinctively when they have a headache.

Use your thumbs to massage the frontalis muscles along the muscle fibres from the top of the eyebrows, as shown, straight up past the hairline. Think about stretching the muscle upwards. Repeat several times.

To massage the occipitalis muscles, find the bony ridge above the base of your skull with your thumbs and move them upwards about 5 cm (2 inches). Press your fingertips in and pull downwards to stretch the fascia. Repeat several times.

Then massage the connective tissue from the centre of the top of the skull outwards, towards the ears on each side as shown in the photo on the right.

Massaging the scalp muscles and fascia, together with moderate pressure on the sub-occipital muscles at the base of the skull, is what makes having your hair washed at the hairdressers so wonderfully relaxing.

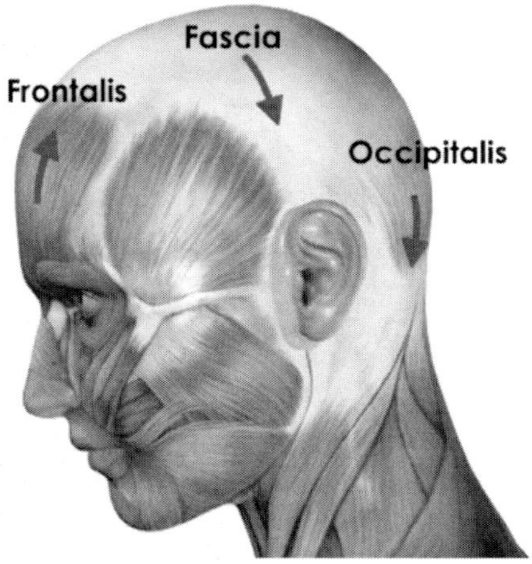

Figure 15.16 – Massage scalp muscle and fascia

In Figure 15.16, arrows show the directions in which massage should be carried out for the frontalis, occipitalis and connective tissue.

Once you have massaged your scalp, you can treat any muscular trigger points in the frontalis and occipitalis muscles using mild static pressure or very small movements along and across the muscle fibres. See Figure 15.15 for their approximate locations.

Figure 15.17 below shows the position of several muscular trigger points in the brow region that are worth treating. The muscles concerned are the circular orbicularis oculi or squinting muscle around each eye and the corrugator and procerus, frowning muscles between the eyebrows.

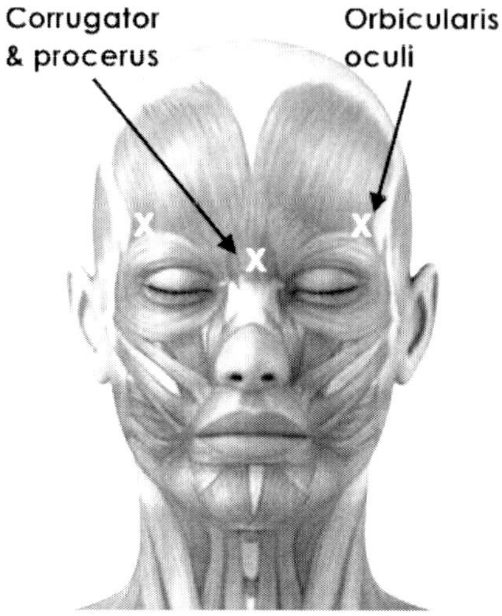

Figure 15.17 – Brow trigger point locations

Muscular trigger points in the orbicularis oculi are indicated with '**X**'s in Figure 15.17. The location of muscular trigger points in the small muscles between the eyebrows is not known exactly so it's best to treat the whole area.

The orbicularis oculi is treated by applying gentle pressure against the bony part of the eye socket just below the outside edge of the eyebrow. This has to be done cautiously as the tissues around the eye are very delicate.

The corrugator and procerus muscles are 'picked up' and gentle pressure is applied or they are rolled between the thumb and forefinger.

A Few Important Stretches

None of these stretches are difficult and many of them might be familiar to you – the main message here is that they are all extremely effective and worth doing often.

The Chin Tuck (Head Retraction)

The chin tuck moves the upper neck vertebrae into place and realigns the head over the shoulders. It also strengthens the muscles at the back of the neck and stretches tight sub-occipital, scalene and pectoral muscles, strengthens weak muscles in the mid-back and temporarily reduces compression of cervical facet joints.

Do the chin tuck exercise several times each day, especially if your neck and shoulders are starting to feel tired. You can do this stretch sitting at a desk or in a car:

- Sit tall in your chair with your feet flat on the floor. Your chin should be level and your nose pointing straight ahead
- Slow down your breathing and raise your chest towards the ceiling. Keep your head level and hold your chest in this position
- Take a slow breath in and as you exhale move your head and neck straight back as far as you can as shown by the arrow in the photo on the right. You need to give yourself a double chin. Do not use force

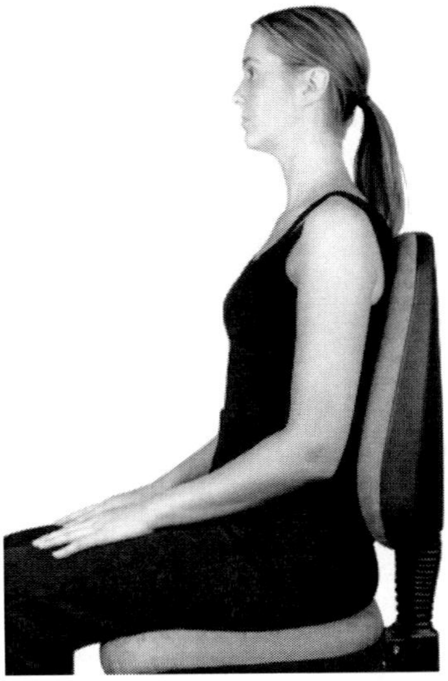
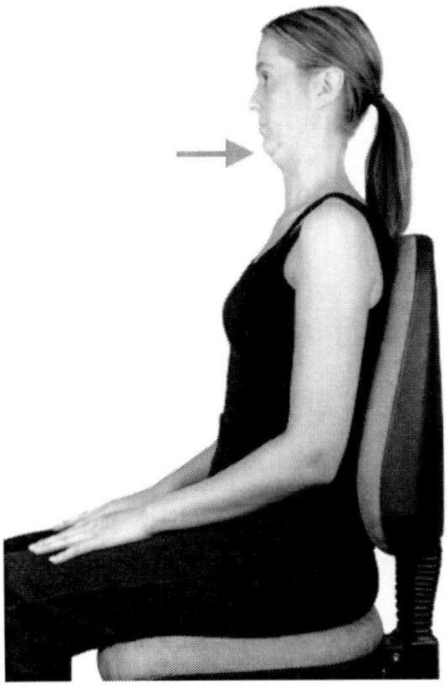

- Hold this position for 10 seconds while breathing normally
- Relax and then repeat the sequence 3 or more times
- Make sure you keep your head level with your nose pointing straight ahead (do not tilt it up or down) and do not open your mouth. It's as if your head was sliding backwards on a railway track
- If you are in the car push straight back against the headrest.

You shouldn't be trying to 'crack' your neck, but don't worry if you hear a few clicks from your neck as you move it. However, there shouldn't be any pain.

To guide and assist the movement you can apply a small amount of pressure horizontally on your chin – see the arrow on the photo.

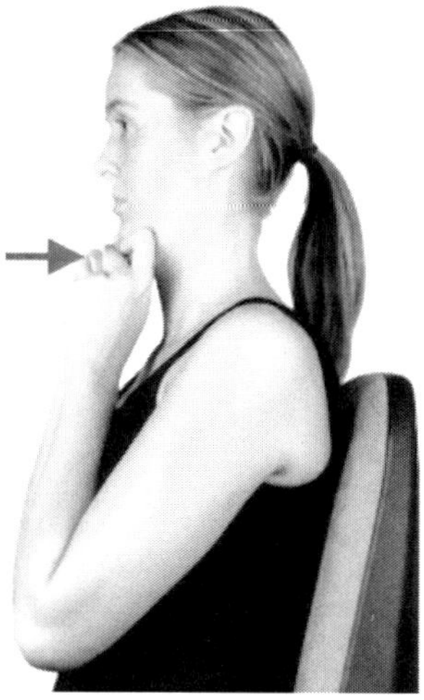

Side-Bending the Head and Neck (Ear to Shoulder)

Side-bending the head and neck stretches the upper trapezius, middle scalene and, to a lesser extent, the levator scapulae muscles on the opposite side of your neck.

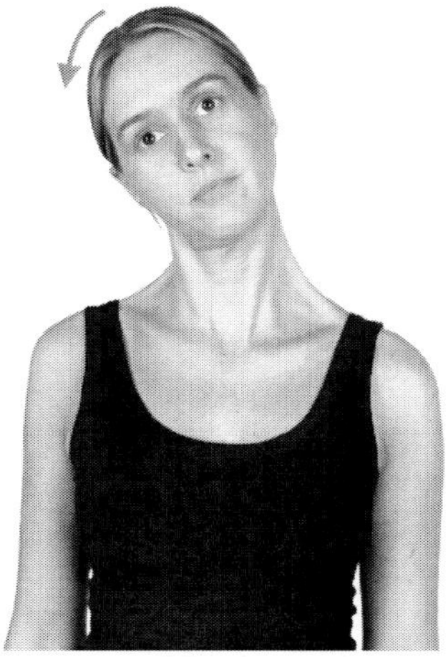

This stretch can be done anytime – sitting at your desk, in your car at the traffic lights or while standing in line. It is performed progressively in 3 stages, each of 10 seconds duration. Each stage follows an exhalation which helps the muscles to relax:

- Sit tall in your chair with your feet flat on the floor as before
- You should be looking straight ahead with your chin level. Keep your neck long and your head slightly retracted
- Let your arms hang loosely by your sides or rest on your thighs. Your shoulders should be back and down
- Slowly bend your head and neck sideways as far as it will comfortably go – your ear moves closer to your shoulder
- You should feel a mild to moderate pain-free stretch along the side of your neck, between your ear and shoulder on the opposite side
- Inhale, then, as you exhale, increase the stretch. Continue to breathe using your diaphragm while you hold the new position for a total of 10 seconds
- Repeat the process two more times using an exhalation to progressively increase the stretch
- Inhale, and as you exhale return your head to the upright position
- Stretch the other side for a total of 30 seconds using the same procedure.

Make sure during the stretch, you don't bend your neck forwards, let your chin drop down or lift your shoulders.

Here are two variations on the stretch:

- Use one hand to apply gentle over-pressure to your head to guide and slightly increase the stretch. Be careful not to pull on your head
- Holding onto the side of the chair seat will deliver a stronger stretch.

Shoulder Shrug and Backward Roll

The shoulders accumulate a lot of stress and tension during repetitive activities like typing. Shoulder shrugs and rolls are a great way to release tension and improve circulation:

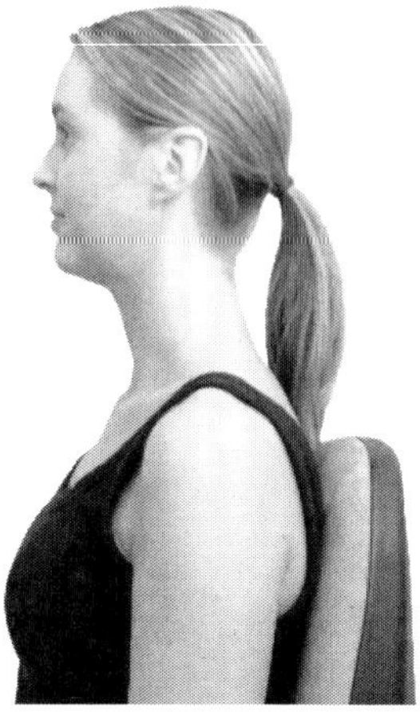

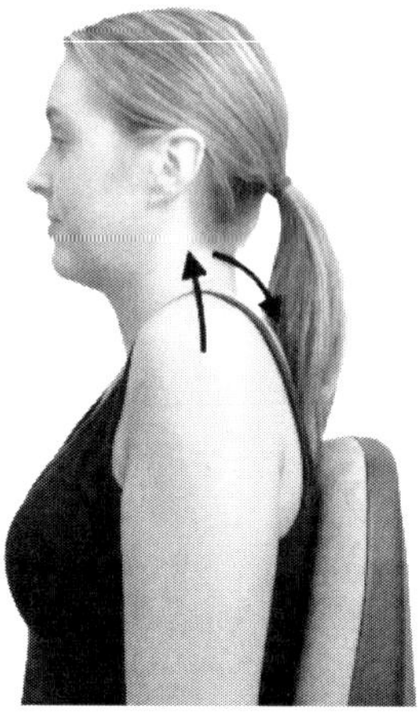

- Sit tall in your chair with your feet flat on the floor as before. Move forward on the seat until you have enough room
- Keep your neck long, your head slightly retracted, and look straight ahead with your chin level
- Inhale and lift your shoulders up towards your ears, pushing them up as hard as you can. Hold for 2 – 3 seconds
- Then exhale and very slowly roll your shoulders back down
- Repeat 8 –10 times.

Chest Muscle (Pectoral) Stretch

Chest muscles get very tight with prolonged sitting and with holding your arms out in front of you, during activities like driving. This can hamper your ability to breathe properly and cause nerves and blood vessels to be compressed.

Here is a chest stretch you can do while seated:

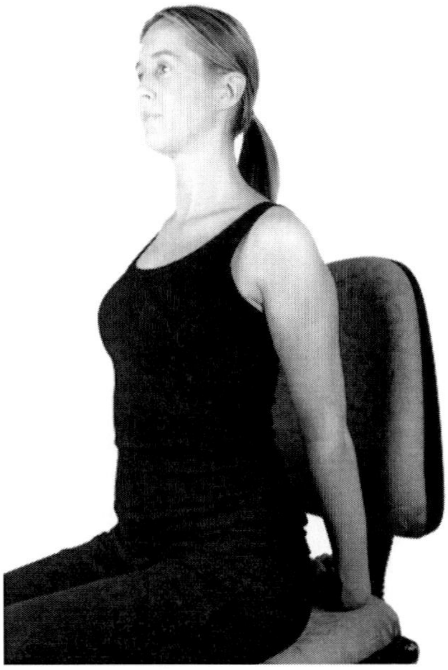

- Sit tall in your chair with your feet flat on the floor as before. If your chair has arms move forward on the seat until you have enough room
- Keep your neck long, your head slightly retracted, and look straight ahead with your chin level
- Bring your hands behind you and clasp them together if you can
- Breathe in, and as you exhale, slowly draw your shoulders back and try to pinch your shoulder blades together as shown in the photo
- Keep your body upright and continue to breathe slowly. You should feel a stretch across your upper chest
- Hold the stretch for 30 seconds and then return slowly to the starting position. Repeat the stretch once.

Self-Traction and Stretch for the Back of the Neck

This stretch is a good way to stretch the muscles at the back of the neck, apply pressure to the sub-occipital muscles and provide some traction to the neck joints, all at the same time. It's similar to the method Andrew Taylor Still, the founder of osteopathy, discovered for treating his childhood migraines:

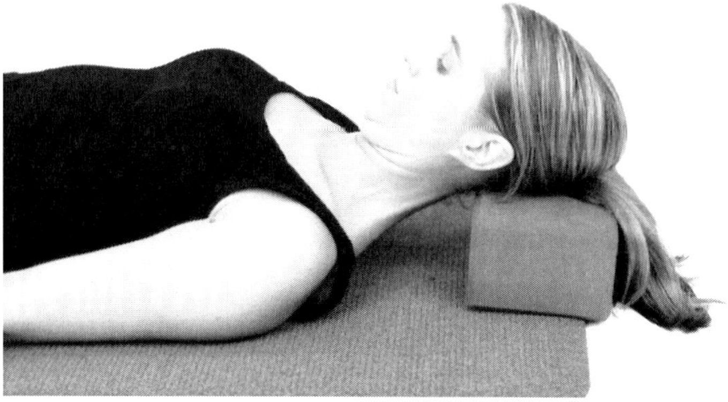

- Lie on the floor with your knees bent
- Lengthen your neck and then place a yoga foam block or a book under your head so that the bony ridge in the middle of your skull will rest on it.
- Focus on the muscles at the back of your neck releasing. Feel your chin dropping towards your chest
- If you wish you may be able to slide a hot water bottle into the gap between your neck and the floor, to warm the back of your neck and increase muscle relaxation and blood flow
- Close your eyes and relax for five minutes or so, breathing slowly and deeply. You can gradually increase the time up to 20 minutes.

Release Tension in Your Paraspinal Muscles

The tennis ball sock can also be used to release tension in your paraspinal muscles. It's particularly useful to help restore mobility in the thoracic region of your spine where several important neck and shoulder girdle muscles attach.

- Lie on your back with your knees bent
- Starting with your upper back, position your body over the sock so that you are resting with one tennis ball on each side of your spine. Let yourself relax down onto the balls for 30 seconds
- Lift up and reposition yourself over the sock so the muscles beside the next lower vertebra are being treated
- Continue this process all the way down to the end of your spine.

Key Points

- Self-massage and stretching are great additions to your professional treatments.
- Relaxed breathing is necessary for correct stretching technique – exhale as you increase the stretch.
- In between professional manual therapy treatments, it is important to be mindful of your posture, avoid prolonged sitting and to stretch regularly.
- You should practice self-massage and stretching techniques when you don't have a headache, so you are ready to use them when you are in pain.
- The Chin Tuck and Chest stretches are two of the most beneficial stretches you can perform.

16

Advanced Stretches

The stretches we covered earlier were for immediate relief when a headache strikes. The stretches in this chapter are more comprehensive, aimed at reducing the incidence of musculoskeletal problems in your neck and shoulders.

There are so many benefits to regularly stretching your muscles. It enables muscles to progressively lengthen, restoring their normal range of motion and improving their internal circulation, which makes it much less likely that treated muscular trigger points will recur or new ones develop.

Stretching helps loosen tight facet joint capsules and shortened ligaments in the neck and relieves pressure on the intervertebral discs. Your neck becomes more flexible, reducing the contribution to headache pain from restricted motion in the three uppermost neck joints. You will find it easier to bend your head forward, backward and sideways and to turn your head from side to side.

Stretching can also help correct the muscle imbalances that perpetuate bad head and neck posture.

Precautions

- All the stretching exercises in this book should be considered as a general guide only.
- You should seek professional advice before performing these stretches to make sure they are suitable for you.
- Do not continue to perform any exercises that cause pain, numbness, and / or tingling. If these symptoms occur, consult your therapist or doctor.
- Depending on how tight your different muscles are, some stretches may need to be modified or you might need to find alternatives to make them effective.
- If you haven't stretched for a long time, start slowly and gently.
- You should stretch to the point of feeling resistance, but no further. Do not use force – you should not feel pain.
- If you are not used to stretching, it can be hard to judge the passage of time, so initially you should either look at the clock or count, or work out how many breaths to take. With a little practice, you won't need to do this, making it a lot easier to relax mentally.

Getting the Most from Your Stretches

Keep Your Jaw, Mouth and Tongue Relaxed

Before you start, check your jaw to make sure it's relaxed. Clenching your teeth can become a habit you don't notice after a while. Teeth clenching is a common cause of muscular trigger points in the jaw muscles and damage to the jaw joint.

An effective way to relax the jaw and prevent teeth clenching is to keep the tip of your tongue on the roof of your mouth behind the upper teeth. This keeps the teeth apart. Keep your lips loosely closed, teeth slightly apart, and breathe through your nose.

Use Correct Diaphragmatic Breathing and Don't Rush

All these exercises should be performed in a slow and controlled manner while breathing slowly using your diaphragm. Correct diaphragmatic breathing is especially important for stretching to be effective. (See Chapter 17 for a full description of Diaphragmatic breathing.)

Slow exhalation while stretching sends a signal from the nervous system to the muscles that encourages them to relax and lengthen further.

In my experience many people don't breathe while they are stretching – they actually hold their breath. Incorporating correct breathing into the stretching is the 'missing key' to unlocking tight muscles. That's why many people say that stretching doesn't help. They aren't breathing and they rush through the sequence.

Repeated Versus Progressive Muscle Stretching

Muscles should be stretched for at least 30 seconds in one of two ways:

- **Repeated stretching:** Each stretch is held for at least 10 seconds. After returning to the starting position, the same stretch is repeated twice over. This is best for the neck and abdominal muscle stretches
- **Progressive stretching:** Each stretch has three continuous stages, with each stage being held for least 10 seconds. An exhalation is used as the signal to progressively increase the stretch. Shoulder, upper back and chest muscles are stretched this way.

Progressive Stretching On Exhalation

- Move the target muscle to the end of its range, which is as far you can go comfortably. You should feel a gentle stretch.
- Take a deep slow breath in, then, as you slowly exhale, gradually increase the stretch until you reach a barrier to further stretching. Do not overstretch.
- Hold this position for a minimum of 10 seconds while continuing to breathe normally. You should feel the muscle gradually releasing.
- Take another deep slow breath in, then, as you slowly exhale, gradually increase the stretch further until you reach a new barrier. Again, do not overstretch.

- Hold this new position for a minimum of 10 seconds while continuing to breathe normally.
- Repeat the last two steps, increasing and holding the stretch one more time to give a total of 30 seconds stretching.
- Slowly return the muscle to its normal position.

How Often Each Day Should You Do the Exercises?

It's better to do an exercise once a day with proper technique, rather than rush through three sets.

Separate sets are also more effective if spread throughout the day.

Here is a suggested program that is hopefully a balance between effectiveness and not being too time-consuming. It can easily be done in small blocks of time and takes less than 30 minutes overall.

- Forward head posture correction: every 1 – 2 hours (minimum of 6 per day).
- Neck and shoulder stretches: 2 – 3 times per day.
- Standing back bend: 2 times per day.
- Shoulder blade stretch: 2 times per day.
- Chest stretch: 2 times per day.
- Neck strengthening: 2 times per day.

For Every Stretch

Good neck and shoulder posture makes these exercises more effective and helps prevent injuries. These six steps should be performed before beginning any and every stretch.

The following instructions apply to every stretch:

- Sit or stand tall, thinking about lengthening your entire spine and especially your neck
- Lift your breastbone (not your shoulders) slightly so your shoulders move back and down
- Slightly retract your head
- Look straight ahead
- Make sure your chin is level
- Gently move your head straight back so your ears are more in line with your shoulders. This is the same movement as in the head retraction exercise in Chapter 14, but do not take your head back so far. You should only feel the beginnings of a double chin.

Exercises to Correct Posture

Two-Part Exercise to Correct Forward Head Posture

The exercise for correcting forward head posture on the following two pages is a combination of two separate exercises:

- A modified shoulder blade squeeze which corrects the muscular imbalance that causes rounded, hunched shoulders and excessively rounded mid-back. This squeeze stretches tight muscles in the chest and the front of the shoulders and strengthens weak mid-back muscles
- A head retraction or chin tuck which moves the upper neck vertebrae into place and realigns the head over the shoulders. It also strengthens the muscles at the back of the neck.

Some things to remember:

- Use correct diaphragmatic breathing to allow stretched muscles to relax
- Keep your head level with your nose pointing straight ahead (do not tilt your nose up or down) and do not open your mouth
- Keep your jaw relaxed, your lips loosely closed and your tongue resting on the roof of your mouth.

Modified Shoulder Blade Squeeze

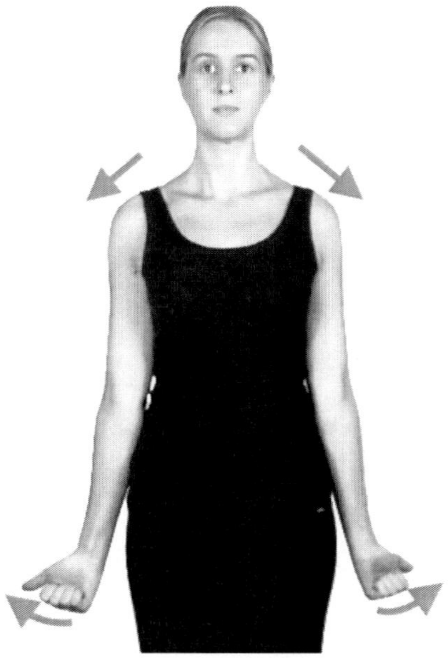

- Stand tall with your feet about 10 cm (4 inches) apart, arms at your side, thumbs pointing forward as usual.
- Tighten your buttocks to stabilise your lower back.
- As you inhale, rotate your thumbs, arms and shoulders out and back as shown in the photo.
- Squeeze your shoulder blades together – imagine cracking a walnut between your shoulder blades.
- Maintain this position of your shoulder blades and as you exhale, pull your shoulders down.
- Hold this position while breathing normally and then continue to the head retraction step which follows.

Head Retraction / Chin Tuck

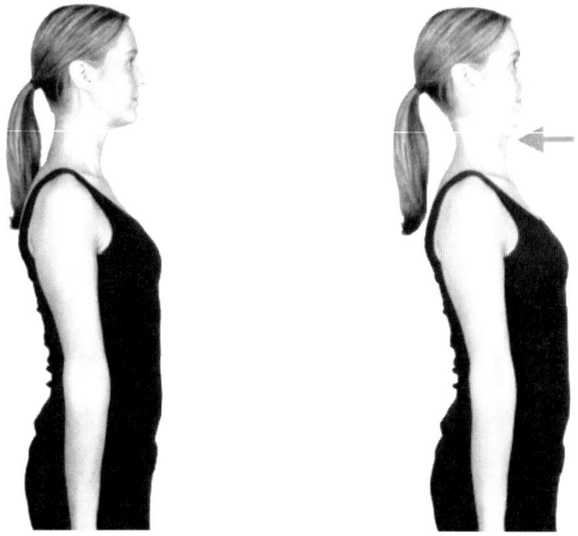

- Take a deep breath in and as you exhale, gently move your head straight back as far as you are able to, as if it is sliding backwards on a railway track. You will feel yourself producing a double chin.
- Do not use force. You should feel the movement along your neck up to the base of your skull.
- Don't worry if you hear a few clicks from your neck as you move your head, but there should be no pain.
- Make sure you keep your head level with your nose pointing straight ahead (do not tilt it up or down) and do not open your mouth – the close-up at the right shows what this should look like.
- To guide and assist the movement you can apply a small amount of pressure horizontally on your chin.
- Hold this position for 10 seconds while breathing normally.
- Relax, but concentrate on retaining good posture.

It's a good idea to check your shoulder posture with the wall test before and after doing the forward head posture exercise. Do you notice any improvement?

If you repeat the exercise to correct forward head posture every 1–2 hours or so (about 6 times total) you will soon start to see real benefits. It is much better to spread it out during the day than to do several sets following each other.

The chin tuck part of the posture correction exercise is beneficial on its own.

You can do the chin tuck while sitting down. There are many opportunities – for example while sitting at your desk at work or in your car while waiting at the traffic lights.
However, before you start, slow down your breathing and raise your chest towards the ceiling.

This will automatically cause your shoulders to move back and down. Hold your chest in this position while you move your head back. Make sure your nose points straight ahead.

Stretches for Neck and Shoulders

In this section, I have grouped related neck and shoulder stretches next to one another to make them easier to remember. All of them can be done standing or sitting.

Each of the stretches should be done 2–3 times every day. Think of it as preventative maintenance, just like brushing your teeth. Once you get into the habit and start to enjoy the feeling of releasing tension in your neck and shoulder muscles, you will probably begin to find new opportunities to fit in a few extra stretches.

You may choose to do some of the stretches during a short break at your desk, others in the car while waiting for the traffic lights, on the bus or train, or while waiting in a queue. The shower is a great place to do the stretches that require you to bend your neck forwards or to the side, as the warm water will loosen the muscles to be stretched.

Good Posture for Neck and Shoulder Stretches

For all the stretches in this section, the following four points apply:

- Sit or stand tall
- Make sure that you don't lift your shoulders – it is a good idea to stand with your hands clasped behind your back or sit on your hands
- Keep your neck long and your head slightly retracted
- Start by looking straight ahead, keeping your chin level.

It's important to maintain good shoulder posture during the neck and shoulder stretches. Both your shoulders should be aligned and down and you need to make sure you don't lift them when you move your head.

There are several ways you can make sure you maintain good shoulder posture and give tight muscles across the top of your shoulders a bit more of a stretch at the same time. If you are standing you can simply stretch your arms down behind your buttocks and interlace your fingers as shown in the photo.

To achieve the same effect while sitting, let your arms hang straight down by your sides and then either sit on your hands or hold onto the sides of your chair seat – this gives a slightly stronger stretch. These methods can be used for all the neck and shoulder stretches.

Once your neck becomes more flexible, you can increase the neck stretches by applying gentle over-pressure to your head. This should only be done when you are bending your head forward, or to one side as shown in some photos below.

Rotate Head and Neck (Left and Right)

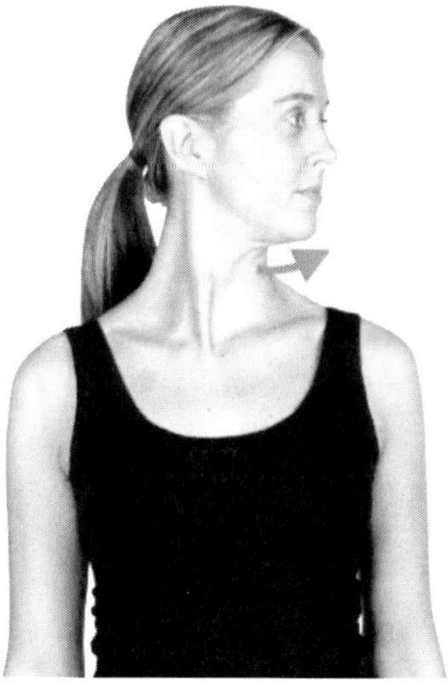

This movement stretches the SCM and upper trapezius muscles on one side of your neck, plus several muscles at the back of your neck. It's one of several stretches that requires extra care with your head and neck posture.

CAUTION: Muscular trigger points in the SCM muscle can make you feel dizzy. Dizziness might also mean the blood vessels in your neck are being squeezed, especially if you are older, in this case it would be wise to get a medical check-up.

- Turn your head slowly round to one side so your chin moves towards your shoulder as far as it will easily go, as shown in above. Keep looking in the direction your head is moving. You should feel a mild to moderate pain-free stretch along the side of your neck and top of your shoulder.
- Exhale, and turn your head slightly further towards your shoulder. Do not use force.
- Hold the stretch for a total of 10 seconds, breathing all the time.
- Inhale and return to the starting position.
- Repeat two times giving a total of 30 seconds of stretching to that side. Do not go from one side to the other or roll your neck about.
- Repeat all steps on the other side for a total of 30 seconds of stretching.

Bend Head and Neck Straight Back, Chin towards Ceiling

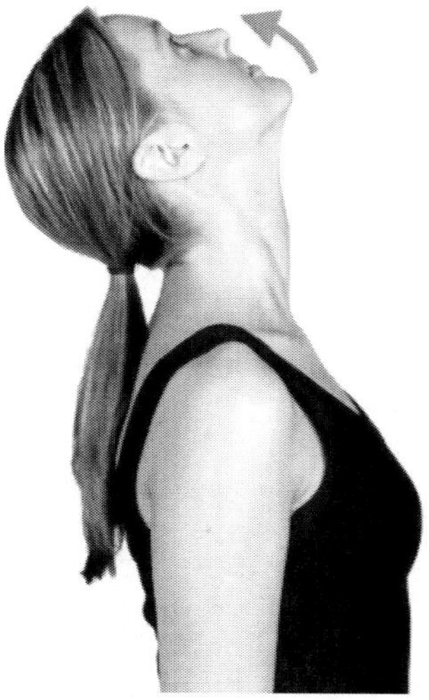

Taking your head straight back as shown stretches the SCM and scalene muscles on both sides of the neck and the deep muscles at the front of the neck.

This is another stretch where you need to take particular care with your head and neck posture before you start, to avoid crunching your neck.

CAUTION: The same cautions about dizziness apply as in the previous stretch. Again, if you feel dizzy doing this stretch it would be a good idea to have a medical check-up.

- Leading the movement with your chin as shown, gently roll your head straight back until your face is looking directly up at the ceiling. You should feel a mild to moderate pain-free stretch along the front of your neck and under your chin.
- Exhale, and allow the weight of your head to increase the stretch. If you want to increase the stretch still further, jut your lower jaw forward and put your lower lip over your top lip. This sounds strange but it works.
- Hold the stretch for a total of 10 seconds, breathing all the time.
- Inhale, and moving your chin first, bring your head back down to the starting position.
- Repeat the procedure two times giving a total of 30 seconds stretching.

Now continue to the angled form of the stretch.

Bend Head and Neck Back on Angle, Chin towards Ceiling

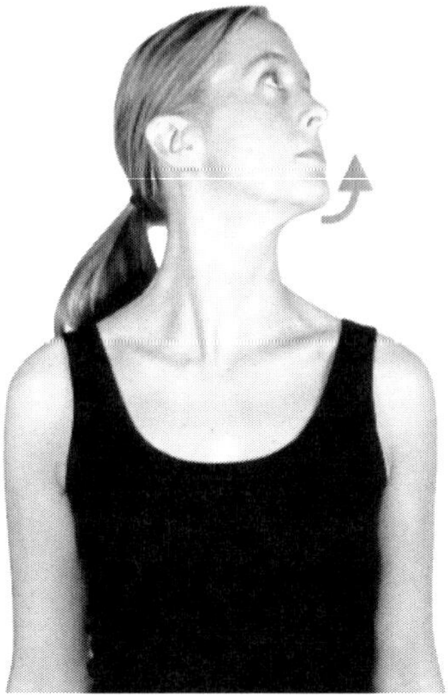

The photo above shows the head and neck bent back at an angle. To perform the stretch you first turn your head and then take your head back.

This angled stretch focuses the stretch on the SCM muscle on only one side of your neck. Both sides need to be stretched equally.

CAUTION: The same cautions about dizziness apply as in the previous two stretches.

- Turn your head to one side as far as you can comfortably go.
- Gently roll your head backwards so your chin moves upwards towards the ceiling as shown. You should feel a mild to moderate pain-free stretch along the opposite side of the front of your neck and under your chin.
- Exhale, and allow the stretch to increase. As before, if you want to increase the stretch still further, jut your lower jaw forward and put your lower lip over your top lip.
- Hold the stretch for a total of 10 seconds, breathing all the time.
- Inhale, and moving your chin first, bring your head back down to the upright position. Then turn your head back to the starting position.
- Repeat the procedure on the same side 2 times giving a total of 30 seconds stretching.
- Now repeat on the opposite side for a total of 30 seconds of stretching.

Bend Head and Neck Forwards, Chin towards Chest

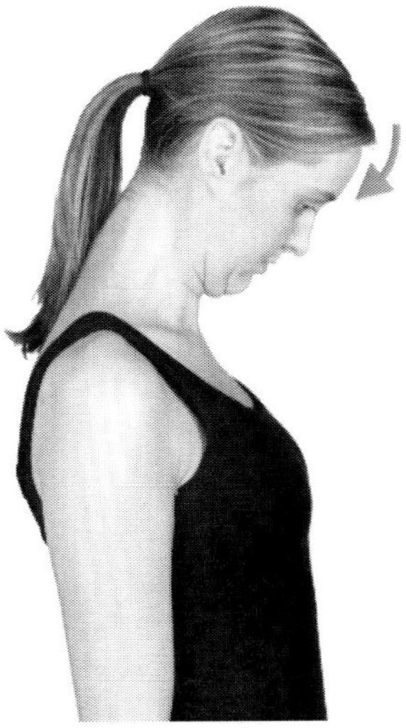

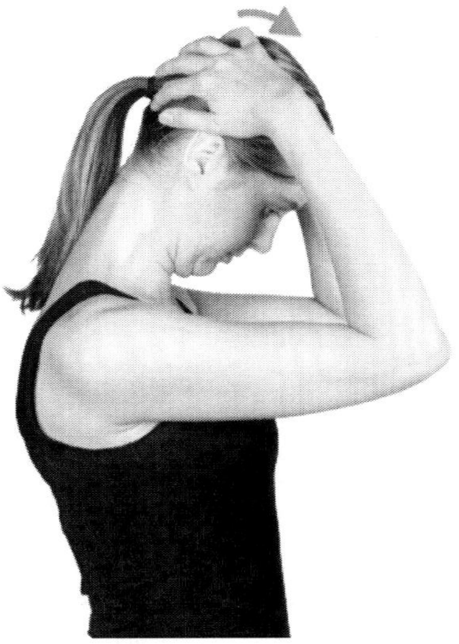

This movement stretches the muscles at the back of the neck, including the sub-occipital and upper trapezius muscles.

- Bend your head forward towards your chest, with your chin leading the movement as shown. You should feel a mild to moderate pain-free stretch along the back of your neck, and possibly as far down your spine as your mid-back.
- Exhale, and allow the stretch to increase.
- Hold the stretch for a total of 10 seconds, breathing all the time.
- Inhale and return to the starting position.
- Repeat the procedure 2 times giving a total of 30 seconds of stretching.

Once you are comfortable with this stretch, you can increase it by providing gentle over-pressure to the back of your head, with one or both hands as shown at right. Make sure you don't pull on your head.

Bend Head and Neck Sideways, Ear towards Shoulder

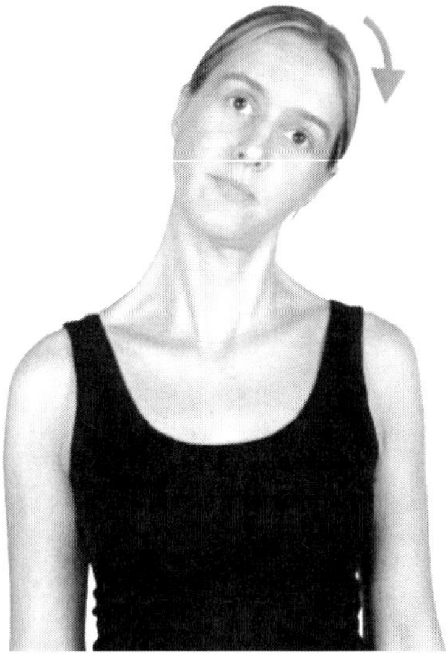

This movement stretches the upper trapezius muscle, the middle scalene muscle and, to a lesser extent, the levator scapulae muscle on one side of your neck.

Both sides need to be stretched equally.

The photo shows the simplest version of the stretch.

- If the stretch feels too strong, move your arms back by your sides until your muscles get looser. If your arms are by your sides, pay extra attention to keeping your shoulders down.
- Move one ear towards the shoulder on the same side as far as it will comfortably go. Do not lift your shoulders. You should feel a mild to moderate pain-free stretch along the side of your neck, between your ear and shoulder.
- Exhale, and allow the stretch to increase.
- Hold the stretch for a total of 30 seconds in 3 stages, using an exhalation to progressively increase the stretch after each 10 second hold. Continue to breathe using your diaphragm.
- Inhale, and return your head to the upright position.
- Stretch the other side for 30 seconds using the same procedure.

The following demonstrate four variations to the basic upper trapezius stretch. Two variations you can use while sitting down and two while standing.

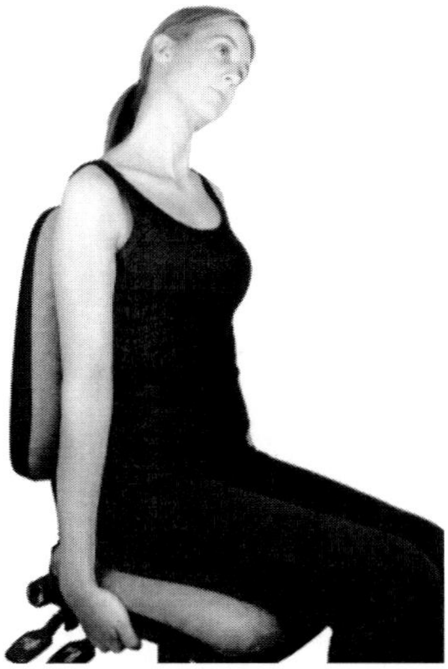

(i) Sitting, holding side of chair to maintain shoulder posture

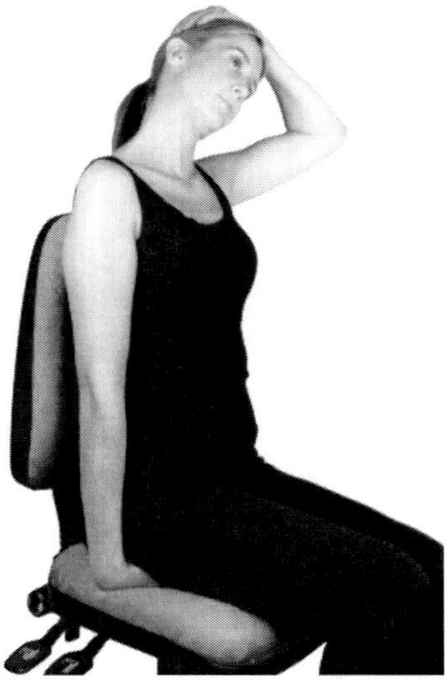

(ii) Sitting on one hand to maintain shoulder posture, plus overpressure

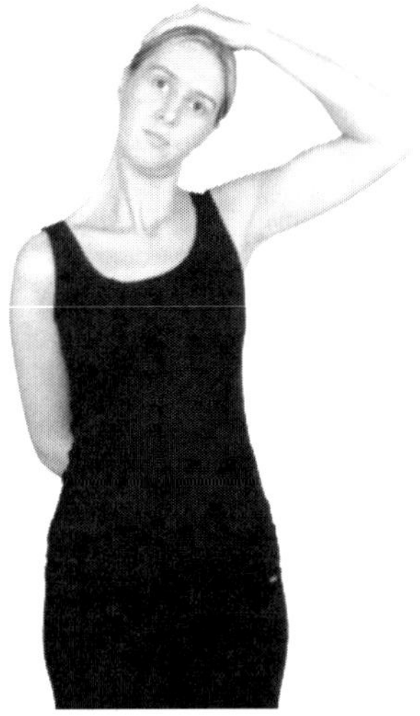

(iii) Standing, arm behind back for shoulder posture, plus overpressure

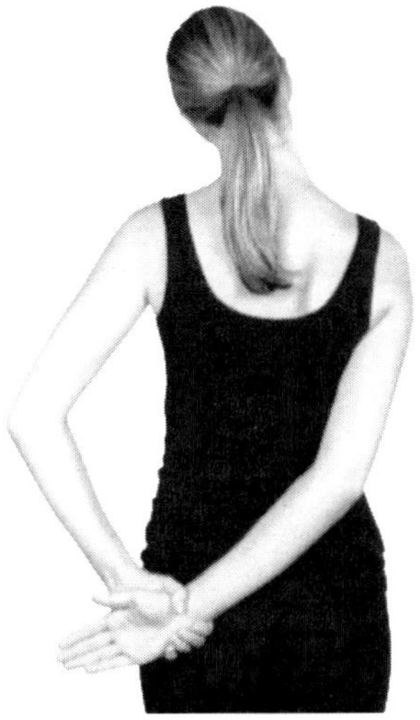

(iv) Standing, pulling on your arm to increase stretch and keep shoulder down

- Sitting on one or both hands or holding onto the seat of the chair with one or both hands as shown in (i) and (ii) helps anchor the shoulder on the side being stretched. It also provides some additional stretch.
- Standing with one or both arms behind the back, as in (iii) and (iv) has the same effect.
- Applying gentle over-pressure on the head with the one hand increases the stretch further. Overpressure can be used when either sitting (ii) or standing (iii). Make sure you don't pull on your head.
- The photo in (iv) shows an alternative to over-pressure to increase the stretch. You pull down on your arm on the side being stretched. This also keeps the shoulder being stretched in place.

Bend Head and Neck Sideways and Turn Face Up

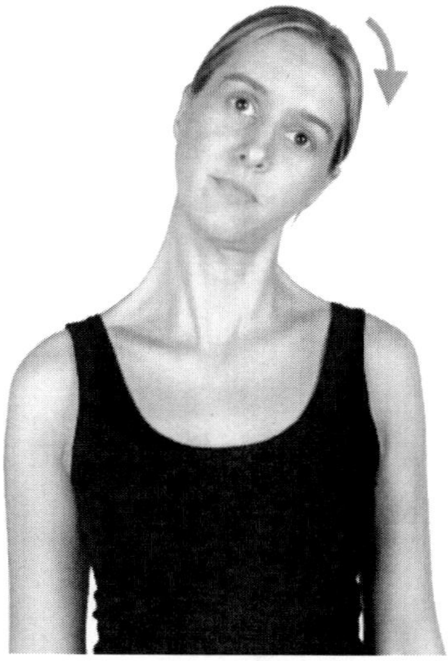

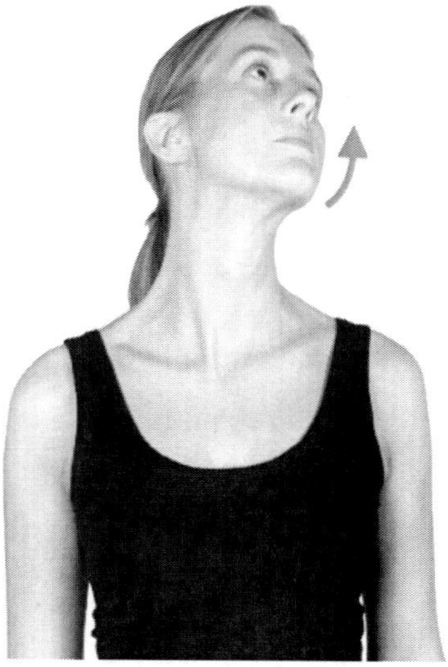

Bending the ear towards the shoulder while looking straight ahead stretches the middle scalene as well as the upper trapezius on one side of the neck.

To stretch the front scalenes, after the neck is bent sideways the face has to be turned up (but make sure you don't bend your neck backwards). You need to take care as you turn your face. Stop if you feel any dizziness or pins and needles.

Both sides of your neck need to be stretched equally.

- Move one ear towards the shoulder on the same side as far as it will comfortably go – see the photo on the left.
- Now turn your face to look up towards the ceiling as in the photo on the right – you should feel a mild to moderate pain-free stretch along the side of your neck, roughly from the collar bone to under side of the side of the jaw.
- Exhale, and allow the stretch to increase.
- Hold the stretch for a total of 30 seconds in 3 stages, using an exhalation to progressively increase the stretch after each 10 second hold. Continue to breathe using your diaphragm.
- Inhale, turn your face to look straight ahead again and then move your head and neck back to the upright position.
- Stretch the other side for 30 seconds using the same procedure.

You should feel the front scalene stretch more towards the front of your neck than the upper trapezius and middle scalene stretch.

Bend Head and Neck Sideways and Turn Face Down

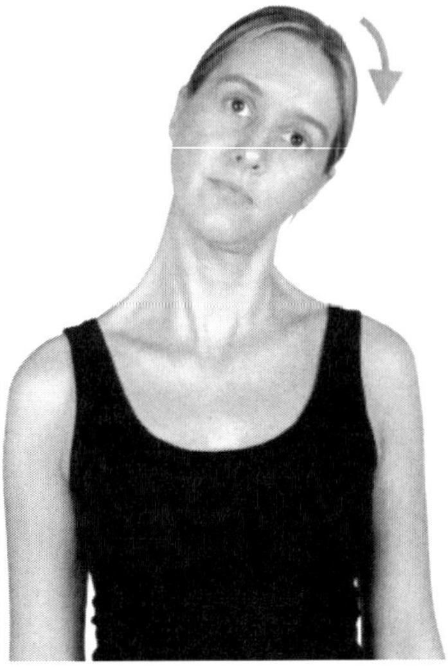 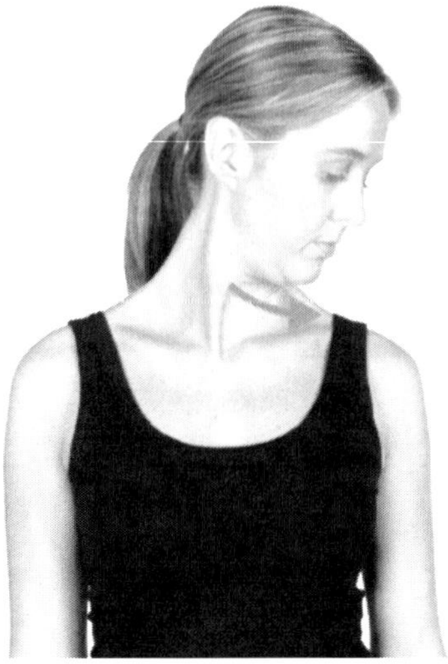

Bending the ear towards the shoulder while looking straight ahead stretches the middle scalene as well as the upper trapezius on one side of the neck.

To stretch the rear scalenes, your face has to be turned down after your neck is bent sideways (but make sure you don't bend your neck downwards). You need to take care as you turn your face. Stop if you feel any dizziness or pins and needles.

Both sides of your neck need to be stretched equally.

- As before, move one ear towards the shoulder on the same side as far as it will comfortably go – see the photo on the left.
- Now turn your face to look down towards your shoulder as in the photo on the right – you should feel a mild to moderate pain-free stretch along the side of your neck, further towards the back of the neck than for the front scalene stretch.
- Exhale, and allow the stretch to increase.
- Hold the stretch for a total of 30 seconds in 3 stages, using an exhalation to progressively increase the stretch after each 10 second hold. Continue to breathe using your diaphragm.
- Inhale, turn your face to look straight ahead again and then move your head and neck back to the upright position.
- Stretch the other side for 30 seconds using the same procedure.

Bend Head and Neck Down on Angle, Turn Head to Armpit

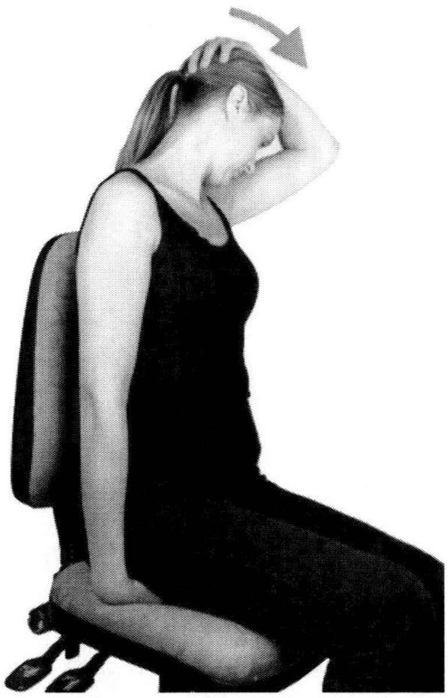

This movement stretches the levator scapulae muscles on one side of the back of the neck.
Both sides of your neck need to be stretched equally.

The photo shows the stretch being done while sitting on one hand to help stabilise the shoulder position, and with gentle over-pressure on the head to increase the stretch.

Begin initially with the simplest form of the exercise without over-pressure on the head (not shown). Even if you don't exert pressure, just placing your hand on your head can help. Exposing the armpit is a good reminder of the final direction to aim for with the stretch.

- Turn your head and neck about 45 degrees to one side and then bend forwards on this angle as far as you can comfortably go.
- Next turn your face so that you are looking towards your armpit as far as you can comfortably go. You should feel a mild to moderate pain-free stretch along the back of your neck and the top of your shoulder on the opposite side.
- Exhale, and allow the stretch to increase.
- Hold the stretch for a total of 30 seconds in 3 stages, using an exhalation to progressively increase the stretch after each 10 second hold. Continue to breathe using your diaphragm.
- Inhale, and reverse the previous set of movements to return to the starting position. (Start by turning your face back to neutral, then move your neck to the upright position and finally turn your head to look straight ahead.)
- Stretch the other side of your neck for 30 seconds using the same procedure.

- If the stretch feels too strong, move your arms back by your sides until your muscles get looser and pay extra attention to keeping your shoulders down.

Alternatives

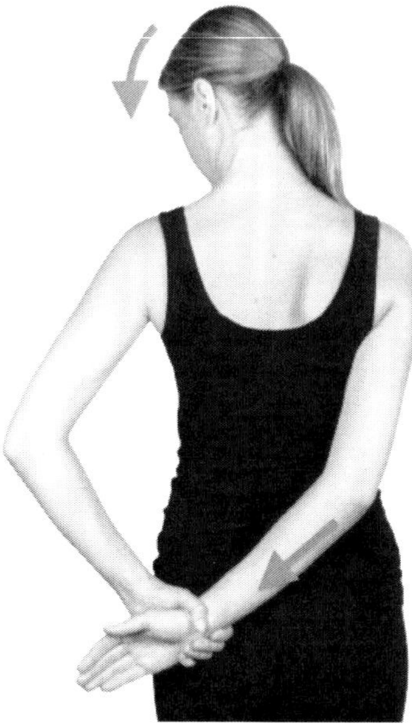

The photo above gives one of several alternative ways of preventing the shoulder from lifting while increasing the levator scapulae stretch. This variation involves pulling down on the arm on the side being stretched.

This looks very similar to the alternative upper trapezius stretch (iv). However, the head position, the direction of movement and the muscles being stretched are different.

Once you're familiar with how the levator scapulae stretch should feel, try various ways to increase the stretch. You can adapt the other upper trapezius stretches.

Stretches for the Upper Torso

Stretch between the Shoulder Blades

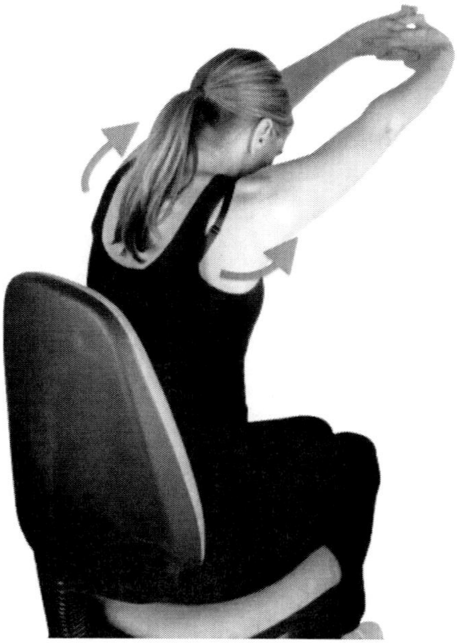

This exercise stretches the muscles of the mid-back, especially between the shoulder blades. These muscles tend to get very tight with lots of sitting, especially doing desk work, and with emotional stress.

- Sit or stand tall. Make sure you keep your shoulders down and back.
- Keep your neck long and your head slightly retracted.
- Start by looking straight ahead, keeping your chin level.
- Interlace your fingers, then turn your palms to face outwards.
- Straighten your arms out in front of you at shoulder height and push your hands away as shown in the photo. You should feel a mild to moderate pain-free stretch across your mid-back between the shoulder blades and in your arms, hands, fingers and wrists.
- Exhale, and push your hands a little further away to increase the stretch. You can allow your mid-back to round slightly
- Hold the stretch for a total of 30 seconds in 3 stages, using an exhalation to progressively increase the stretch after each 10 second hold. Continue to breathe using your diaphragm.
- Relax and drop your arms.

Do this stretch two times per day or more if you feel like it. This is one that feels great to do any time.

Standing Back Bend (Counteracts being Bent Forward)

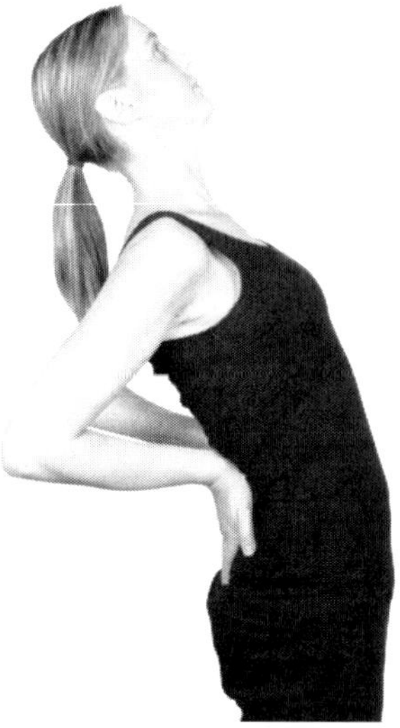

The standing back bend shown in the photo stretches out your upper abdomen, chest and the front of your neck, all which get very tight if you spend a lot of your time bending forward.

This may be the result of standing at surfaces which are too low or due to lengthy periods of sitting – with muscle fatigue, we all tend to gradually lean further forward.

Remember to do correct diaphragmatic breathing and you will feel an increased stretch in your abdominal muscles.

CAUTION: If you suffer from low-back pain check with your therapist or doctor before doing this stretch.

- Stand tall with your feet shoulder width apart and knees slightly bent.
- Slightly retract your head and keep your lips loosely closed, tongue on the roof of your mouth.
- Tighten your buttocks to protect your lower back.
- Place your palms on the back of your pelvis with fingers pointed downward.
- Take a deep breath in and as you exhale, lean back from the hip joints (not the waist), slowly dropping your head back at the same time.
- Squeeze your shoulder blades together.
- Gently push your hips forward and puff your belly out to increase the stretch.
- To increase the stretch at the front of your neck and under your chin, jut your lower jaw forward and put your lower lip over your top lip.
- Hold the stretch for 10 seconds while breathing normally.
- Breathe in, slowly return to an upright position and relax.
- Repeat the sequence twice for a total of 30 seconds stretching.

This stretch should be done two times per day.

Chest Stretch – Preferred Version with Bent Arm

Tight chest muscles play a major role in perpetuating forward head posture. Gradually loosening your chest muscles can help correct rounded shoulders and make a big improvement to your head and neck posture.

It is more effective, and safer for your shoulder, to stretch each side of your chest separately.

The chest is best stretched with the arm bent while standing next to a wall.

Stretching your chest muscles properly requires separate stretches with three different hand positions and elbow placement as shown in the photos. Each position stretches different parts of the chest muscles, where muscle fibres run in different directions.

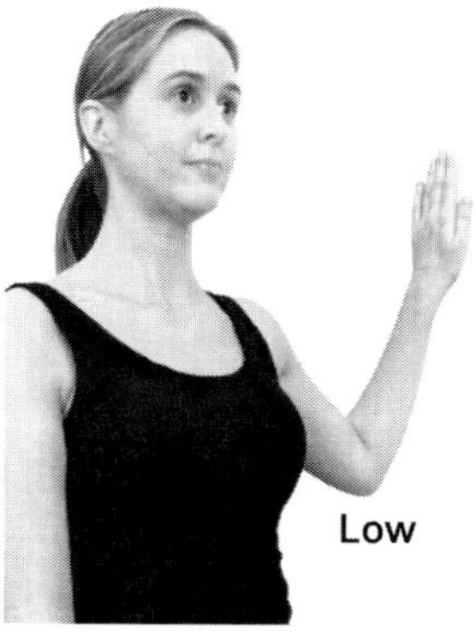

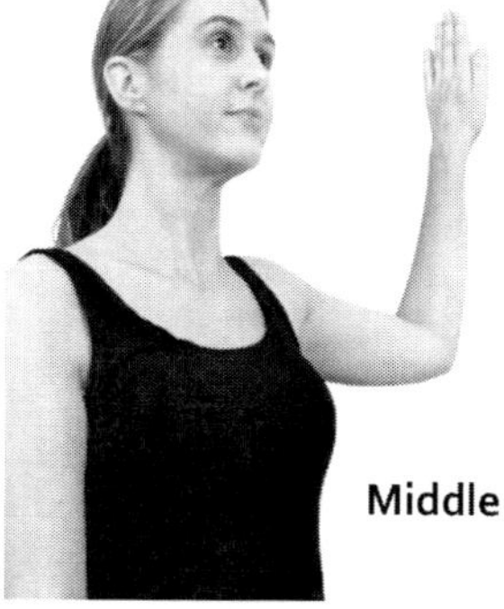

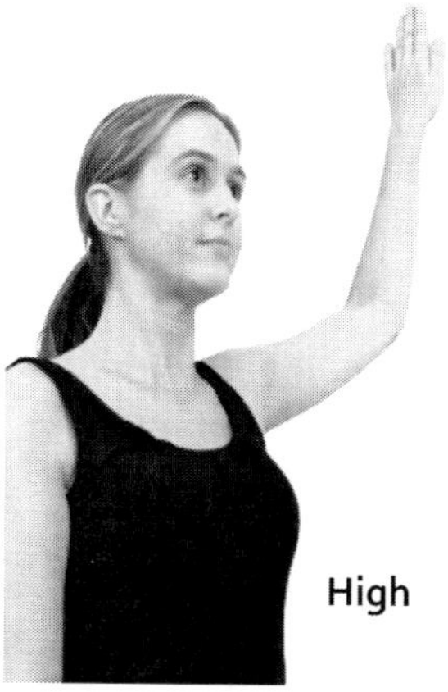

The middle hand position with your elbow bent is at 90 degrees stretches the middle section of the large pectoralis major muscle or 'pecs'.

The low hand and elbow position stretches its upper section and the high hand position with the arm only slightly bent stretches its low section.

However the main purpose of the high hand position is to stretch the pectoralis minor muscle which lies beneath pectoralis major.

The pectoralis minor muscle plays the largest role in causing your shoulders to round forward. In addition, when it is tight it can lead to compression of major nerves and blood vessels.

The next two photos show what the start and end of the bent arm chest stretch looks like when viewed from the back. In this case the hands are in the middle position.

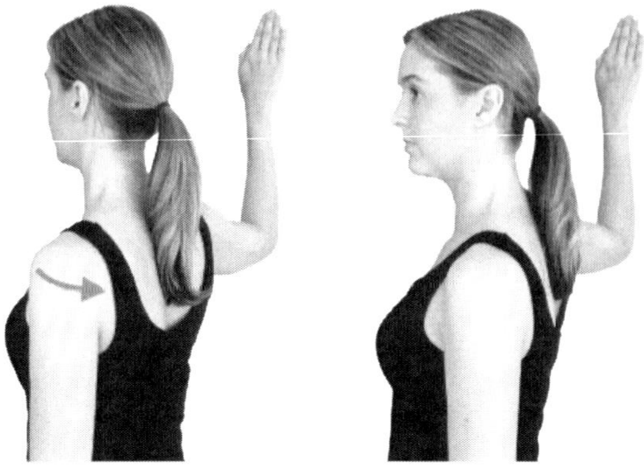

Do the chest stretch sequence for each hand position two times per day.

CAUTION: If you suffer from shoulder problems check with your therapist or doctor before doing these chest stretches.

- Stand tall facing towards a wall with your neck long and your head slightly retracted as usual.
- Make sure you keep your shoulders down and back and your chin level.
- Start by placing your hand, the inside surface of your forearm and your elbow flat against the wall.
- Raise your hand until your upper arm is horizontal and your elbow is bent at 90 degrees. Lightly press your elbow and forearm against the wall.
- Now move your feet around to turn your whole body away from the wall. Keep your hand, forearm and elbow fixed in position while you do this.
- Stop when you feel a gentle pain-free stretch across your mid-chest and upper arm.
- Inhale, and then as you exhale, cautiously turn your body a little further away from the wall to increase the stretch.
- Hold the stretch for a total of 30 seconds using an exhalation to progressively increase the stretch after each 10 second hold. Continue to breathe using your diaphragm.
- Repeat the whole procedure with the middle hand position to stretch the middle portion of your chest on the other side of your body.
- Repeat the whole procedure for both sides of the chest with your hand and elbow as high as possible and your arm almost straight. This is the upper hand position. You will feel the stretch in a different area than before, more towards the outside of your chest and armpit.
- Repeat the whole procedure once more for both sides of the chest, this time with your hands below head height and your elbows bent to about 45 degrees. This is

the lower hand position. Again, you will feel the stretch in a different place, especially across the upper chest from your collar bone.

Chest Stretch – Alternative Version with Straight Arm

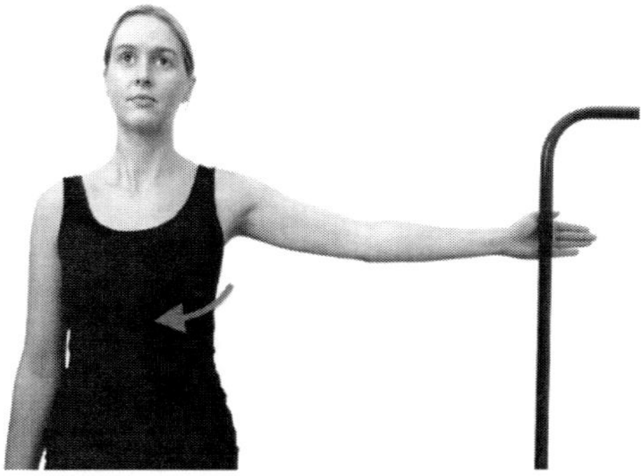

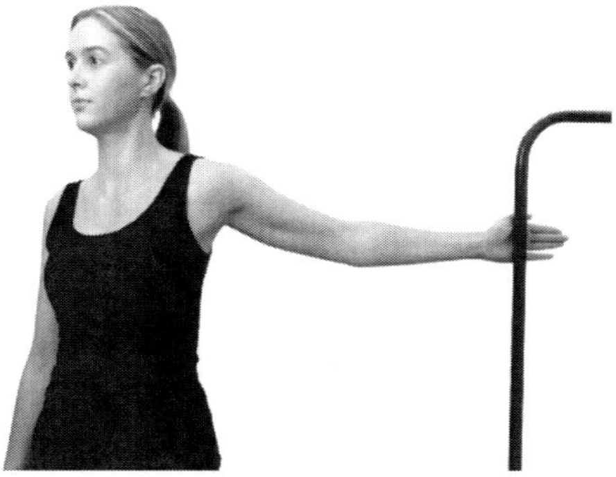

The bent arm version of the chest stretch is the most effective standing stretch for the chest muscles, but sometimes tightness around the shoulder can make it hard to feel the stretch where you should. If you think this is the case, try the straight arm version shown in photos for the middle hand position.

- Stand tall with your neck long and your head slightly retracted as usual. Make sure you keep your shoulders down and back and your chin level.
- Start by placing your hand flat on a post or doorframe with your arm horizontal. This is the middle hand position.
- Slowly move your feet around to turn your whole body away from your outstretched arm.
- Stop when you feel a gentle pain-free stretch across your mid-chest and upper arm.
- As you exhale, slowly turn your body a little further to increase the stretch.
- Hold the stretch for a total of 30 seconds using an exhalation to progressively increase the stretch after each 10 second hold. Continue to breathe using your diaphragm.
- Repeat the whole procedure for the middle hand position on the other side of your body.
- Repeat the whole procedure for both sides of the chest with your arm angled diagonally upwards – this is the upper hand position.
- Repeat the whole procedure for both sides of the chest with your arm angled diagonally downward – this is the lower hand position.

Extra 'Feel-Good' Chest Stretch, Hands behind Head

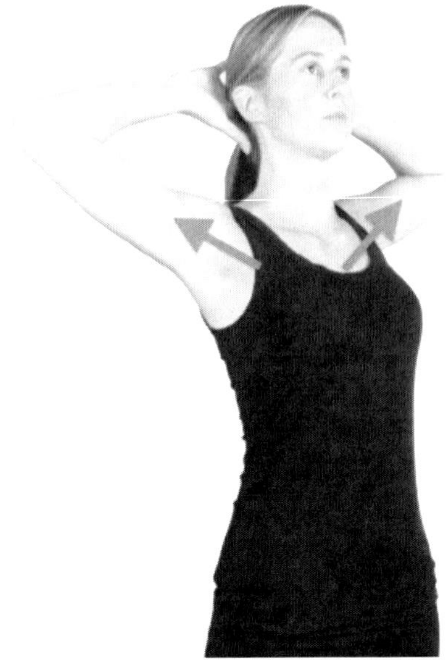

The photo shows an additional feel-good stretch you can do at your desk any time to help open your chest. It's a good accompaniment to the stretch for the tight area between the shoulder blades.

- Sit tall. Make sure you keep your shoulders down and back.
- Keep your neck long and your head slightly retracted.
- Start by looking straight ahead, keeping your chin level.
- Put both your hands behind your head, interlocking your fingers, and with your elbows pointing to the sides as shown.
- You should feel a mild pain-free stretch in the front of your shoulders and in your arm pits.
- Exhale, and cautiously push your elbows back a little to deepen the stretch. Hold the stretch for 10 seconds, continuing to breathe using your diaphragm.
- Relax and drop your arms.
- Repeat this stretch whenever you feel like it.

Isometric Neck Strengthening Exercises

The following three neck strengthening exercises are designed to improve the strength of the muscles in your neck and help you maintain good head and neck posture. In each case, you press your head against your hand, using your neck muscles to resist the pressure. No movement occurs – the exercises are isometric.

Do each exercise twice a day.

- Sit or stand tall.
- Make sure that you don't lift your shoulders – keep them back and down.
- Keep your neck long and your head slightly retracted.
- Start by looking straight ahead, keeping your chin and gaze level.

Pushing Backwards with the Head

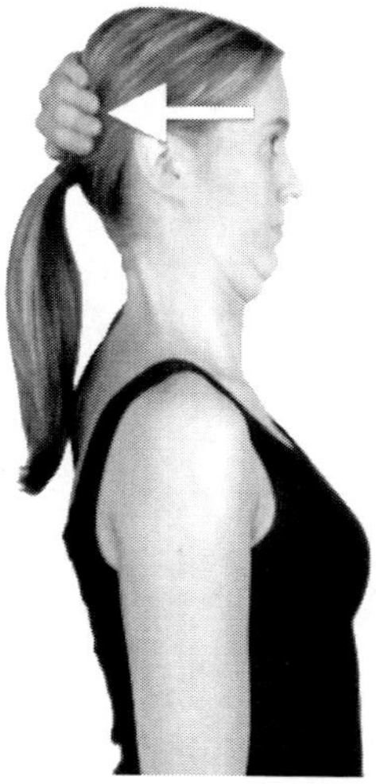

- Place your hand behind your head and slowly push your head back against your hand as shown using no more than about 20% of your maximum possible effort.
- Hold the muscle contraction for 10 seconds while continuing to breathe using your diaphragm.
- Relax.

Pushing Forwards with the Head

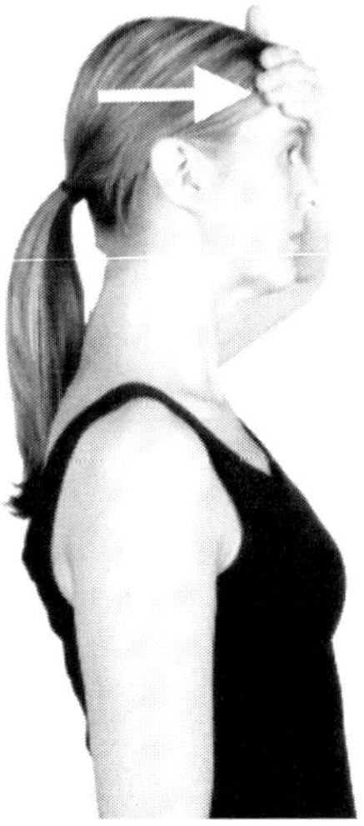

- Place your hand on your forehead and slowly push your head forwards against your hand as shown using no more than about 20% of your maximum possible effort.
- Hold the muscle contraction for 10 seconds while continuing to breathe using your diaphragm.
- Relax.

Pushing Sideways with the Head

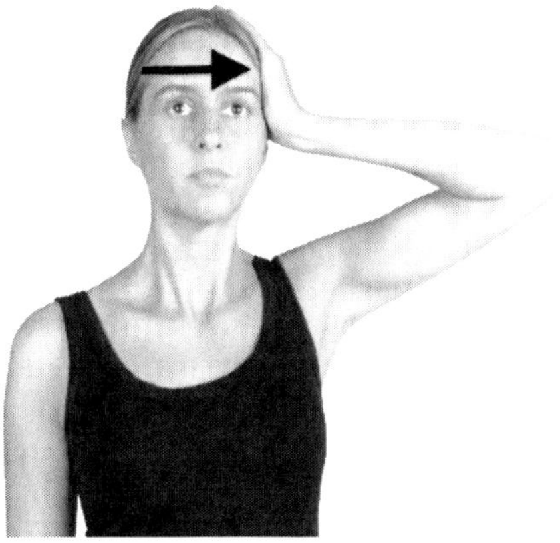

- Place your hand on the side of your head and slowly push your head sideways against your hand as shown, using no more than about 20% of your maximum possible effort.
- Hold the muscle contraction for 10 seconds while continuing to breathe using your diaphragm.
- Relax.

- Repeat the whole procedure for the other side of the head.

Overview of All Stretches

The table below lists all the exercises that have been described in this chapter, set out as a daily practice.

The exercise to correct forward head posture takes about 15 seconds in total. It should be done every 1–2 hours (minimum of 6 per day). Combining this exercise with two sets of each of the stretches and neck strengthening exercises takes less than 30 minutes in total. Of course, you can do them as a group, or start to incorporate them into your daily routine.

Separate sets of exercises are more effective if they're spread throughout the whole day.

All the stretches are held for a total of 30 seconds, except for the neck strengthening exercises, which are held for 10 seconds.

- The entry 10s x 3 indicates holding the stretch for 10 seconds, returning to the starting position and repeating the procedure another two times.
- (10s+10s+10s) indicates progressively increasing the stretch on an exhalation after each 10 second hold.

Table of All Stretches as a Daily Practice

Exercise	Frequency
Posture Correction Exercises	**6 Times per Day**
Wall test for overall spinal posture	10s
Forward head posture	15s
Neck and Shoulder Stretches	**2–3 Times per Day**
Neck rotation	10s x 3 each side
Chin to ceiling straight	10s x 3
Chin to ceiling diagonal	10s x 3 L and 10s x 3 R
Chin to chest	10s x 3
Ear to shoulder	(10s+10s+10s) L and (10s+10s+10s) R
Ear to shoulder plus face up	(10s+10s+10s) L and (10s+10s+10s) R
Ear to shoulder plus face down	(10s+10s+10s) L and (10s+10s+10s) R
Head to armpit	(10s+10s+10s) L and (10s+10s+10s) R
Upper Torso Stretches	**2 Times per Day**
Shoulder blade stretch	(10s+10s+10s)
Standing back bend	10s x 3
Chest stretch middle hand position	(10s+10s+10s) L and (10s+10s+10s) R
Chest stretch upper hand	(10s+10s+10s) L and (10s+10s+10s) R

position	
Chest stretch lower hand position	(10s+10s+10s) L and (10s+10s+10s) R
Neck Strengthening Exercises	**2 Times per Day**
Pushing head backwards	10s
Pushing head forwards	10s
Pushing head sideways	10s R and 10s L

Key Points

- Stretching can bring immediate relief when a headache strikes but its main aim is to reduce the incidence of musculoskeletal problems in your neck and shoulders.
- Maintaining a regular routine of thorough stretches should be an important part of your headache pain management strategy.
- Correct diaphragmatic breathing is especially important for stretching to be effective.
- These stretches are most effective if they are spread throughout the day.
- It's better to do an exercise once a day with proper technique, rather than rush through three sets of stretching.

Part F

Preventing Headaches:

Strategies

17

Strategies

In this chapter, you'll find a range of simple strategies to treat your headaches. The aim is to reduce one or more of the musculoskeletal, neurovascular and emotional contributions to your headache pain and thereby reduce the intensity of your pain. Most of these methods are suitable for both tension headache and migraine. I have also included several methods that are specific to the symptoms of migraine, such as compression of the scalp arteries.

I don't expect you will use all the methods in this chapter. You should select those that work best for you by trial and error. This particularly applies to heat and cold therapy – what works for one person doesn't work so well for another. Your choice of methods will also depend on what is convenient for you at the time – whether you are at work, out somewhere, or at home.

Two of the simplest and most effective – rehydration and slowing down your breathing – can be done anywhere.

Hydration

One of the simplest and most beneficial things you can do if you sense a headache attack approaching is to drink some water.

Dehydration is a common headache trigger and can lead to a headache even in people who rarely get them. It's quite easy to become mildly dehydrated during normal everyday activities and not be aware of it. Part of the problem is we don't sense thirst until we've have lost 1% to 2% of our body mass as water.[92]

If you already have a headache, there is a lot anecdotal evidence, and an increasing body of scientific evidence,[93] that suggests drinking water can ease headache pain, whereas continued dehydration can prolong it.

As a habit, you should drink water regularly during the day – how much water per person per day is a surprisingly controversial subject, but a good indicator of hydration is the colour of your urine. The volume should be much the same as usual and the colour should be a very pale yellow, almost but not completely colourless.

If you feel a headache coming on, drinking a glass of water containing an oral rehydration product is more effective than drinking water alone. The major components of oral rehydration products are glucose and electrolytes (sodium and potassium salts), so the solution is absorbed into the bloodstream more quickly and more completely than plain water. Oral rehydration products are available from pharmacies. They are specially formulated for treating loss of water and electrolytes due to diarrhoea, vomiting and excessive sweating. When dissolved, they create a solution with a similar electrolyte concentration to the intravenous saline drip used in hospitals. They may not be suitable for people with certain medical conditions, so check with your pharmacist before you take them.

The most convenient forms of oral rehydration to use and store are effervescent tablets. They're handy to take with you when travelling – you lose approximately 1.5 litres (50oz) of water during a three-hour plane flight. Oral rehydration products can also help counteract the effects of vomiting that often accompanies a migraine attack. Water and salts both need to be replaced and the glucose will boost blood sugar levels depleted by lack of food.

If you are feeling nauseous, sip the liquid slowly and if vomiting is prolonged or excessive you should seek medical help.

Walk

Sometimes a short, gentle walk may be all you need to head off an approaching headache attack. Contraction and relaxation of the calf muscles squeeze and release the deep veins in the lower legs, which pumps venous blood out of the muscles and back towards the heart.

If you spend a lot of time sitting or standing without movement, blood will pool in your lower legs and feet, reducing the blood supply to your brain. Sitting hunched forward with your arms in front of you can also restrict blood flow to and from the brain, and it will certainly make muscular trigger points in your neck and shoulder muscles more irritable. If you can't get out for a walk, getting out of your chair and moving about will help alleviate stress on these muscles and get your circulation going again.

Migraine sufferers are understandably cautious about exercise when they sense an attack is on its way, but you don't have to take a long or vigorous walk – it could be just up and down the corridor a few times. Even a trip to the water cooler might help (nothing like killing two birds with one stone!) If you already have a migraine, it's important to rest. Bending forward or fast head movements generally aggravate pain. On the other hand, tension headache sufferers may benefit from more vigorous exercise, even after a headache attack has already started. It will help to relax tense muscles, reduce stress and increase blood oxygen levels. If you can manage to find a pleasant place outdoors, so much the better.

Diaphragmatic Breathing

Another simple and effective thing you can do if you sense a headache is about to start is make a conscious effort to slow down your breathing.

If you are like most people, you probably haven't given much thought to the way you breathe.

Common examples of incorrect breathing include:

- Chest breathing (breathing high into your chest)
- Shallow breathing
- Irregular breathing
- Failing to breathe out fully
- Forgetting to breathe out at all for a while and holding your breath
- Breathing too rapidly or too deeply (hyperventilation)
- Breathing through your mouth rather than your nose.

Correct breathing is essential for optimal physical and emotional well-being. Incorrect breathing patterns can have some surprising effects. Habitual chest breathing could cause muscular trigger points to develop in the neck and shoulder muscles.

Fast, shallow breathing high in the chest is a common reaction to feeling stressed, which can happen when you have a headache. However, it causes levels of carbon dioxide gas in the blood to fall below normal values, which means blood vessels, including those taking blood to and within the brain, constrict and the brain's oxygen supply drops. Not surprisingly, this type of breathing pattern has been shown to worsen migraines.[94,95] Other effects include dizziness, visual disturbances, fainting, muscle cramps and a heightened sense of anxiety.

Slow diaphragmatic breathing can make a significant contribution to reducing the frequency and severity of your headache attacks. Consciously slowing down your breathing will help relax your muscles, reduce emotional stress and get more oxygen to your brain and replacing chest breathing by diaphragmatic breathing plays an important part in preventing muscular trigger points from recurring. The best way to slow down your breathing is to use your diaphragm.

Diaphragmatic breathing, also called abdominal or belly breathing, is the most efficient way to breathe, requiring the least physical effort and almost completely filling the lungs with air. A sleeping baby breathes with its diaphragm, its abdomen rising and falling with each breath.

Diaphragmatic breathing involves drawing air deeply into the lungs while keeping the belly relaxed and using the diaphragm to do most of the work, which causes the abdomen to expand rather than the chest.

The Mechanics of Diaphragmatic Breathing

The diaphragm is a thin dome-shaped layer of muscle and tendon, attached to the bottom of the rib cage, the breast bone and the lumbar spine. It acts as a partition between the organs of the chest and the abdomen.

When we inhale (breathe in), the diaphragm contracts and flattens as it descends in the chest cavity and presses down on the abdominal organs beneath (see figure 17.1). The belly (just under the ribs) protrudes slightly and the lower part of the rib cage moves outwards. Both actions also enlarge the chest cavity.

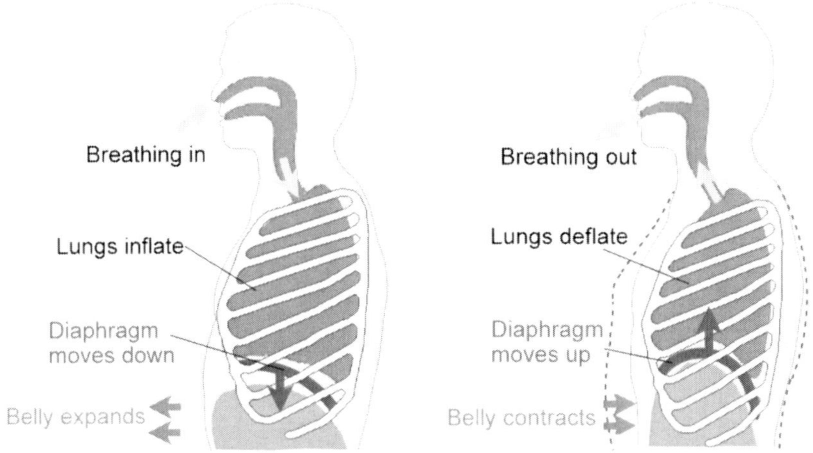

Figure 17.1 – Diaphragmatic breathing

The lungs expand into this increased space creating a suction effect, drawing in fresh, oxygen-rich air through the nose and mouth. The upper part of the rib cage hardly moves. During quiet breathing, the movement of the diaphragm provides about 75% of the force needed to inhale.

The remaining 25% is provided by small muscles between the ribs which move the rib cage like a bellows and neck muscles which help to lift the front of the rib cage. The diaphragm is a large muscle and its main function is breathing, so inhalation should feel relatively easy.

It is only if we need more air, for example if we are exercising vigorously, that we need to expend more energy to further enlarge our chest cavity. To do this, we use the neck muscles and more of the muscles between the ribs to increasingly expand and lift the upper part of the rib cage.

When we are breathing quietly, exhalation (breathing out), unlike inhalation, is mainly a passive process requiring little energy. It depends instead on the elasticity of the lungs. As the diaphragm relaxes, it returns to a dome shape causing it to rise upwards.

This releases the pressure on the abdominal organs and reduces the volume of the chest cavity. The belly falls and the lungs and chest wall, which were stretched during inhalation, deflate, like a balloon that is released. Stale air containing carbon dioxide is forced out through the nose and mouth.

When the abdominal muscles contract, they raise the pressure in the abdominal cavity, pushing the relaxed diaphragm against the lungs. This empties the lungs more completely, so that more air can be drawn in with the next breath.

Check Your Usual Breathing Pattern

If someone asks you to take a deep breath, do you suck in your stomach, puff out your chest and raise your shoulders? This is a very common response and unfortunately also an example of chest breathing and of what not to do. Not only does it take a lot of effort, it's not actually deep breathing – you are only getting air into the top portion of your lungs. Sucking the stomach in moves the abdominal organs up towards the chest cavity, blocking the downward movement of the diaphragm.

To check your usual breathing pattern, make sure you are rested and not out of breath from exercise or activity.

- Sit upright in your chair.
- Place one hand on your belly just above your belly button and the other hand on your breast bone in the middle of your chest.
- Relax and breathe the way you usually do for a couple of minutes.
- Then, without changing anything, look down and notice what happens as you breathe in. Which hand moves more?
- If the bottom hand moves more then you are breathing with your diaphragm. If it is the top hand, or there is not much difference, you are breathing with your chest.

If you can't tell, try repeating the test lying on your back on the floor. It can be easier to see what's happening in this position.

If you are doing diaphragmatic breathing correctly, whether sitting or lying down, your belly should move out when you inhale and move in when you exhale and there should be little movement of the upper part of the chest.

Relaxed Diaphragmatic Breathing

Diaphragmatic breathing is taught as part of a diverse range of disciplines and traditions including yoga, tai chi, singing, physical therapy, Pilates, Alexander technique, martial arts, meditation and respiratory medicine. Not surprisingly, there are variations in the way it is taught and in some of the details, plus more than a little controversy about what is the 'right' way, but here is a basic set of instructions to get you started:

- Sit upright in your chair or lie on the floor with your neck supported. Your clothes should not be too tight around your waist. (If you are lying down you may want to try having your knees bent or a pillow under your knees.)
- Place one hand on your belly just above your belly button and the other hand on your breast bone in the middle of your chest as before.
- Breathe as you usually do for a short time and allow your belly to relax.
- Now breathe all the air out of your lungs.
- Breathe in slowly through your nose in such a way that the hand on your belly rises but the hand on your chest hardly moves.
- Breathe out slowly through your nose and watch as your belly falls. Aim to make the exhalation take longer than the inhalation.
- Repeat these two steps, observing your belly rising and falling. Aim initially for several five-minute sessions during the day.

The more you practice, the more natural it will seem and the more benefit you will gain. Your aim is to make relaxed diaphragmatic breathing your usual breathing pattern when you are not moving about.

Although diaphragmatic breathing has many undeniable health benefits, our first objective is to reduce the overload on your neck and shoulder muscles caused by habitual chest breathing, so it's important to be able to do relaxed diaphragmatic breathing during normal activities, such as working at your desk, and use it as much as possible during your day.

You may prefer to learn the technique sitting in a chair. Alternatively, you may find it easier to feel what is happening if you start off lying down and then move to a chair when you become more proficient. The belly movement should not be forced or exaggerated – try to keep a mental picture of your diaphragm moving down as you inhale and up as you exhale.

To verify that it is not just your belly that is moving, put one hand on each side of your waist and press tightly. Now breathe in. Feel your fingers on the front of your waist and your thumbs at the back both move outwards as the entire lower part of your rib cage expands up and out. Then breathe out and feel how your lower rib cage contracts.

Slow diaphragmatic breathing is also an extremely effective way of reducing emotional stress. When we are feeling stressed we tend to take rapid, shallow breaths or inhale and hold our breath. Slow diaphragmatic breathing will help you achieve a sensation of relaxation and release excess muscle tension. It's particularly important to prolong the exhalation phase. Ideally it should be at least double the length of the inhalation. Only then does the brain signal the body that it can switch from a state of 'fight or flight' to 'rest and digest'.

If you are having trouble slowing down the exhalation sufficiently, instead of breathing out through your nose try breathing out through pursed lips, it helps to regulate the release of air.

Diaphragmatic breathing is done somewhat differently when part of a progressive relaxation session at home or in a quiet place. You breathe in slowly through your nose, hold the breath for a short time and then breathe out through your mouth even more slowly.

What If My Belly Doesn't Move?

To do diaphragmatic breathing, your belly must be relaxed.

If you find after several attempts you are still not able to allow your belly to expand when you inhale, check that you are not inadvertently holding your muscles tight due to nervous tension. Other possible reasons include adhesions and scar tissue in the abdominal wall or tight, overworked abdominal muscles.

Your abdominal muscles are very likely to be tight and short if you always keep your stomach sucked in to look slimmer, you do lots of crunches and other 'ab work' or you excessively 'brace your abs' in Pilates classes.

Unfortunately, habitual chest breathing will also cause your abdominals to tighten up in a self-reinforcing cycle. Just like tight, overused muscles anywhere in the body, the abdominal muscles can develop muscular trigger points and thickened adhered fascia which prevent them from stretching. Fortunately, these problems can be treated very effectively by remedial massage.

Tight abdominal muscles lead to the same problems as from corsets from centuries gone by. Not only do they restrict your breathing, they cause your back muscles to be overworked, contributing to lower back pain, and they compress your abdominal organs.

Breathing Through Your Nose

It is considered normal to breathe through the nose when resting and during light exercise, but simultaneously through the nose and mouth during vigorous exercise when more oxygen is required.

For our usual everyday activities, nose breathing has several health benefits compared with breathing through the mouth. When we breathe in through the nose, the air is filtered, warmed and humidified before it enters the lungs. Filtration helps remove allergens, dust and disease causing organisms.

Breathing out through the nose slows the whole exhalation process down so that more oxygen can be extracted. It also promotes relaxation. Finally, breathing through the mouth can cause muscular trigger points in one of the muscles that opens the jaw. However, if you suffer nasal and sinus congestion due to allergies or frequent upper respiratory tract infections you may find it very difficult to breathe through your nose. There are two simple but effective ways of relieving this congestion that don't involve taking medication.

The first method involves using some type of nasal and sinus rinse product available from your local pharmacy. Most consist of individual sachets which contain a pre-measured amount of solid salt and sodium bicarbonate.

You mix the contents of a sachet with a specified amount of warm water. Then you either pour the warm liquid into the nasal passages using something called a neti pot, which looks like a small teapot, or squirt it through using a plastic squeeze bottle.

Another alternative is to breathe steam into the nasal passages. You can put your head over a bowl of hot water and cover yourself with a towel to stop the steam escaping. You may like to try adding a drop or two of eucalyptus oil to the water. This helps clear congestion and kill viruses and bacteria.

If you don't want your whole face to get overheated you can purchase an inhaler consisting of bottle with a funnel that fits over your nose and mouth. These are available from many pharmacies.

You may find that by relieving sinus congestion you reduce the frequency of your headaches. Although true sinus headaches are much less common than is generally believed, sinus conditions and allergies can act as headache triggers for many people.

Deepening Your Breathing for an Energy Boost

Once you have started to get familiar with relaxed diaphragmatic breathing, you may want to try extending the technique to breathe more deeply.

This will fill and empty your lungs more completely so you will get more oxygen to your brain and muscles. As with relaxed diaphragmatic breathing, it is important to breathe in and out slowly through the nose, and to prolong the exhalation.

For deeper diaphragmatic breathing, go through the same first four steps as in relaxed diaphragmatic breathing. Then:

- Breathe in slowly and deeply through your nose taking in more air than before. Your belly will rise further and the hand on your chest will move up somewhat as the upper part of your rib cage starts to expand
- Breathe out slowly through your nose
- At the end of the exhalation gently contract your abdominal muscles and pull your belly button in towards the spine. This forces some more air out of the lungs. Then relax your abdominal muscles ready to inhale again.

If you have been cooped up in a stuffy room, taking a short walk and spending a few minutes doing some deeper diaphragmatic breathing can be a great energy booster. It is even better if you can get some fresh air outside.

Deeper diaphragmatic breathing is appropriate when more oxygen is needed while exercising. It is also the foundation for exercises designed to improve your core stability and overall spinal posture. However, it's not appropriate for normal everyday activities – relaxed diaphragmatic breathing is the breathing pattern to aim for here.

Hot and Cold Therapy

Broadly speaking, heat, particularly moist heat, is best for relaxing muscles and reducing muscle pain. Heat also assists mental relaxation and improves blood flow. Cold is best for reducing pain from inflammation of blood vessels, nerves and surrounding tissues.

Heat Therapy

From what we know about the mechanism of headaches, heat is best applied to the muscles of the back of the neck and the top of the shoulders. Muscular trigger points in these muscles are a significant source of headache pain.

Warmth will reduce muscle tension, improve blood flow and make muscular trigger points less irritable. It will also stimulate feelings of comfort and mental relaxation. Heat therapy used early enough may prevent a headache from developing. If the headache is already underway, heat therapy will help to relieve the pain. During a migraine attack, just reducing the level of pain may be sufficient to prevent distressing symptoms like vomiting.

A hot water bottle will stay warm for at about 30 minutes. A cover will make it more comfortable and stop you burning your skin, however, it is not practical if you want to sit in a chair or move about.

Commercial heat packs come in many different shapes and sizes, but there are only three main types:

- Electrically heated packs. These are like a small electric blanket – some are shaped to fit the neck.
- Instant heat packs where the heat is generated by a chemical reaction. Most are single use and include self-adhesive products which can be worn under clothing. Reusable instant heat packs are available but need to be regenerated by boiling for a few minutes and allowing to cool.
- Reusable heat packs which you heat up, usually in the microwave although some may be heated by immersion in hot water. Packs are filled with a variety of materials including wheat, liquid gel and patented beads. Look for one that drapes across your neck and shoulders and has some type of fastener to keep it in place.

Whatever type of heat pack you use it's important to follow the manufacturer's instructions. Check the temperature – you may need a layer of clothing between your skin and the pack.

Some heat packs will produce moist heat, which is more effective than dry heat in desensitising muscular trigger points and reducing muscle pain. Alternatively, try standing under a hot shower with the water massaging the back of your neck. Better still, take a hot bath and let yourself relax. Try propping a hot water bottle against the back of the bath so you can rest the back of your neck on it. Alternatively use a hot damp towel or wash-cloth (run it under the hot tap and then wring it out).

Adding Epsom salts can make your bath more effective. This is an old home remedy for easing muscle pain which is still widely used today. It is not just an old wives' tale – there are good reasons for thinking it will help your muscles and your headaches.

Epsom salts act as a source of magnesium ions. These play an essential role in body chemistry, including the maintenance of normal functioning of nerves and muscles.

Many headache sufferers have lower than normal levels of magnesium ions in their blood and brain[96,97,98,99] and intravenous magnesium will often quickly relieve a headache attack.[100]

Magnesium ions can also enter the bloodstream by absorption across the skin[101] A small study showed that soaking in an Epsom salt bath for 12 minutes two times a week should be sufficient to restore normal levels.[102] The effects on headaches have not been studied but it seems well worth trying.

You will need about 2 cups of Epsom salts in a standard sized bath tub.

If you suffer from migraines, you may have noticed that your hands and feet tend to get colder before and during an attack. For many people this is a reliable early warning sign. A warm bath taken at this stage will help prevent the attack from progressing further by drawing blood away from your head towards your extremities.

Cold Therapy

Cold therapy is generally used to treat pain once a headache has started. Cold tends to aggravate muscular trigger points, so you need to be careful about applying it to the back of your neck.

It's more useful for constricting dilated arteries beneath the scalp and reducing inflammation. The pulsation of these arteries with each heartbeat causes the throbbing pain that accompanies a migraine attack.

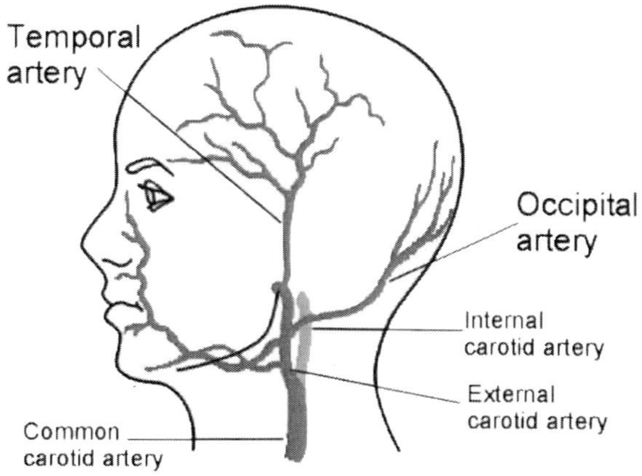

Figure 17.2 – The main arteries of the scalp

Figure 17.2 shows the most important scalp arteries. They are the temporal arteries, which lie under the skin of the temple at the side of the head, in front of each ear, and the occipital arteries beneath the skin at the back of the head. These start just above the base of the skull not far from the mid-line.

Applying cold to the side of the head may also help to reduce pain from inflamed dura on the surface of the brain. The skull bone in this region is very thin and one of the arteries that supply the dura lies close beneath it. Cooling the blood which flows through the dura will reduce the sensitivity of the surrounding tissue.

There are different ways to apply cold to your head. If you have nothing better available, a cold wet cloth wrapped around your head will help. An ice pack or even a packet of frozen vegetables will be more effective, but make sure to wrap them in a cloth to protect your skin.

A cold gel pack is easier to use and mould to shape and will lead to more rapid cooling. Whatever you use, don't leave any sort of cold pack on your head for longer than 20–30 minutes at a time.

Concentrate on cooling the side of your head. Adding pressure will make cold therapy more effective. Press the cold pack against your temporal artery. It is just in front of your ear. This will provide some additional pain relief.

If you have a second cold pack you may also be able to arrange to rest the back of your head on it (not your neck) so you can cool the area around the occipital artery at the same time.

Reusable gel cold packs should be kept in the freezer until needed. Instant cold packs don't need refrigeration but they can only be used once. I would avoid patches marketed for migraine treatment which you stick on your forehead. These produce cooling by evaporation of a gel and won't get as cold. In any case, cold therapy should be applied to the side of the head, not the front. This will cool the area lying above the temporal artery and at least part of the area above the occipital artery.

Cold therapy has been shown to reduce the severity of pain during a migraine attack.[103,104] Some therapies are quite drastic, but there is one relatively pleasant way of rapid cooling to relieve migraine pain which works for some people. It may possibly even end an attack.

It involves holding something cold in the back your mouth against your palate. What you use doesn't matter much, as long as it's cold – ice cubes, ice water and ice cream all get a mention. Some have even dubbed it the ice cream cure – hold several spoonfuls of ice-cream against the roof of your mouth with your tongue while they melt.

A small placebo controlled trial on 35 migraine patients provides scientific confirmation of patient reports.[105] Small steel tubes chilled with recirculating ice-cold water were used to chill the palate. Interestingly, the trial found that 40 minutes of chilling was better in reducing pain and nausea than sumatriptan (a triptan and the most commonly used migraine abortive medication) at all times tested. At 24 hours there was some recurrence of pain and nausea with the medication, but not with chilling.

Transfer of cold through the roof of the mouth will reduce inflammation and swelling of nearby blood vessels, nerves and dura. One of the nerves affected is a branch of the trigeminal nerve system which plays an important role in migraine.

Nothing seems to have been published on the effect of cold therapy on tension headache. The neurovascular contribution to pain is less important for tension headaches, so I wouldn't expect cold therapy to be as useful as heat applied to neck and shoulder muscles. However, one small study, which used a specially constructed device, found that cold encircling the head combined with heat on the very top of the head reduced pain in 6 out of 7 tension headache sufferers.[106]

If you already have a tension headache and heat doesn't help, you may like to try cold as well as, or instead of, heat. A wet cloth across the forehead may be useful.

Combined Cold and Heat Therapy

A combination of cold and hot treatments may be useful for treating a migraine attack. In theory, we would expect that putting a heat pack on your neck and shoulder muscles together with a cold pack on your head would be an effective way to relieve migraine pain. It will simultaneously treat head pain referred from irritable muscular trigger points and local pain from inflamed scalp arteries. It is relatively convenient to carry out and I think it's well worth trying.

If you can, it may be more effective to lie in a warm bath with a cold pack on your head. Warming the whole body promotes deeper relaxation. It also causes blood vessels in cold hands, feet and ankles to dilate, drawing blood away from the head. Both will provide some additional pain relief.

Some migraine sufferers exploit this last effect by sitting with their feet soaking in hot water while applying cold to the head. It may also help to put a heat pack on neck and shoulder muscles.

Compression

Compression of the scalp arteries has been demonstrated to alleviate pain during a migraine attack in research going back to 1905.[107] For example, for one group of 94 migraine sufferers, over half experienced a large reduction in pain after applying 3–6 minutes of finger pressure to the scalp arteries.[108]

Pressing firmly enough on the temporal arteries to stop blood flow lessens pain in the front half of the head; pressing on the occipital arteries lessens pain in the back half. Pressure should be maintained for several minutes or pain will return when it is released.

Usually the temporal and occipital arteries on both sides of the head need to be treated. Even though migraine pain is most often one-sided, the arteries on the left and right sides of the head are interconnected by many smaller blood vessels.

It's a good idea to practice finding these arteries and working out where you need to press when you don't have a migraine.

For the temporal arteries use the flats of your first and second fingers to explore the area of your cheek. You should feel a pulse just in front of your ear, above the bone. The occipital arteries are harder to find, although during a migraine attack you will feel them pulsating strongly near the base of your skull, not far from the mid-line.

If a migraine attack starts, press very firmly on the pulse of the temporal artery you feel on both sides of your head. Maintain the pressure for 30 seconds and then release it but don't shift your fingers.

If the pain first eases but then quickly returns it is worth continuing compression for a longer time, say 3 minutes. This is quite hard on the fingers – try swapping between your first and second fingers.

If pain is little improved you may like to test positioning your hands so you can apply pressure to your temporal and occipital arteries at the same time. This is not easy, but it is possible – use your fingers and thumbs.

Temporal Artery Massage

An alternative to compression is temporal artery massage. A study of 15 patients suffering from migraine with aura found that vigorous massage of both temporal arteries successfully blocked 34 of 42 attacks (81%), provided massage was started at the first sign of the aura and continued until it ended.[109]

Key Points

- Hydration is one of the key elements in headache management.
- You should drink water regularly throughout the day, not all at once.
- Diaphragmatic breathing is essential for optimal physical and emotional well-being and is important for headache management and needs to be practiced.
- Heat therapy will reduce muscle tension, improve blood flow, make muscular trigger points less irritable and reduce pain.
- Cold therapy is generally used to treat pain once a headache has started and tends to aggravate muscular trigger points.
- Walking and compression can also help manage headache pain.

18

Good Posture

Manual therapy and stretching can help release the existing tension from your muscles and get you started towards better posture, but it's our everyday actions that play the most significant role in maintaining good posture.

The Main Culprit – Forward Head Posture

If you have been sitting for a few hours in front of your computer without getting up to move around, it's very likely that you will have a muscle overuse injury. Although it may seem like you haven't been using your muscles at all, the muscles in your neck and shoulders have been working hard just to hold your head up against gravity.

This is because your head is not perfectly balanced on top of your spine. It has slightly more weight towards the front of the body, which is why your head falls forward when you fall asleep sitting up – your muscles relax, and your heavy, unbalanced head falls forward towards your chest.

The head is a lot heavier than you might expect. It weighs around 5 kg (10 pounds), about the same as a bowling ball. Imagine holding a bowling ball still with your elbows bent. Now think about lowering the weight a little and continuing to hold it up. The effort involved in counteracting the force of gravity is much greater than before.

In the same way, the stress on your neck and shoulder muscles is far greater if you crane your head forward to look at a screen, as shown in the photo below. For every 3 cm (1 inch) that your head moves forward from a neutral balanced position, it increases the effective weight your neck muscles must support by an extra 5 kg (10 pounds).

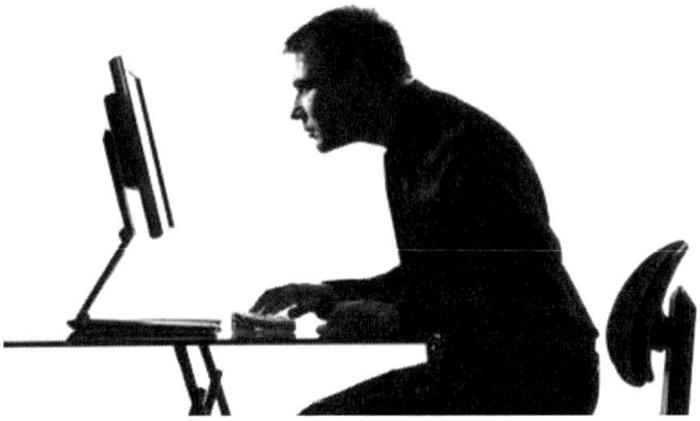

Not only are you holding up a heavy weight, but when you are in forward head posture, which often tends to go with rounded shoulders, you are using muscles that weren't designed to hold up your head and therefore, get tired easily.

Forward head posture is a potent cause of muscular trigger points in many muscles of the neck, jaw and upper shoulders, including the trapezius, sub-occipital and sternocleidomastoid muscles. Projecting your head forwards also compresses the joints and intervertebral discs of your neck, causing pain and accelerating the normal processes of wear and tear, and it alters the alignment of your jaw joint. These stresses are compounded by the need to tilt the chin upwards to be able to see.

The Whole Body

Improving your head and neck posture is likely to be one of the most effective things you can do to reduce the frequency and severity of your headache attacks. It's important to consider the head and neck as part of the whole body. Tight joints in the lower or mid-back and tight, shortened postural muscles will cause compensatory changes in the muscles and joints of the neck. Similarly, forward head posture will change the alignment of the other regions of the spine. It is very hard to determine which problem came first.

Correcting forward head posture is therefore unlikely to be successful in the longer term unless it is done in conjunction with improving overall spinal posture. Improving overall spinal posture will also reduce any indirect musculoskeletal contribution to headaches from irritation of nerves and blood vessels and stretching of the dura of the brain and spinal cord.

The first step in improving your overall spinal posture is to be aware of your posture during different activities and at different times of the day and knowing what good spinal posture looks like.

What is Good Spinal Posture?

When viewed from the side, the healthy spine consists of three gentle curves, linked together in an overall S-shape. The spine curves inward at the neck (cervical spine), outward at the mid back (thoracic spine) and inward again at the lower back (lumbar spine). This combination is referred to as a neutral spine. Good posture means maintaining a neutral spine while you're standing, sitting and sleeping and moving from one position to another.

When the spine is in a neutral position, the heaviest areas of the body, the head, rib cage and pelvis, are stacked directly above one another. Your ear, the bony bump on the outside of your shoulder and your hip joint should all line up (see Figure 18.1).

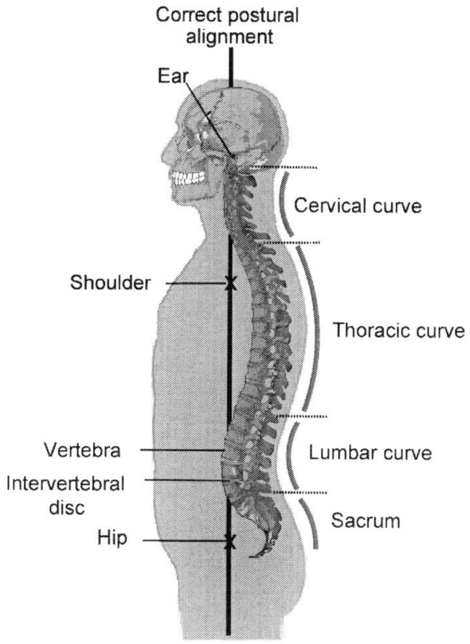

Figure 18.1 – Good posture: side view – the neutral spine

Weight should be evenly distributed between the back and front of the body. This leads to maximum stability. It minimises the amount of work the muscles and spinal ligaments have to do to keep the spine upright against the force of gravity and it reduces stress on facet joints and intervertebral discs.

Having good posture means maintaining the three natural curves of your spine while you are standing, sitting, sleeping and when moving from one position to another.

Good standing posture requires weight to be equally distributed between the left and right sides of your body. When viewing the spine from the rear, it should appear vertical, and ears, shoulders, pelvis and knees should be level as shown in Figure 18.2

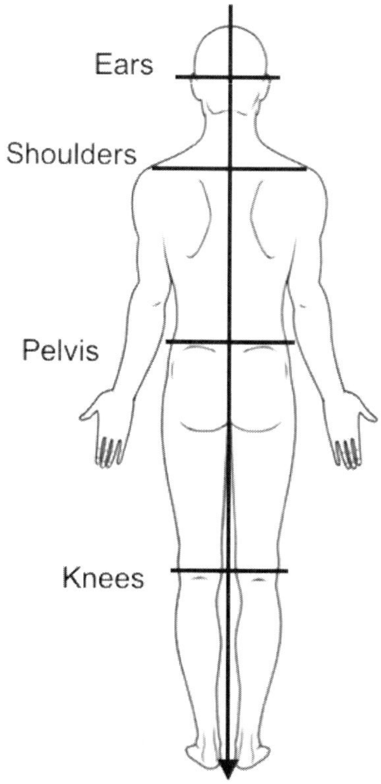

Figure 18.2 – Good posture: rear view

Common Problems

Standing

If you study the people around you, you will see many different ways of standing.

The young man in the photo below shows what good standing posture with a neutral spine should look like. Notice his ears are positioned directly above his shoulders.

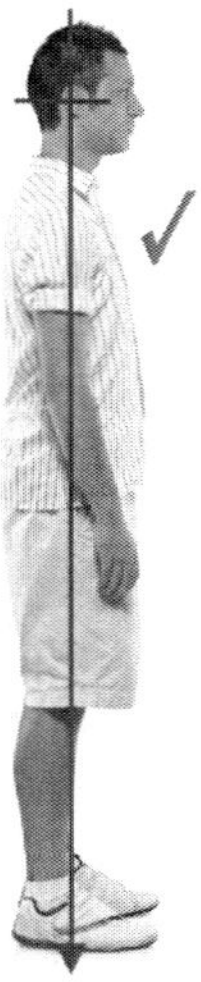

If we use his posture as a standard for comparison, we see that only two people in the group below have reasonable posture. These are indicated by tick-marks. The remainder with 'X's have one or more postural faults.

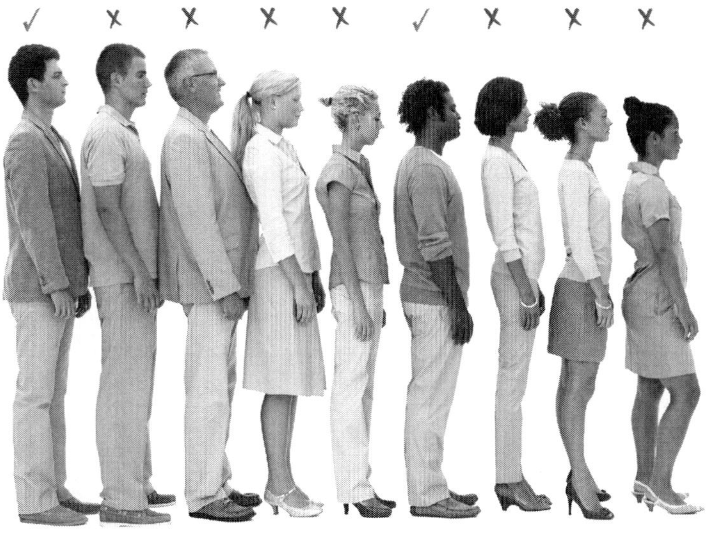

Figure 18.3 below gives a closer look at two of the most common faults.

The slouched posture of the woman in Figure 18.3(b) is very common. Her ears are positioned well forward of her shoulders – she has pronounced forward head posture. In the photo she is looking down. However whenever she needs to look straight ahead she will be have to tilt her chin upwards, kinking the back of her neck in the process. She is also holding her shoulders hunched forward, causing an excessive rounding of her mid-back.

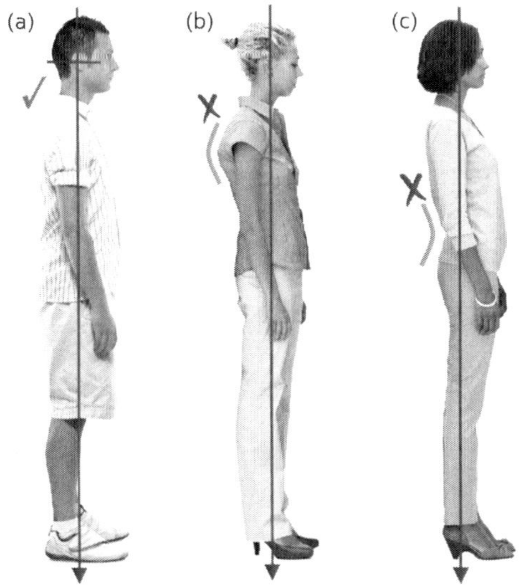

Figure 18.3 – Good and bad standing posture

The posture of the woman in Figure 18.3(c) shows a different but equally common fault. Her lower back has an excessive inward curve (in other words a large hollow) which is often referred to as a 'sway back'.

It forces her to lean backwards with her entire upper body to compensate. An excessive lumbar curve can often be an adaption to carrying extra weight around the mid-section. This may due to pregnancy or a carrying extra weight around the waist.

Standing in high-heeled shoes is another major contributing factor. It is equivalent to standing on a slant rather than on level ground and the body has to make significant postural adjustments to cope, otherwise people in high heels would topple forwards. The higher the heels, the greater their effect.

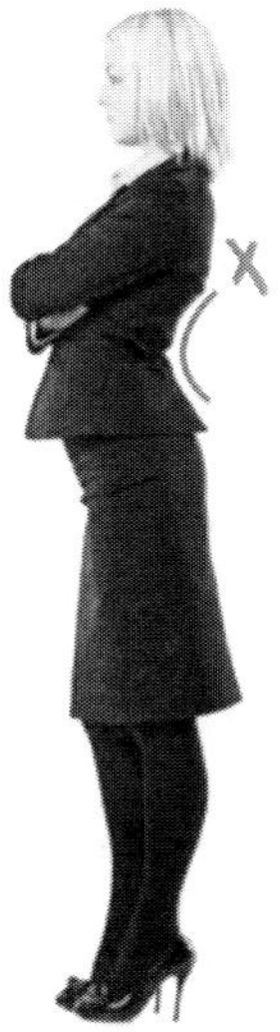

The young woman in black has a very exaggerated curve in her lumbar spine for which her high-heeled shoes are at least partly responsible. She also has hunched shoulders and an excessively rounded mid-back. These three postural faults, and forward head posture, tend to occur together.

Sitting

As we move from standing to a seated position, the pelvis rotates backwards, reducing the lumbar curve, which means an excessive lumbar curve is seldom a problem during sitting. However other postural faults tend to be magnified, due to a combination of bad habits, bad ergonomics, insufficient movement and muscle fatigue.

The longer we sit without moving, the more tired our muscles get and the harder it becomes to maintain the three natural curves of the spine.

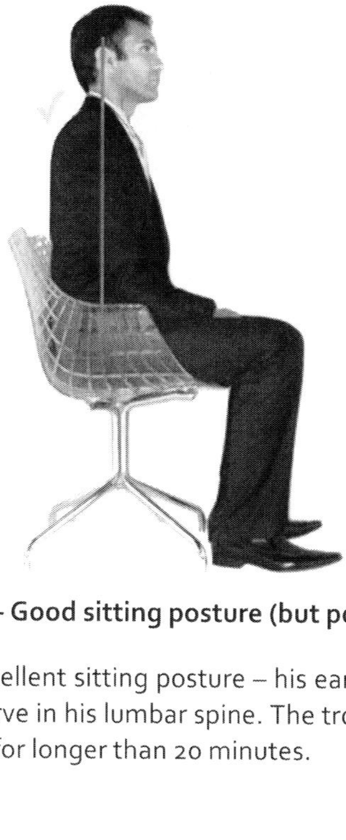

Figure 18.4 – Good sitting posture (but poor chair)

The man in Figure 18.4 has excellent sitting posture – his ear, shoulder and hip are all in line. He has a gentle inward curve in his lumbar spine. The trouble is, he won't be able to maintain this posture if he sits for longer than 20 minutes.

The chair he is using provides insufficient back support making it even harder to sit correctly, but even with a good chair, most people tend to slouch after sitting for a while, even those who are generally conscious of their posture.

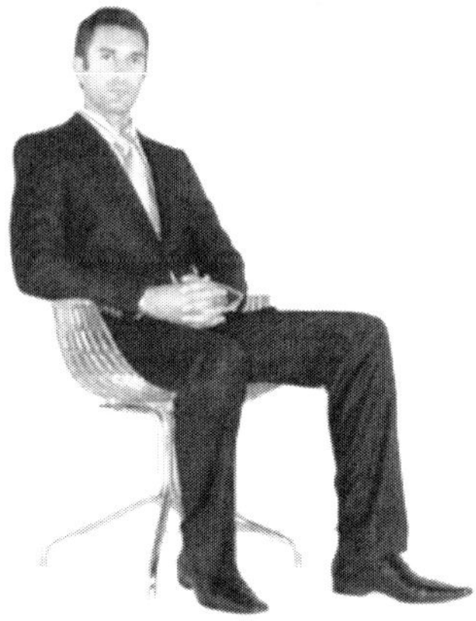

Without noticing, they slide down and forwards in the chair, rounding their entire back in the process. Rounding the back reduces the usual inward curve of the lumbar spine, giving what is known as a 'flat back' posture and it's not possible to sit with a flat back and keep the head and neck upright. Gradually, the head and neck start to protrude forwards.

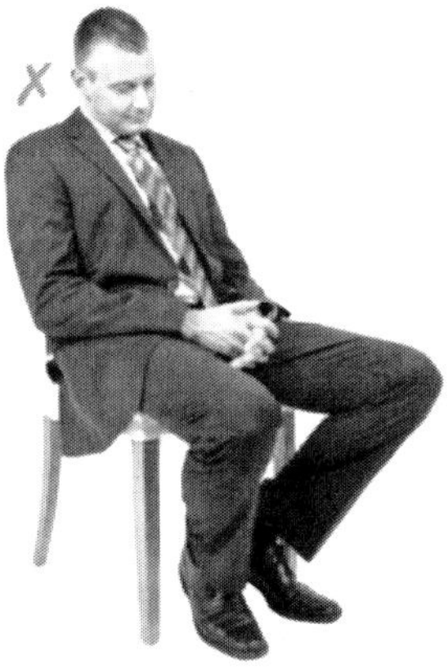

After sitting for too long, some people will often lean forward and prop their elbows on their thighs or on a desk for extra support.

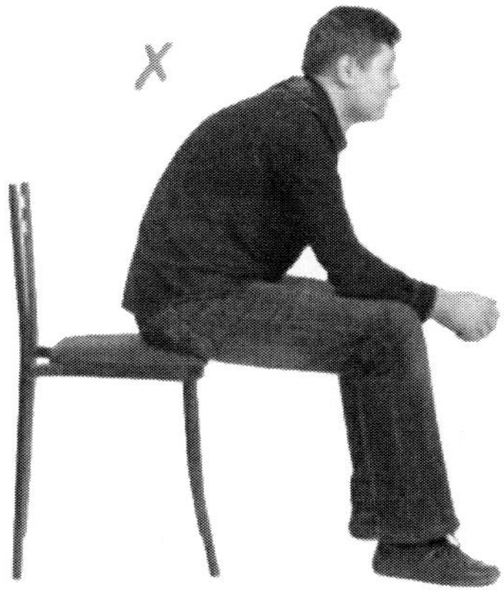

Notice how the man sitting on the edge of his chair is poking his head and neck forward and the way he is kinking the back of his neck. His mid-back is excessively rounded, his shoulders are hunched forward and his lower back curves outwards – the normal inward lumbar curve has reversed giving his back a C-shape rather than an S-shape.

This is a further progression of the flat back mentioned above, and it causes excessive wear and tear on lumbar joints and discs. It also restricts breathing and compresses the abdominal organs. This is the posture some people adopt in front of their computer for many hours each day.

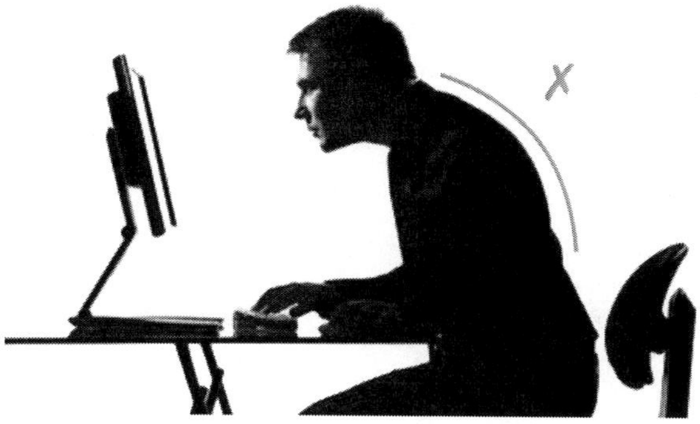

The key to sitting with correct head and neck posture is to maintain the inward curve of lumbar spine. Your chair needs to prevent you sliding down and forwards. It should also provide adequate lumbar support. However no chair, no matter how well designed, will stop you slumping if you don't use it properly, and if you sit without moving for too long.

Checking Your Own Spinal Alignment

You can check your spinal alignment quickly by standing in front of a mirror and looking at yourself side-on. If your spine is in the neutral position, your ear, shoulder, hip bone, knee and ankle should all be in line. Similarly, when sitting with a neutral spine, your ear, shoulder and hip bone should line up.

A photograph will give you a more accurate analysis. You don't have turn your head and you can rule a vertical line through your ear to help you make the assessment. Either ask a friend or use the camera self-timer to take your photo while you stand and then sit next to a blank wall.

Loose clothes make it harder to spot postural faults. It's best to wear something tight fitting such as gym gear or strip down to your underwear. Make sure you adopt your usual standing posture by walking up and down on the spot to relax before the photo is taken. For the sitting test, sit on the chair you use most often.

The other postural test you should do for your standing posture is the 'Wall Test'.

The Wall Test

This test can be used to assess your standing posture and improve it at the same time. It's a good idea to repeat the wall test several times a day.

- Stand with your head, shoulder blades and buttocks touching a wall.
- Your feet should be shoulder-width apart and your heels about 5 cm (2 inches) away from the wall.
- If you can, put the back of your head comfortably against the wall.
- Keep your eyes and chin parallel to the floor. Don't tilt your chin up or retract your head so much that you get a double chin. (If you can't do this part of the test it means your shoulders are rounded forward. There are specific exercises you can do to redress this problem.)
- Reach back and slide the back of your hand behind the curve in your lower back.
- If your posture is ideal, you will just be able to fit the knuckles of your hand between your back and the wall, as shown in the photo.
- If there is too much space, you have a sway back (this is common). Draw in your lower abdominal muscles to flatten the curve in your back.
- If there is too little space (this is uncommon), you have a flat back. Your lower back has too little curve. Arch your back more so that your hand just fits comfortably behind you.
- Once you are in alignment, walk away from the wall while maintaining your new, more optimal back posture.

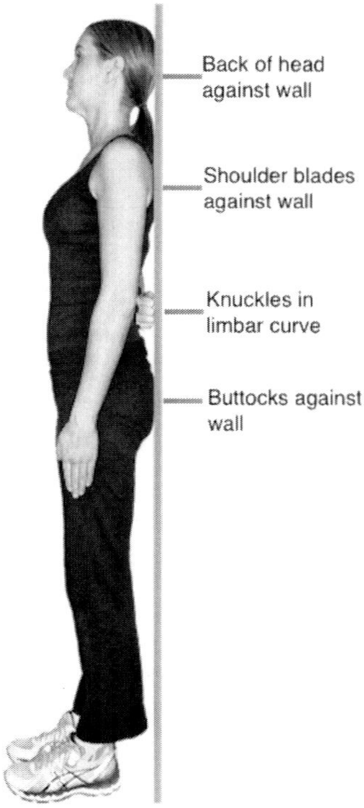

Wall Test

Maintaining Your Posture

Awareness and persistence are the two most important factors for improving your overall spinal posture.

Good posture is achieved by lengthening the spine. This isn't a forceful action. It involves re-educating your brain to let go of unnecessary tension in your muscles as you become used to what this feels like.

Letting go of tension in your neck muscles is particularly important. Various mental images can be used to help you do this. You may like to try imagining a string attached to the top of your head pulling your spine upwards and lengthening it or a balloon attached to your head floating it upwards off your shoulders.

It can be quite difficult to form an accurate impression of your own body alignment, especially when you are changing long-term postural habits. Several mind-body exercise disciplines focus on developing awareness of posture, body use and breathing and a few lessons in one of these would provide useful feedback. Two such systems which take a western perspective are Pilates and Alexander Technique.

Good Standing Posture

- Stand with your feet parallel about hip-width apart.
- Weight should be borne equally by both feet.
- On each foot, distribute your weight evenly between the heel, the inside of the front of the foot and the outside of the front of the foot.
- Knees should be very slightly bent, not locked.
- Let your arms hang naturally down beside your body.
- Lift your breastbone (not your shoulders) slightly. As you do this, your shoulder blades will move downwards in your back.
- Gently tighten the muscles in the lowest part of your abdomen above the pubic bone. This is to support your lumbar spine and prevent you arching your back excessively or leaning backwards, especially with prolonged standing. You should maintain a small hollow in your lower back.
- Think about lengthening your entire spine including your neck (see mental images).
- Relax your jaw. With the mouth closed, rest your tongue on the roof of your mouth.
- Check your chin is level and facing forward.
- Check your shoulders are relaxed and down away from your ears.
- Check your standing posture from time to time during the day with the wall test.

Good Sitting Posture

Chair Choice and Lumbar Support

No chair or seat, no matter how well designed, will ensure good posture, but some are obviously better for your posture than others.

A good quality ergonomic office chair will provide adequate support for your lumbar spine, provided it is correctly adjusted. Unfortunately, many commercial seats and most domestic chairs have very poor lumbar support. Couches, car, bus and plane seats are among the worst offenders.

One of the most effective things you can do to improve your seated posture is to purchase or make a lumbar roll. This is a foam roll you place in the curve of your lower back. It will maintain the inward curve of your lumbar spine and help keep you upright.

You can also use a small rolled up towel, a small pillow or part of your jacket if necessary. Whatever you use, make sure it has the right width to feel comfortable.

A chair with adjustable height makes it easier to maintain good posture. An adjustable chair for home use is a worthwhile investment, especially if you work from home.

Most couches provide very little in the way of lumbar support, or postural support of any kind. The end of the day is the most dangerous time for your posture. It's all too easy to sink into a soft couch and forget all about your spine, especially if you are tired. A couch also gives you enough room to adopt various awkward positions in which you are partly sitting and partly lying down. Keeping your head turned to one side or lying out flat with your head propped up on the arm-rest, as in the photos, are two sure-fire ways to strain your neck.

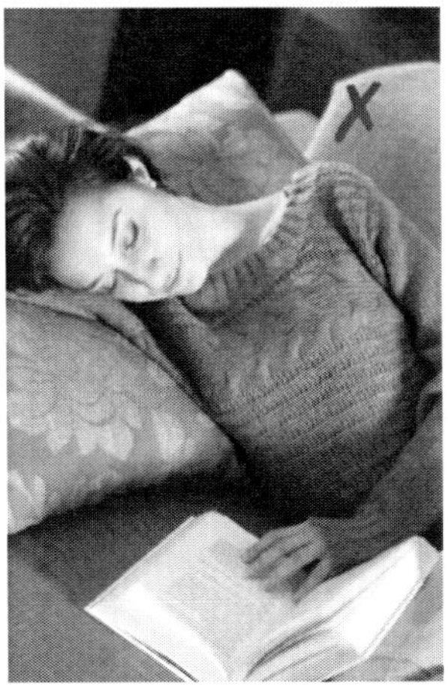

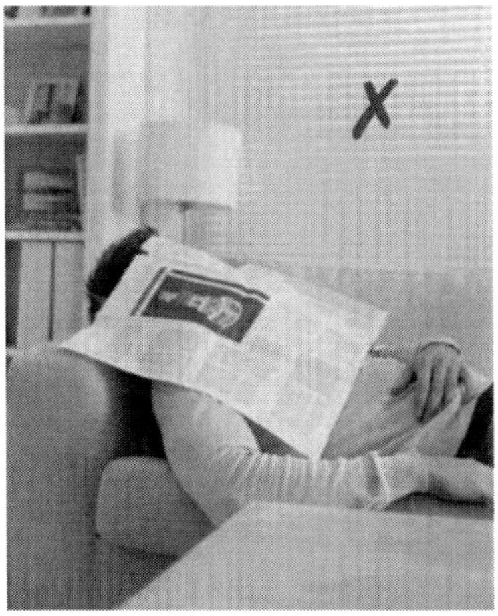

A firm upholstered chair is the best choice for anyone who suffers headaches, or from back and neck pain. The chair should have arm rests and a slope of about 25 degrees for comfort. The armrests do need to be the right height for you, so that your arms and shoulders are relaxed. Too high and your shoulders will be forced up towards your ears (more muscular trigger points), too low and you won't use them. Depending on how much lumbar support the chair provides, you may still need a lumbar roll or a rolled-up towel to help stop you rounding your lower back.

Good Posture When You Sit

The following advice applies equally to sitting in a chair at your desk, in a plane or car seat, or in an easy chair.

- Sit with your bottom as far back as it will go on the seat, even if you are only sitting down for a little while. The bones of your pelvis, which you can feel just below your waist, should be right up against the backrest. This is important to help prevent you from slouching.
- Make sure you have good lumbar support. If you are sitting on an ergonomic office chair, the lumbar support must be correctly adjusted. In most other chairs and seats you will probably need a lumbar roll. Place it in the curve of your lower back near the belt line.
- Sit with your mid-back resting against the back of the chair.
- Both feet must be able to rest flat on the floor. If your feet don't reach the floor, and you can't adjust the height of the chair, you should use a footrest, or some other support for your feet. Your body weight should be evenly distributed on both feet.
- Bring the chair close to the edge of the desk or table. When seated, your navel should be 5-7cm away from the edge.
- Your arms should be relaxed and supported. Rest your arms, hands and wrists on the desk or table.
- Avoid using arm-rests. They get in the way when placing the chair close to the desk or table and they encourage you to lean on one elbow.
- Your thighs should be roughly horizontal, depending on the type of seat. There should also be a small gap between the back of your knees and the front of the seat. These factors help ensure that the seat doesn't cut into the back of your legs and interfere with your circulation.
- Don't cross your legs or wrap them around the legs of the chair.
- Check your shoulders are relaxed and down.
- SIT TALL. Think about lengthening your entire spine including your neck
- Lift your breastbone (not your shoulders) slightly. As you do this, your shoulder blades will move downwards in your back.
- Check your chin is level and facing forward.
- Relax your jaw. With the mouth closed, rest your tongue on the roof or your mouth.

Once you've done all this, remember, even perfect sitting posture is bad if you stay in it too long. Take frequent short breaks. Stand up and move to relieve muscle fatigue and get your circulation going.

You and Your Posture Against the World

Most modern jobs and leisure activities are a recipe for encouraging bad posture and forward head posture. We have to make a deliberate effort to counteract their effects.

With increased automation and advances in technology, most of us now spend a large portion of each working day sitting, often while performing a limited number of repetitive movements. When we get home, we usually do more sitting while eating, watching TV, reading, studying, surfing the web, playing video games or catching up with friends.

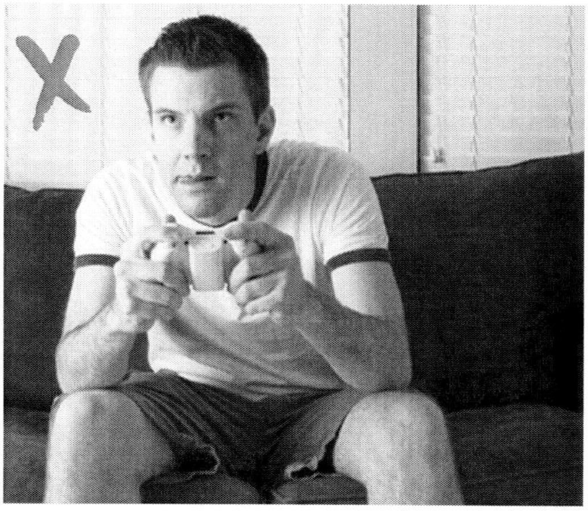

Our bodies aren't suited to sedentary activities. In our hunter-gatherer past, we were continually on the move and our movements were much more varied. Even with the best possible posture, if you sit regularly for a long time without moving or changing position, various muscle imbalances will inevitably develop in your body.

Muscle imbalance occurs when one group of muscles pulls more strongly on a joint than the opposing muscle group, changing its normal resting position. If you regularly hold your arms out in front of you, whether sitting or standing, muscle imbalances will develop in your upper body. Typical activities include typing at a keyboard, hairdressing, carrying a baby, sewing, using a computer mouse and scanning items at a supermarket checkout. Often the activity will affect one side of the body more than the other. If you habitually slouch, or poor ergonomics force you to work in an awkward position, these and other muscle imbalances will develop, but much more quickly.

Prolonged sitting shortens and tightens the muscles at the front of your hip and lower back, as they work against the opposing muscles of your buttocks and abdomen. The short tight muscles win out in this tussle. When you stand up, the front of your hips will be pulled down, increasing the curve of your lumbar spine.

In a similar way, keeping your arms held out in front of you makes the muscles of your chest and the front of your shoulders shorter and tighter than the opposing muscles in the upper part of your middle back. Again, the short tight muscles dominate, making your shoulders round forwards. Unfortunately, once your shoulders are rounded it is hard not to project your head and neck forward as well.

Unless you correct this accumulating list of muscle imbalances at an early stage by stretching the tight muscles followed by strengthening the weak ones, they will become more pronounced and increasingly difficult to remedy. And it is not just muscle imbalance that needs to be corrected. Once established, poor posture causes other changes that help make it self-perpetuating.

If we repeat a particular posture or movement pattern often enough, eventually the brain and muscles learn to adopt it as an automatic response to a particular situation, without us making a conscious decision. This is similar to what happens once you have learned to ride a bike.

To improve your posture, you have to become aware of and continually monitor the way you're holding our body. Every time you notice you've slipped back into your old postural habits, you must consciously replace them with new and better ones, until these, in turn, become automatic.

Over time, the fascial network moulds itself according to how the body is used. If you sit slouched at your computer for eight hours a day your fascia will alter to make this posture easier to support. Some parts will stretch, while other parts, such as the fascia at the front of the neck and chest, will become shorter, thicker and tighter. Formation of adhesions will reduce flexibility further. Fortunately the short, thickened fascia can be gradually stretched to help the body return to a more optimal posture.

If you've had bad posture for a long time, it will take time and a concerted effort to fix it. When you first try to switch to a better posture, it will probably feel rather strange and uncomfortable for a while. However, it is important to persevere. Improving your posture has many benefits for your physical and emotional health.

Bad posture isn't just bad for headaches. It causes pain elsewhere in the body, as well as altered movement patterns, stiffness and reduced mobility. It accelerates arthritic changes in the spine, interferes with breathing and compresses the abdominal organs.

Bad posture also affects your mood and self-image and transmits a powerful message to others. When we're sad, we round our shoulders and our head droops. Slouching in your chair can project an uncooperative and lethargic attitude.

Good posture makes you feel and look more positive and confident. It can help you regain some lost height. In fact, it's sometimes said that good posture can make a person look 10 years younger and 10 pounds lighter. For many of us, this is a nice bonus!

Situations When it's Hard to Sit Correctly

Reading or Writing

The major challenge with achieving good sitting posture while reading or writing is that you have to bend your head down to a certain extent to be able to see properly.

If you are sitting at a desk, you can minimise this by moving your chair in very close. It also makes sure that you don't have to bend your body forward to reach your work, which rounds your whole back.

It's important to take frequent breaks, whether you're studying or engrossed in the latest best-seller. You should also do regular neck and shoulder stretches to counteract the effects of postural stress.

Here are some suggestions to help you maintain good posture while you're reading or writing:

- When you are sitting at your desk, move your chair in very close so you don't round your back. Rest your arms on the desk
- When you are reading at your desk try propping your book up at an angle by putting something beneath it, like a thicker book
- Leave space on your desk next to your computer for writing and doing paperwork. It should be on the same side as the hand you write with. This will reduce the amount of twisting and reaching you need to do
- If you are reading in an easy chair, put a pillow on your lap under the book to raise it closer to your eyes and provide a better angle
- A chair with arms of the correct height is best for your posture and makes it less tiring to hold the book
- Make sure you can see clearly or else you are automatically going to bend your head forwards
- Check you have enough overhead light. Supplement the room light with a desk or standard lamp if necessary. There should be no dark patches, glare or reflections
- Do eye exercises to reduce eye strain:
- Look away from your screen and focus on something in the distance
- Change focus from a distant to a near object and back several times
- Rest your eyes by covering them with your palms
- Blink a lot.
- If you wear glasses for reading have them checked. The angle of the lenses and the shape of the frames may be partly obstructing your vision when you look downwards through your glasses, causing you to tilt your head down more than you need to
- You may be able to hold your book up for a short time just to give your neck a break. Make sure your neck is straight, and your shoulders are level

- A good book support that holds a book open at a similar angle to a document stand would go a long way towards improving reading posture
- An inclined writing surface like those used by draftsmen and medieval monks will reduce how much you bend your head when you write. A range of different portable inclined surfaces, known as slant boards or desk slopes, which you can place on your desk are available online.

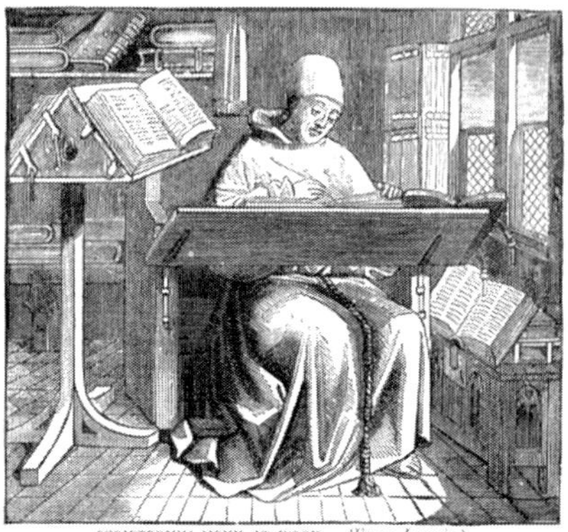

SCRIPTORIUM MONK AT WORK. (From *Lacroix*.)

Flying

As far as spinal posture is concerned, most economy class plane seats are an ergonomic nightmare and seats on buses and trains are not much better. Backrests are narrow and curved, with wings at the side which don't leave enough room for your arms. This forces your shoulders forward and makes you round your entire back just so you can fit into your seat. Then the headrest pushes your head and neck forwards.

To fix these problems, you need two additional supports.

Sit right back in your seat and place a pillow or a lumbar roll in the inward curve in your lower back. This will move your shoulders away from the sides of the seat.

Place another pillow higher up to fill the space behind your upper back. Sit tall and then lean back. You should now be able to rest the back of your head against the headrest.

Driving

Like plane seats, the majority of modern bucket-style car seats are bad for your overall spinal posture, and especially for your neck. They have narrow backrests with large wings on the side that get in the way of your arms.

The aim of this design is to enclose your body to help limit sideways movement when the car changes direction or if it's involved in a collision. However, it also makes you round your shoulders and upper back. The two other common problems are that lumbar support is generally insufficient or incorrectly placed and head-rests (head restraints) protrude so far that they stop your shoulder blades reaching the back-rest and force your head and neck forwards at an unnatural angle.

Unless your car seats are fitted with an adjustable lumbar support, some form of external lumbar support, such as a lumbar roll, is essential. Proper lumbar support will stop you sliding down in your seat and rounding your lower back. It will also move your shoulders and arms clear of the sides of the seat and your head a little further away from the headrest. This will stop you rounding your shoulders and upper back and will help with your head positioning.

If your head is still too far forward, you have some more work to do. All recent model cars enable you to alter the height of the headrest but this won't help. You must leave the headrest positioned high enough to protect your neck against whiplash injury. In the event of a collision, the headrest should contact your head, not your neck. It should therefore sit squarely behind your head, as in the photo, and no more than 5 cm (2 inches) away from it.

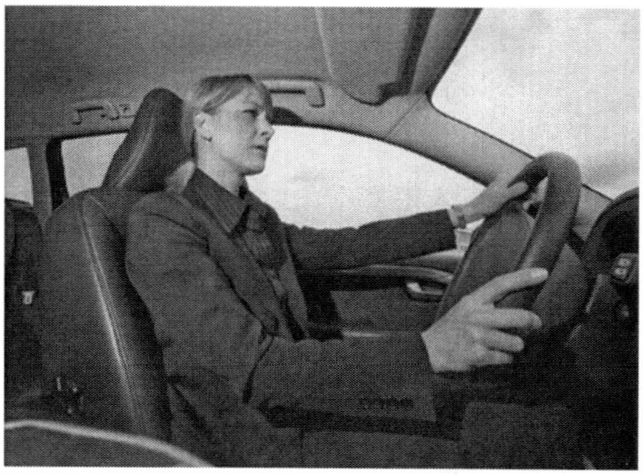

The headrest doesn't need to be right up against the back of your head and it certainly shouldn't be pushing your head forward. Altering the tilt of the headrest will help but unfortunately few cars are fitted with this control. Otherwise there are not many really satisfactory solutions.

If you have a problem with your car headrest that sitting up tall and providing satisfactory lumbar support doesn't fix, it may be worth trying:

- Reclining your seat at a slightly greater angle to give you more room behind your head
- Looking for a long support cushion that fills the gap between your upper back and the seat, in addition to providing lumbar support
- Having your seat altered to fit you better
- Using a mesh back support which moves you further away from the back-rest than a lumbar roll.

Vehicle seat design can contribute to poor posture, however the main causes of poor driving posture are incorrectly adjusted seats and bad postural habits, such as slumping in the seat or driving with one hand, or a combination of both.

You should adjust your seat to suit your body, including when you switch between vehicles. The two most important parameters to set for good driving posture are the distance between the seat and the pedals, and the angle of the backrest. Adjustments available in most modern cars allow you to raise or lower the seat above the floor, tilt the front of the seat downwards and adjust the position of the steering wheel. These can be used for fine tuning your driving posture.

To achieve good driving posture:

- Slide your bottom all the way back in the seat when you get into the car
- Sit tall as with any other type of seat. Raise the height of your seat if you need to but make sure your feet still reach the floor
- Move the seat forward to a position where you can depress all the foot pedals completely while still leaning against the backrest. Vary the seat position forward and back slightly until your thighs are roughly horizontal. Your knees should be about the same height as your hips
- If there is too much pressure on the underside of your thighs either tilt the front of the seat forward (if this control is available) or experiment with sitting on a wedge cushion. The cushion will also reduce the amount of vibration transferred to your spine through the seat and hence the risk of low back pain
- Check there is a small gap between the edge of the seat and the back of your knees. If there isn't, an external lumbar support will help by moving you further forward on the seat
- Adjust the angle of the backrest so that you are reclining slightly. It should feel comfortable
- Unless the seat comes with an adjustable lumbar support, position a lumbar roll or other external support in the curve of your lower back
- Check your arms can reach the steering wheel comfortably without you having to hunch forward – you should be able stay leaning against the backrest. Your arms should also be slightly bent. If necessary, reduce the backrest angle a little
- If necessary, adjust the height of the steering wheel and its distance from you so that your arms feel relaxed. With your hands on the wheel, your elbows should be bent and your upper arms relaxed and close to your side. If the steering wheel is too low it will be too close to your legs or stomach and interfere with your driving. If it is too high it will force you to hold your arms up, putting strain on your neck and shoulder muscles. It will also obscure your view of the instrument panel and the road
- Hold the sides not the top of the steering wheel – the 9 and 3 o'clock positions are ideal – and try to keep your wrists straight. How you hold the steering wheel while you are driving is very important for avoiding muscular strain
- Adjust the height of the headrest (head restraint). The middle of the headrest should be at eye level
- Finally adjust your seat belt and your rear and side view mirrors. You should be able to see your mirrors without excessive twisting of your neck and upper body.

Now check your posture. Sit tall. Lean against the backrest of the seat. Make sure you are not projecting your head forward out of habit. Check you are facing straight forward in the seat and holding the steering wheel with both hands. When some people drive, they tend sit partly twisted to one side, with one hand on the steering wheel and their elbow on the door rest or the console between the seats. This twisted position is a major cause of muscular trigger points in the SCM muscles.

Case Study Learnings

After a consultation with Tony, a patient of mine, I now ask my patients about the way they sit when they drive. Tony had been referred to me because he regularly suffered from severe headaches. Tony had a high-pressure job and spent a lot of time bent over, looking at charts, both headache risks. When I treated trigger points in the SCM muscles in his neck, Tony experienced an immediate and dramatic relief of his headaches. However, they returned after a while.

When I first treated Tony, I noticed that the muscles on one side of his neck were much tighter and more tender to pressure than the other and had asked him about his posture.

It took a few more sessions before Tony mentioned that he often drove with one hand, sitting slightly across the seat so he could lean his elbow on the door rest. He asked if this would make any difference. It certainly did make a difference. After a small number of additional treatments and changes to his driving position, with no other changes to his lifestyle, Tony's headaches improved.

Extra Tips for Lessening the Effect of Driving on the Body:

- On a long trip, take a ten-minute break from driving every hour. Walk around to get your circulation going and do some neck and shoulder stretches.
- Don't forget to RELAX. Consciously relax your jaw and don't grip the steering wheel too hard. Your shoulders should be down and relaxed, not held high towards your ears.
- If you are stuck in traffic it is especially important to relax. Do some slow deep abdominal breathing and some neck and shoulder stretches while sitting in your seat.
- Wear a suitable pair of sunglasses. Frowning and squinting because of glare can cause muscular trigger points in some of the smaller muscles of the face, causing pain that we perceive as headache. Glare is also a commonly reported migraine trigger.

Sleeping

We've all woken up with a stiff neck or sore back and immediately thought I must have slept the wrong way.

Most people are aware that poor sleeping posture can cause neck, shoulder and back pain. However, the significant role it can play in provoking headache attacks tends to go unrecognised.

A good mattress and pillow can certainly help your sleeping posture. However, the most important factor is to look at the way you lie in bed.

Although we change our position many times while we are asleep, we all have a favourite position. This is the position that we adopt automatically as we drift off to sleep, the one we continually return to during the night and the position we spend the most time in. Video studies have shown almost everyone can identify it reliably.[110] Having good sleeping posture means your pillow and mattress should support your head and body so that your spine retains its three natural curves, just as when you are sitting or standing and your spine, and especially your neck (cervical spine), should not be twisted to one side – your shoulders and hip bones should be aligned.

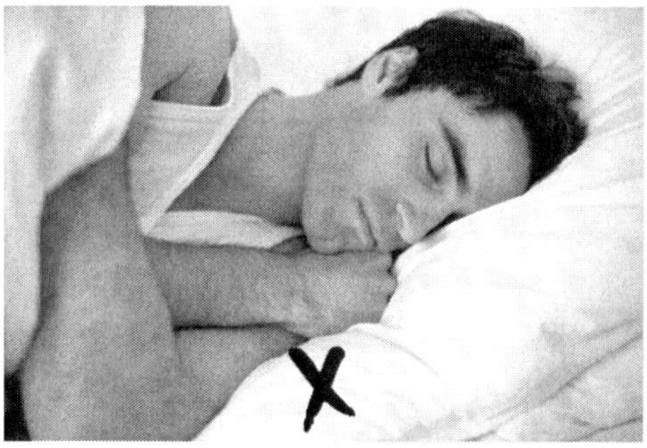

The position of your arms and legs should not put any muscles in either an overly shortened or overstretched state. For example, avoid crossing your arms tightly against your chest as shown in the photo. Awkward positions such as this, when held for hours on end during sleep, will cause or reactivate muscular trigger points and worsen existing muscle imbalances.

There is some disagreement among scientists and doctors as to whether sleeping on your side or your back is better for the spine. However, all agree that sleeping on your stomach is very bad for the spine and should be avoided.

Stopping sleeping on your stomach may be one of the most effective things you can do to stop your headaches. When you sleep on your stomach, your face is turned to one side, rotating your neck almost as far as it can go and tilting it backwards.

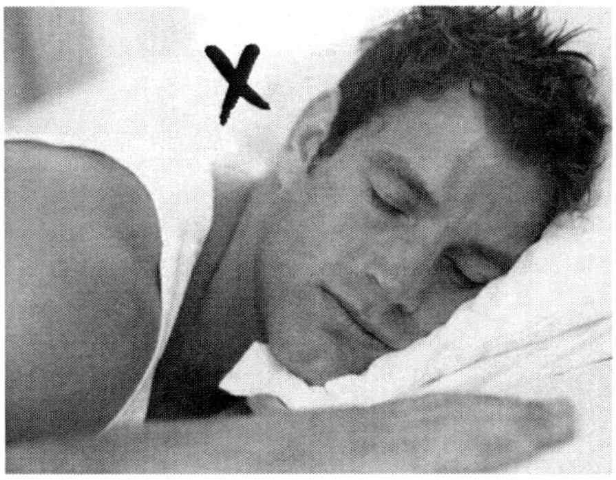

This type of posture puts a tremendous amount of strain on the joints, muscles and ligaments of the neck, including those which are a direct source of headache pain. Kinking the neck can also irritate nerves and blood vessels and so trigger a headache attack. It may be one possible cause of migraines that often strike when you wake up. Sleeping on your stomach causes other problems too. It twists the rib cage, increases the curve of your lower back leading to back pain, puts stress on your jaw joint and impairs breathing.

If you are a stomach sleeper, and especially if you suffer headaches or pain in the neck, back or shoulder, you should train yourself to sleep on your side. It takes perseverance but it is possible to do, and the benefits make the effort well worthwhile.

Changing from Stomach to Side Sleeping

When you get into bed, start out on your side and do a relaxation exercise. It will initially take longer than usual for you to feel comfortable enough to fall asleep, so remember to be patient.

Each time you wake up during the night and find yourself on your stomach, reposition yourself on your side. If you go through the same process each night, with sufficient repetition your body and brain will gradually become accustomed to the new position.

If you are having difficulty making the change, start by sleeping half on your side and half on your stomach. A large body pillow may be more comfortable and help you stay on your side. Bend one knee up and place a medium firm pillow under your stomach and hip on the bent knee side. This reduces the stress on your neck and lower back and helps with breathing. When you are comfortable with this intermediate position, switch to sleeping fully on your side.

Our postural habits are so ingrained that we are mostly unaware of them. It is a good idea to demonstrate the way you usually lie when you go to sleep to your manual therapist and ask them to comment on any possible problem areas that they notice.

Your Mattress

Choose a mattress that is firm but has enough cushioning to distribute your body weight. It should be both supportive and comfortable, but not too firm.

The illustration shows a mattress with the right amount of support. It allows the parts of your body that are in contact with the mattress to sink in sufficiently. There should be no gaps left between your body and the mattress, otherwise sections of your spine will be unsupported.

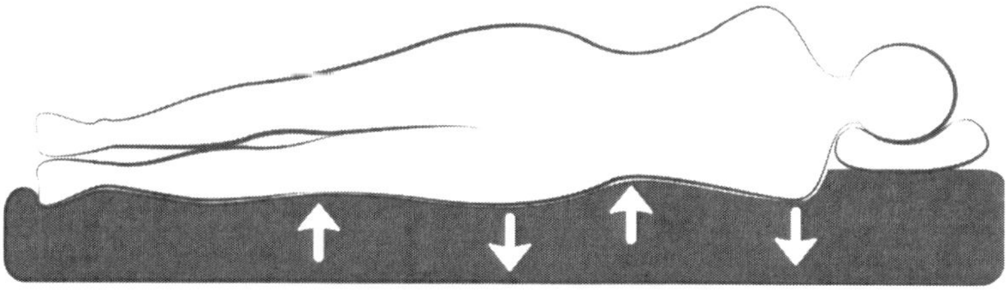

If you have already bought a mattress that you now find is too firm, adding a good quality foam mattress topper about 2.5 cm (1 inch) thick may possibly solve the problem.

A mattress which is too soft or which is getting old and has started to sag in the middle will not support your spine in its neutral alignment. Your back and neck will be forced into unnatural positions, straining muscles, joints and ligaments. A plywood bed board placed between the mattress and its base will make a soft mattress firmer and provide a temporary reprieve for a sagging mattress.

Your Pillow

Sleep with one pillow under your head. Never use more than one pillow and make sure you do not pull it under your shoulder. Your pillow should support your neck as well as your head and so should fill the space between your head and shoulders.

Your pillow should also be the right thickness – not too high or it will force your head upwards and not too low or it will allow your head to tilt downwards.

Pillow too high
Neck kinked up

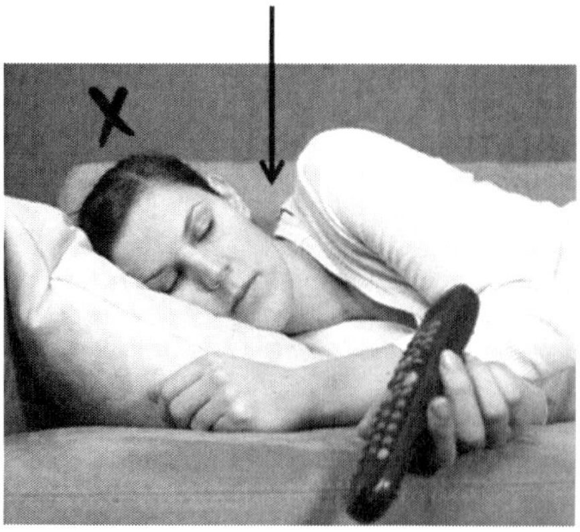

No pillow (or pillow too low)
Neck tilted down

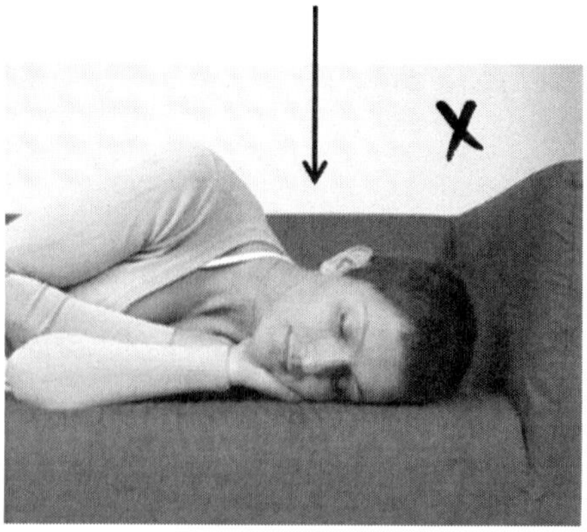

Whether you sleep on your side or your back, your head should be aligned with your spine in the same way it is when you are standing. Your neck shouldn't be twisted to one side, as this will create or reactivate muscular trigger points in the SCM (sternocleidomastoid) and trapezius muscles.

Your head should rest in a small hollow in your pillow to hold your neck straight.

Pillows come in a bewildering array of styles, shapes and filling materials. Basically, your pillow shouldn't be too springy. A contoured pillow made of latex or memory foam will provide good neck support provided it's the right thickness and profile for your build and the way you sleep.

Memory foam has the advantage that it moulds to the shape of your head and so helps stop your neck from twisting. If your existing pillow doesn't have a contoured shape you can use a soft foam neck roll inside the pillow case to support your neck. There are many neck rolls available. Experiment with positioning the roll about a quarter of the way up from the lower border of the pillow.

Additional Postural Support

Although you shouldn't use more than one pillow under your head, you may need some additional pillows to support other parts of your body so your spine is properly aligned and your muscles aren't under stress. Even though these pillows are likely to move during the night they will at least help for a while.

Lying on your side with your knees somewhat bent helps counteract a sway back and can relieve back pain. Depending on the proportions of various parts of the body, some people will need a pillow between the knees to maintain the spine in a neutral position. A pillow in this position will also counteract any tendency for the top leg to roll across and down onto the mattress, which twists the spine.

It's also a good idea to wrap your arms around a soft pillow in front of you to support your uppermost arm and shoulder. It will stop them from dropping forward towards the mattress and pulling on your neck and upper back. You may be able to use a full body pillow to perform both these functions.

Avoid tucking your knees up close to your chest in a foetal position or crossing your arms tightly against chest as this puts various muscle groups in a shortened state. Lying on your back with your legs straight can cause low back pain. If you sleep on your back, bend your knees slightly and place a pillow under them for support. This keeps your spine in a neutral position. Alternatively, use a lumbar roll under your lower back.

Keep Moving

Muscles kept in a contracted state develop muscular trigger points because they restrict their blood supply. Lack of movement to keep the blood flowing to the muscles only compounds this problem. We also know that anything that impairs blood flow to the brain can provoke a headache attack. These are both reasons why movement is important for preventing headaches.

Whether you're sitting or standing, remaining in a fixed position for a lengthy period of time without moving causes muscle fatigue and after a while, your posture inevitably deteriorates

It's best if you can vary your activities so that you swap frequently between sitting, standing and walking around. If that's not possible or practical, you should take regular breaks to change position, which uses some different muscles, and, most importantly, move around.

Some Tips for Coping Better with Prolonged Standing

If you have to stand for a long time, say in a slow moving queue, shift your weight from your toes to your heels and back, and from one foot to the other, pedal your feet up and down, or walk up and down on the spot.

If your job requires lots of standing in the one position, occupational health and safety organisations[111] strongly recommend that you schedule frequent short regular breaks, such as a five-minute break after 15 minutes of standing, to combat muscle fatigue.

During the break, sit for a short time to rest your muscles and then walk around to restore circulation. Other recommended actions to lessen the effects of prolonged standing on the body include using a sit-stand stool or a portable footrest. A sit-stand stool enables you to work in a semi-standing position while resting most of your weight on a padded and adjustable seat. A portable footrest allows you to shift your body weight from both legs to one leg and back again to relieve tiredness and help prevent excessive curvature of the lumbar spine.

Certain tasks in the home, such as food preparation, dish washing and ironing, also involve a lot of standing. Don't forget to think tall. Look down with your eyes rather than bending forward, move about as much as you can and take lots of short breaks.

If you cannot avoid bending forward because work-surfaces are too low, try to bend from the hip joints (just above the top of the thighs), not the waist and lightly brace your lower abdominal muscles to protect your lower back.

Offsetting the Effects of Prolonged Sitting

The amount of time we spend sitting continues to increase.[112] It's very easy to underestimate the amount of time you spend sitting each day, and, more importantly, to become so engrossed in your computer or a show on TV that you forget to move.

The only way of counteracting the effects of prolonged sitting is to break the time up into smaller chunks. The most important thing to do is to schedule regular breaks. Whether you are sitting on your couch, in front of a computer or in the car, you should take a break to stand up and move around.

Whenever possible, you should get out of your seat at least once every hour. Find some way of reminding yourself that works for you. If you spend all day sitting at your job, occupational health and safety organisations recommend that you have a 5–10 minute break for every 40–50 minutes of sitting. This is also a useful guideline to keep in mind if you are sitting at home.

During each break, spend some time walking around to help restore circulation and exercise heart, lungs and muscles. Do several of the exercises from the stretching and strengthening routine given in this book, and the exercise to correct forward head posture. These exercises are designed to counteract the effect that sitting has on your head and neck posture.

Here are some extra suggestions for getting more movement into your day:

- Always try to get away from your desk during lunch breaks. If you can manage to get outside, so much the better
- While you are sitting down, move around in your seat and shake out your arms and legs
- Pedal your feet up and down on the floor. Do some of the neck and shoulder stretches, such as turning your head from side to side
- Try sitting on a fit ball (Swiss ball, physio ball) as a break from sitting on a chair. The fit ball will help you move around more while sitting. Once you get used to it you can do small bounces up and down and hip circles.

A Note on Fit Balls

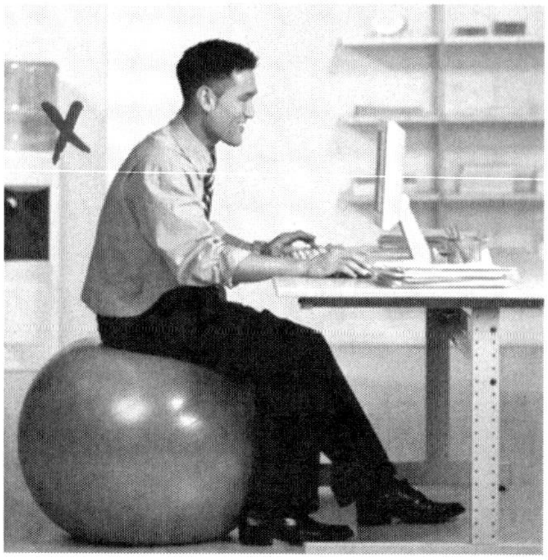

Sitting on a fit ball can help strengthen some of the postural muscles that support your torso because you have to work to maintain your balance. However, you have no back support so you need to pay even more attention than usual to maintaining correct posture. Your posture on the ball should look the same as when you are sitting correctly on a chair.

If you are using the ball in front of the computer make sure you move it close into your desk as usual. Your legs must be able to fit under the desk.

Start off by sitting on the ball for a few minutes at a time until you get used to it. Once you get tired, switch back to your usual chair. A useful guideline[113] is to start with 15 minutes and gradually build up in 15 minute blocks to a maximum of 1 hour at a time. After this, alternate every hour between the fit ball and the chair.

The ball should be a suitable diameter for your height and weight. You can adjust the height of the ball further by varying the inflation pressure. Make sure the ball is made of an anti-burst material so that it will only deflate slowly if punctured. And don't believe the hype – it is even easier to slouch on a fit ball than a chair, especially when you get tired.

Avoiding Muscle Strain

I have already emphasised the importance of maintaining correct posture so that any musculoskeletal problems that contribute to your headache pain don't recur. However, the way we move and use our bodies as we go about our daily activities and our various unconscious habits can also place unnecessary stress on our muscles and joints.

Anything that lessens blood flow to muscles can cause muscular trigger points to recur or new ones to form. It may be the result of muscle overuse from repeating the same actions or from holding an awkward posture, from lack of movement or even from wearing constrictive clothing.

Here are some extra potential sources of muscular trigger points in the muscles of the neck, shoulder and face that you need to be on the lookout for.

The Phone

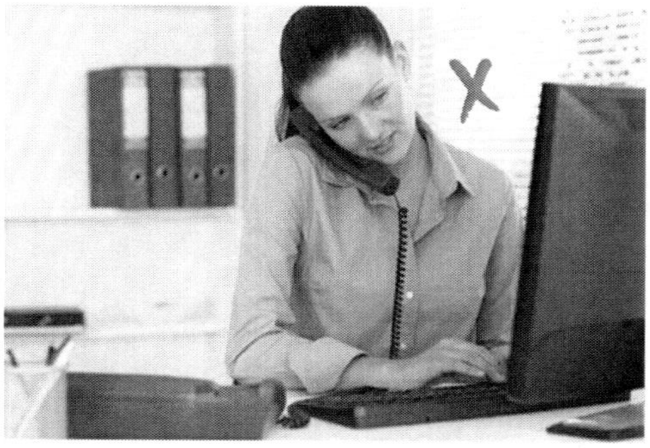

- Cradling the phone between your ear and shoulder is a common cause of muscular trigger points in the upper trapezius muscle.
- If you walk around your house with your cordless phone tucked under your chin while you continue to do chores, cook or write, swap to a phone with a speaker you can put down.
- For longer calls on your cell phone, use a hands-free headset.

Constrictive Clothing

- Avoid wearing a tight shirt collar and tie.
- Avoid wearing a heavy coat that drags on your shoulders. Most people unconsciously tend to relieve the weight by putting their hands in their pockets.
- Make sure you have a well fitted bra. Watch out for narrow bra straps that cut into the top of your shoulders and fasteners that pull tightly across your chest and back. A special note for women with D cup and above: It is even more important to wear a properly fitted bra that provides adequate support and does not restrict circulation.

Bags and Cases

- Avoid carrying heavy briefcases and laptop bags. If you can, spread the load between two smaller bags, one in each hand, or use a backpack.
- Avoid carrying a heavy purse (handbag) or clutching it under your arm. Get a bag with a strap that you can wear diagonally across your chest and try to carry less around with you.
- Don't wear a purse or backpack over one shoulder, even if it's light. You will be holding up that shoulder to keep the bag from slipping off.
- Don't carry a heavy backpack that makes your head and neck project forward to compensate. School children should not carry a backpack that weighs more than 10% of their bodyweight. A chest belt keeps the shoulder straps in place and helps spread the load.

Cold Temperatures and Draughts

- Chilling muscles especially when they are fatigued (for example, after a day at the office) can cause muscular trigger points to develop.
- Watch out for cold draughts from air conditioning blowing on your neck and shoulders. Keep your muscles warm with a scarf. Take a scarf if you are going out at night if it is likely to turn cold.

Eyesight and Glasses

- Check to see if you are bending your head forward or narrowing your eyes to see better. If it's been a while since you had your eyes examined, you may need glasses or a more powerful prescription.
- Watch for habits like bending your head down to look over the top of your glasses – take your glasses off to see without them.

Common Activities, Movements and Postures

- Chewing gum can cause muscular trigger points in the chewing muscles.
- Avoid continually turning your head to one side, for example to speak to someone sitting beside you, to see the stage in a live performance if you have a seat on one side, or to take a breath when swimming the crawl stroke.
- Avoid continually looking upwards while working above head level, for example when painting a ceiling, or during other activities, such as bird watching.
- Avoid continually looking behind you, for example when using a ride-on mower.
- Don't lie down to watch TV or read, whether lying on your side with your head supported on one elbow, lying on your stomach with your head propped up on both elbows (a favourite of children and teenagers) or lying on your back with your neck kinked.
- Avoid holding your shoulders up due to tension or lack of awareness while you work, such as forcefully screwing the lid on a jar.
- Avoid prolonged use of one arm, for example using a mixing spoon or a chainsaw.
- Be wary of reading in bed, something many of us love to do – it can cause a lot of problems if you don't set yourself up properly. A pillow behind the shoulders is not enough. You need good lumbar support or you will inevitably round your back and project your head.
- You could use a lumbar support or several well-arranged pillows. Alternatively, you may want to consider a bed rest or a special wedge shaped reading pillow.
- You also need to check the direction of light so that your head is not turned to one side Have a light directly above you or get a special book light that clips onto your book.
- You need some way of supporting the book at an angle, such as a scrunched up pillow or a book support.

Key Points

- Forward head posture is one of the main culprits of bad posture and causes muscular trigger points.
- Good posture is a crucial element of reducing the frequency and severity of headache pain.
- Good posture means maintaining a neutral spine while you are standing, sitting and sleeping and moving from one position to another.
- The longer we sit without moving, the more tired our muscles get and it becomes very difficult to maintain good posture.
- Even if you have a perfect ergonomic setup and correct sitting posture, sitting for too long is still bad for you. Take frequent short breaks. Stand up and move to relieve muscle fatigue and get your circulation going.
- Sleeping on your stomach is very bad for your posture and plays a significant role provoking headache attacks. You should work to change to side sleeping if you are a stomach sleeper.

19

Screen Time

Mobile Electronic Devices and Forward Head Posture

Portable Computers

Laptops are increasingly replacing desktop computers in the workplace and the home, but even when a laptop is used at a desk, its design is a recipe for postural problems.

Firstly, the screen is way too low. You have to keep bending your head forwards to read it – this is a well-recognised cause of forward head posture and headaches. For a desktop computer, screen height is easy to set correctly, but for a laptop computer, the keyboard and screen cannot be adjusted independently.

There are other problems too. Using the touchpad in the centre of the laptop instead of a mouse and typing on the small keyboard puts your arms in an awkward position. This puts additional strain on your neck and shoulder muscles and makes you round your shoulders forward. It can also cause your wrists to twist outwards.

Finally typing with your hands resting on the hard front of the laptop puts pressure on the carpal tunnel on the underside of your wrists. Laptops were never designed for long term use. As a headache sufferer, you need to be especially careful of how you use them. In spite of its name, never use a laptop on your lap, as the young man in the photo is doing.

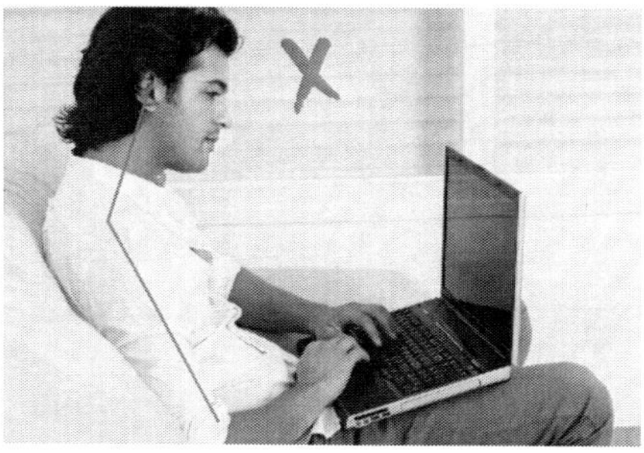

His head and neck posture is even worse than it might otherwise be because he is also sitting on a very soft couch which provides next to no back support. Notice that his spine has adopted a C-shape. Similarly, never rest your laptop on a couch or bed to use it. Put it on a table that is not too high, or preferably on a proper desk.

Getting the screen height right is your priority. If you use a laptop for more than a few minutes at any one time, it is essential that you're able to see the screen without bending your neck. There are two ways of achieving this. You could place the entire laptop on a stand (or if nothing better is available, put it on some books or telephone directories) and add an external mouse and keyboard. To be able to raise the laptop screen sufficiently, you will probably need to purchase a type of tilted stand known as a vertical laptop riser. However, if you intend to use a laptop on your desk as your primary computer, a laptop stand isn't very convenient.

If you can, I recommend connecting your laptop to an external screen. Again, you should plug in an external mouse and keyboard. This will greatly reduce the stress on your neck, shoulders, arms and wrists, especially over the longer term. Sit the external screen on a flat stand. If you need it to be higher, you can always add a thick book. The larger external screen will also be easier to see than the laptop screen.

Whichever alternative you choose for your laptop, you then need to set up your furniture to minimise postural stress in the same way as you would with a desktop computer.

If you carry your laptop around, remember, it's heavy. Carrying a heavy bag over your shoulder is a significant source of muscular trigger points in neck and shoulder muscles. It is a good idea to use a backpack or a bag with wheels instead.

Mobile Phones

Wherever you are, in a restaurant, in shops, at the bus station or just walking along the street, you will see people of all ages hunched over their cell phones, texting.

A recent article[114] highlighted the emerging problem of forward head posture among young people caused by excessive texting. The article cited the case of a girl who, at only 16 years of age, had a reverse curve in her cervical spine and degenerative changes to her neck vertebrae due to spending most of each day texting. More than 15% of people in 12–24 age bracket send and receive over 200 text messages a day![115]

Symptoms of 'text neck' include neck pain, headaches, shoulder pain and arm numbness and tingling.

Adults aren't immune to text neck and adult use of text messaging is on the increase, especially among parents with school age children. The small screen and keypad of mobile phones makes it far harder to maintain correct head and neck posture while texting than while typing on a laptop.

To avoid worsening forward head posture, try to limit the number of text messages you send. When texting or just looking at the screen of your mobile phone, hold it level with your eyes so you don't have to bend your neck. The same advice holds true for using other small hand-held devices.

Tablet Computers and Smart Phones for Internet Access

Unfortunately, the problem of forward head posture is only likely to escalate. People are increasingly turning to smart phones and tablet computers for browsing the internet, social media and answering emails and these types of small mobile devices are even less suitable for prolonged use than laptops or notebooks.

We have already seen how bending over a mobile phone puts a great deal of stress on your neck. The same is true for tablet computers, even though the larger screen makes them easier to read. Whether you hold the tablet in your hand, place it on your lap or on a table, or prop it up with its case, you will still have to bend your neck forwards to some extent to use it.

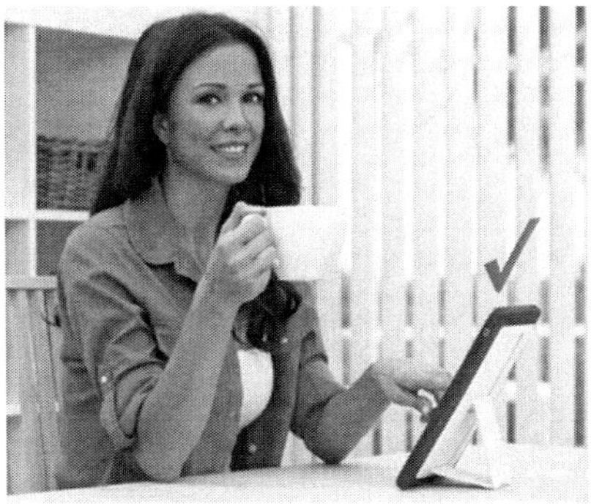

A recent study by the Harvard School Public Health[116] on a group of experienced tablet users confirmed just what we would expect:

- Tablets are worse for the neck than laptops or notebooks, regardless of how they are positioned.
- Postural stress is greatest when tablets are hand held or placed on the lap.
- It is best to place the tablet on a table or desk and use its case to tilt it upwards as far as possible – see the photo on the right. Even so, the screen height is still way too low.
- You need to take rests often – I recommend every 15 minutes.

Setting up Your Computer to Minimise Postural Stress

Maintaining correct sitting posture at the computer is a crucial part of decreasing the frequency of your headache attacks. Relatively minor changes in how you set up your computer workstation can make a world of difference.

In the past, your only option for changing the height of your desk was to use bricks or commercial height risers, but in recent years, height-adjustable desks have been more common and affordable, and are a better option for maintaining a good posture while working at a desk. Many workplaces now offer a couple of height adjustable desks that can be shared within the office. If you're looking for a budget height adjustable desk, manual adjustment, instead of electronic, will save you money.

While height adjustable desks are great for helping maintain good posture, they won't magically solve all your ergonomic problems. A height adjustable desk is not good if you are standing on your feet all day, placing all your weight through your joints. This will open another can of worms, such as knee and hip pain, varicose veins, calf pain and plantar fasciitis. For prolonged standing, consider a mat.

If you use a height adjustable desk, I suggest breaking up an eight hour working day into quarters – sit at an ergonomically sound desk for two hours then raise the desk and stand for two hours and repeat.

The guidelines on setting up your computer in this section assume that your computer is on a simple fixed height desk but that you have an office chair that has some adjustments available. If you use a height adjustable desk, the guidelines for the elbows, shoulders, wrists, head, eyes, keyboard and mouse remain the same except for when you are standing.

First you set up your chair in combination with your desk and then you adjust the position and height of your computer screen. If you use a laptop as your primary computer there are some extra steps. As discussed before, the best way to make sure you have a screen of the correct height is to connect the laptop to an external screen. You will also need to plug in an external keyboard and mouse. For using your laptop in other locations include a lightweight stand, external mouse and keyboard in your bag.

Apart from this, the procedure for setting up desktop and laptop computers to minimise postural stress is identical. Remember, fixing your workstation won't fix everything – you still need to keep a check on how you are holding your body. Any time you notice you are starting to slump down in your seat or project your head and neck forwards you need to correct this. Gradually your posture will improve.

It is also important to avoid sitting for too long and to learn how to recognise and counteract excessive tension in your neck and shoulder muscles.

What Does Ideal Computer Posture Look Like?

It's one thing to follow the guidelines for achieving good sitting posture at your computer workstation but another to know what it should look like. Searching the internet will not be very helpful. Most diagrams you are likely to find are complicated and many are either out-of-date or incorrect in one or more details.

The simple, correct overview of ideal computer posture in Figure 18.1 is a modification of an original image from the web page of Safety and Health at the University of Western Australia (used with permission). This web page is also a useful source of information about types of chairs and other office equipment for workstations.

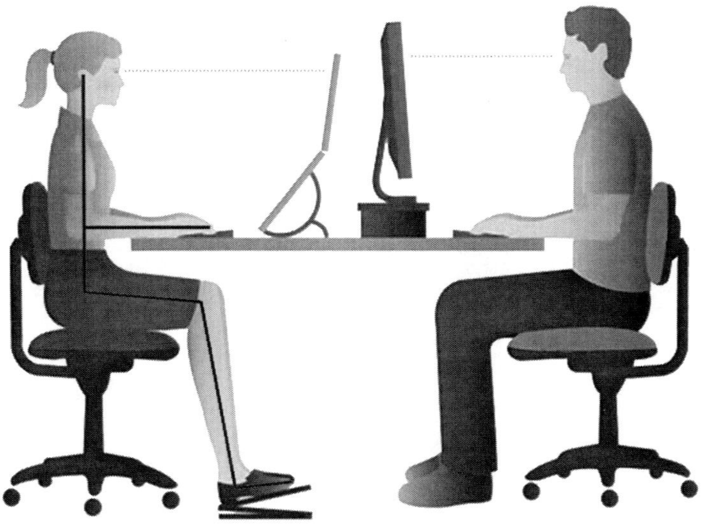

Figure 19.1 – Ideal posture at the computer

The boy and girl sitting opposite each other at the same desk are of different height and are using different types of computer. However they each have the top of the viewable part of their screen near eye level. (She is using a vertical laptop riser and he has a screen stand). Both also have good posture:

- A neutral spine with ear, shoulder and hip all in line
- The curve in their lower back supported by the back of the chair
- Relaxed shoulders, forearms parallel to the floor and wrists straight
- Thighs supported and approximately horizontal with a 90° angle at the knee
- Feet firmly supported (his on the floor, hers on a footrest) A foot-rest is only needed if the required chair height does not allow your feet to firmly touch the floor.

Setting up Your Chair

Whether your office chair is a top of the range model or a budget special, it still should be correctly adjusted to fit your body so you'll be able to sit with good posture in front of your computer.

The screen shot below shows a real-life example of what this should look like. It comes from an interactive guide on the web site of the Department of Labor and Industries, Washington State, which deals with how to set up your computer workstation. This guide is well worth consulting, especially if you are setting up your computer at home. It provides detailed advice on chair adjustment, workstation layout, keyboard and mouse placement, and monitor and document placement.

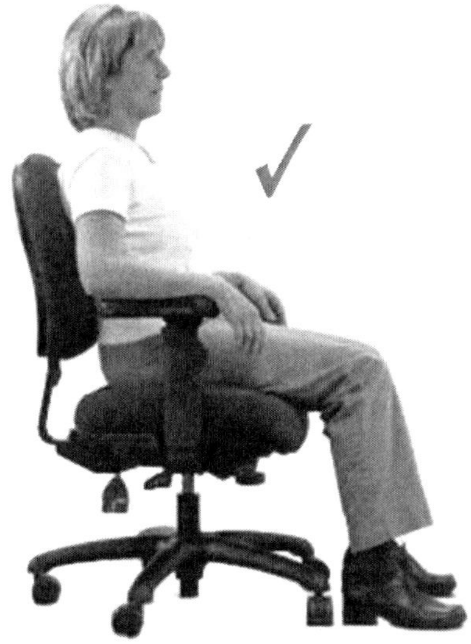

Here are some basic instructions on adjusting your chair. Your chair may not have all the adjustments mentioned – the most important are seat height followed by backrest tilt and height.

- Sit up tall in your chair with your bottom back as far as it will go on the seat and lean against the backrest.
- Adjust the seat height. When the height is set correctly, both feet should rest comfortably flat on the floor. Your thighs should be horizontal, with your knees at the same level as or slightly lower than your hips as shown.
- If necessary, adjust the seat tilt. The seat should be level or else tilt downward very slightly to ease any pressure under your thighs.
- Adjust the backrest tilt so that you are reclining slightly backwards.
- Alter the backrest height so that your lumbar spine is properly supported. The back-rest should also support your mid back.
- Adjust the depth of the seat – it should be deep enough so that it supports your thighs properly but still leaves a small gap behind your knees.

Some chairs allow you to vary the width of the lumbar support region as well as its height. If the amount of lumbar support is not sufficient, experiment with positioning a lumbar roll in the curve of your lower back. For most people and most reasonable quality office chairs, this shouldn't be needed.

If your chair has armrests these should provide comfortable support for your arms and shoulders. Many better quality office chairs have multiple armrest adjustments but in cheaper chairs they are usually fixed. If the armrests don't feel comfortable, remove them.

Ensuring Your Keyboard is at the Correct Height

Your keyboard needs to be at the correct height so you can keep your shoulders relaxed and your wrists straight while typing. The photo shows what your wrists should look like.

The following instructions will assume your keyboard is on a desk or table without any form of built-in height adjustment. This is what most people have at home and it is also common in the workplace.

First make sure you can move your chair in close to the desk so your stomach is nearly against the edge. If you can't do this there is a problem with your furniture. There should be ample room for your knees under the desk. If you can't make room under your desk for your knees, you need to change desks.

If you have already tried adjusting the armrests on your chair, but they are still stopping you from moving close to your desk, you should remove them.

Now you're sitting close to your desk, check your keyboard is at the correct height. You should have your elbows at desk height and your forearms and wrists parallel to the floor (see Figure 18.1). This position puts the least stress on your upper body and wrists when you are typing. It also lets you rest your hands and wrists flat on the desk beside your keyboard.

If your desk is too high, your forearms will be bent upwards. If this is the case, you should raise the height of your chair. If your feet don't reach the floor, you will need a footrest, like the girl in Figure 18.1. If your desk is too low, your forearms will be bent downwards, in which case, you might be able to raise the desk surface sufficiently by putting risers under the legs as discussed above.

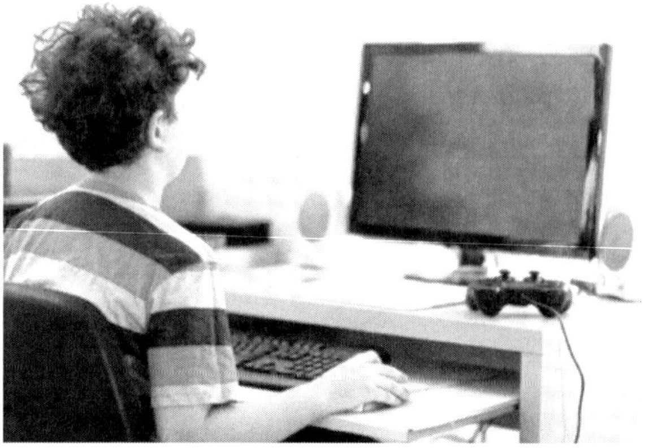

The boy in the photo has his keyboard too high. Notice his elbows are below the height of his keyboard and his forearms are bent upwards. He should first check that his chair has been correctly adjusted. If his keyboard is still too high, there may be room for him to lower his keyboard tray. Otherwise he will need to raise his chair and use a footrest to support his feet.

Positioning Your Keyboard and Mouse

Three general guidelines are:

- Place the keyboard close to the front edge of the desk – it should feel comfortable. You should make sure you are not reaching forward with your arms or bending forward with your upper body to reach the keys.
- Position the keyboard so that the section you use most frequently is aligned with the centre of your body. Don't hit the keys too hard – the average user hits them four times harder than necessary.
- Place your mouse close to the keyboard.

It's hard to see both the keyboard and screen at the same time. Moving your head to look between the keyboard and the screen is a major cause of strain to neck and shoulder muscles. The only real way to eliminate this problem is to learn to touch type so you don't need to look at the keys. Failing this, you can at least minimise the strain if you place the keyboard a little further back from the edge of the desk and keep your neck long and your chin slightly tucked in when you look down.

Using the mouse is an important cause of muscular tension all the way from your hand to your shoulder and neck. There are many different types of mouse you can buy and some may suit your hand better than others, but just modifying the way you use the mouse will help.

- Make sure you are resting your forearm on the desk when using the mouse.
- Let go of the mouse! Don't continue to grip the mouse when you're not using it.

- Train yourself to use the mouse with either hand. When you use the mouse with your left hand your arm is closer to your body, you don't have to reach past the number pad.
- Learn some keyboard shortcuts to lessen the need to use the mouse.
- Watch out for leaning to one side when using the mouse – keep your torso balanced.

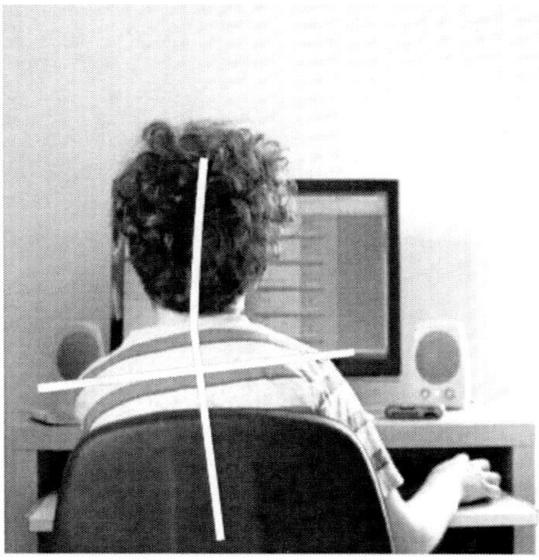

In the photo the young boy's left shoulder is much lower than his right. His back leans to the left and his neck is bent to the right to compensate.

Much of the problem is due to him leaning on his left arm which he has crossed over in front of his body. People often sit like this when using the mouse for browsing the internet.

Setting up Your Computer Screen and Documents

- Distance – place your screen at least one arm's length from your seated position, directly in front of you.
- Position – make sure your head is not turned to one side when you are looking at your screen. Like your keyboard, your screen, should be aligned with the centre of your body.
- Make sure you are sitting square on to your desk with your shoulders level.
- Before you adjust the height of your screen, check that your head is lightly balanced on the top of your neck and your chin is level. Sit tall in your chair, with your neck long and shut your eyes. Make little movements with your head to let your neck muscles relax and stop in the position where you feel most comfortable and the least strain. Open your eyes and continue.
- Height – the top of your screen should be close to eye level when you are sitting upright at your desk (refer again to Figure 18.1).
- The screen should not be too low or you will need to bend your neck forward to see it. If you need to raise the screen, use a flat screen stand, or a book, or both.

With a laptop use a vertical riser. The screen should not be too high either, as then you will have to tilt your head upwards to see it. The main thing is to check that you can view your entire screen by moving your eyes while keeping your head level and your neck and shoulders relaxed. If you wear bifocals or progressive lenses your screen will need to be lower than average. If your screen is large it will probably need to be higher.

- Set your computer to display a font that is easily readable and large enough that you don't have to strain your eyes.
- If necessary, move the screen a little closer so you can see it clearly. It is important to avoid poking your head forward to read the screen. It often occurs out of habit but it's sometimes because the screen is too far away. The screen shouldn't be too close either as this adds to problems with eye strain.
- Use a document stand to hold any papers you need to read while typing. If your papers are on your desk you will need to keep looking down or sideways or both to read them. If possible, place the document stand directly in front of you between the keyboard and the screen. If there isn't enough space here, put it next to the screen on the side of your dominant eye (see below). Otherwise you will be turning your head to read without realising.
- Place your telephone within easy reach so you don't have to keep twisting your body to get to it.
- Don't cradle the handset between your shoulder and ear – this causes muscular trigger points in the upper part of the trapezius muscle. Use a headset or a speaker phone instead.

Find Your Dominant Eye

Once you know which eye is your dominant eye, it makes sense to place all documents on the same side as your dominant eye. If you place documents on the same side as your weaker eye, your eyesight will begin to fatigue, causing you to lean forwards to read the documents, which causes forward head posture.

Your dominant eye has no connection to whether you are right or left-handed. It's the eye you automatically use when looking through a telescope or a camera viewfinder.

To determine which eye is dominant, go through the following procedure:

- Make a small circle with your thumb and forefinger and hold it about 45 cm (18 inches) in front of your eyes
- With both eyes open, look through the circle and focus on a small distant object such as a doorknob or light switch
- Close your left eye. With your right eye open, if the object remains centred in the circle you are right eye dominant
- To check the first test, repeat, this time closing your right eye. If you are right eye dominant, the object will appear to jump outside the circle
- Similarly for left eye dominance, the object will stay centred with your left eye open and jump outside the circle when it is closed.

General Guidelines for Good Sitting Posture – A Reminder

Having set up your chair, keyboard and screen, once you have been using it for 30 minutes or so do a quick check on your sitting posture.

- Is your bottom right back in your chair?
- Are you sitting square on to your desk with your shoulders level?
- Are you sitting in close to your desk?
- Are your hands and wrists relaxed?
- Is your body weight evenly distributed on both feet? Make sure your legs are not crossed or wrapped around the legs of the chair.
- Is your lumbar spine well supported, using a lumbar roll if necessary?
- Is your mid back resting against the back of the chair?
- Are your shoulders and neck relaxed?
- Check you are not projecting your head and neck. Make sure your chin is level and facing forward and your jaw is relaxed.

Glasses and Computer Use

Most people who spend more than two hours on a computer each day suffer problems with their vision. Any work performed close up puts extra demands on our eye muscles compared with looking into the distance.

Our eyes have to work even harder to focus on characters on the screen than on the printed page, causing the muscles responsible to tire more quickly. Eyes commonly feel tired, burning, aching, dry and sensitive to light. Difficulty focussing, including temporary inability to focus on distant objects, blurred vision and double vision are also common. So are headaches.

If you are having vision problems or just finding it more difficult to see the screen as clearly as you used to, you should have your eyes checked. You may need glasses – some people only need glasses for the computer. If you already wear glasses your prescription may need updating.

Although it adds to the expense, it is a good idea to get glasses especially designed for computer use, in addition to your regular glasses. Reading glasses are not suitable for computer use as they focus much too close.

Computer glasses need to be able to focus at arm's length, which is much further than the usual reading distance. Although you can see the screen if you wear bifocal or multifocal glasses, your usual prescription is not suitable for long-term use. These types of glasses provide little vision correction at the typical screen distance and so contribute to eyestrain. They also have a narrow field of view which forces you to tilt your head back and to move it from side to side to see clearly, straining neck and shoulder muscles.

Tips for Minimising Eye Strain

- Tilt the top of the screen slightly backwards to eliminate reflections or glare and to make it easier to read if you wear glasses.
- Install an anti-glare screen filter.
- Close curtains or blinds to prevent glare and reflections from bright outside light. If possible, position your screen so that windows are to the side of it, not in front or behind.
- Keep overall lighting at a moderate level. Many offices are too bright causing glare. However lighting levels should not be too dim. Too much contrast between the brightness of your screen and darker surroundings will cause eye strain through your peripheral vision.
- Alter the brightness and contrast settings on your screen. Reduce the brightness of your screen to a similar level to that of your surroundings. Increase the contrast to make it easier to distinguish the characters from the background.

The following eye exercises should be done regularly throughout the day:

- Look away from your screen and focus on something in the distance
- Change focus from a distant to a near object and back several times
- Rest your eyes by covering them with your palms
- Blink a lot.

Don't Forget Your Home Computer

Once you've set up your computer at work, it's important to set up your home computer. I regularly treat patients for headaches, neck and back pain caused by bending for hours over laptops set up on a corner of the kitchen or dining room table, kitchen bench or breakfast bar.

Most of these surfaces are not the correct height for typing – they're usually too high. Coffee tables on the other hand are way too low. To make matters worse, sometimes the person concerned cannot even to fit their knees underneath. Instead they are forced to sit sideways while twisting their entire upper body around to type.

And all of this is in addition to the postural strain inherent in the design of the laptop.

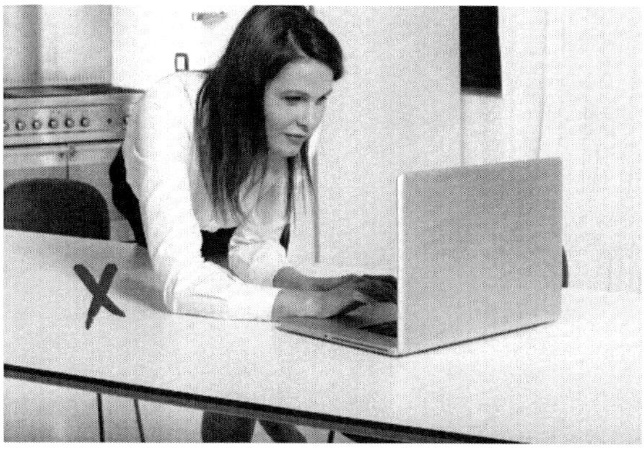

You need to set up a computer workstation somewhere in your home with a desk, an adjustable chair and good lighting. If you use a laptop, put it on a laptop stand or preferably connect it to an external screen, just as in your office. These improvements can help reduce the number of headaches you suffer, especially if you use your home computer regularly.

Key Points

- Laptops, mobile phones and tablet computers are the enemies of good posture.
- Whether it is a computer monitor, laptop, tablet or mobile phone, getting the screen height right is the priority. It is essential that you are able to see the screen without bending your neck.
- Don't stand all day while using a height adjustable desk. Lower the desk and sit at an ergonomically sound desk as well.
- Eye strain is also a consideration when you are setting up your work station.
- Correct computer and laptop use is often overlooked when not at work. You need to take care in setting up your home computers to minimise the impact on your posture.

20

Stress

We often associate stress with feeling overloaded, under pressure, tense, uptight, nervous or worried, but stress is more than just these feelings. Scientifically, stress is the body's normal physical, mental and emotional response to a stressor. A stressor is a situation or event which places demands on us that we feel we cannot meet and which we regard as a threat to our wellbeing.

Whenever we sense danger, real or imagined, an automatic emergency survival mechanism known as the 'fight-or-flight' reaction kicks in to protect us. Our sympathetic nervous system goes into over-drive and our blood-stream is flooded with stress hormones, particularly adrenaline, noradrenaline and cortisol. This leads to changes which prepare our body to fight the danger or run away from it as fast as we can.

- We feel fearful or anxious.
- Heart rate and blood pressure rise.
- Breathing becomes more rapid and shallow.
- Sweating increases.
- Blood is re-routed from less essential areas – our extremities, skin and digestive organs – towards the brain, heart and large muscles. (The skin and the fingers and feet will feel cold and clammy to the touch. We will be aware of our heart pounding and 'butterflies in the stomach').
- We become more mentally alert and more sensitive to sights and sounds in our environment.
- Muscles become tense to prepare for action.
- We get a brief energy surge as glucose is released from liver stores into the blood-stream.
- The immune system and tissue growth and repair are suppressed.

Once the threat has passed, the parasympathetic nervous system takes over. Levels of stress hormones and bodily reactions gradually return to normal and we start to calm down. This is known as the relaxation or 'rest-and-digest' response.

However, if the threat is repeated or prolonged, stress hormones stay elevated, which can have significant effects on our physical and mental health. Too much cortisol depletes the body's energy stores, causes muscle wasting and weakens the immune system. We become more vulnerable to infection and are at increased risk of developing high blood pressure, heart disease and diabetes. It can also increase the risk of headaches.

How Stress Contributes to Headaches

The important role that stress plays in provoking both tension headaches and migraines is widely recognised.[117] Reducing your stress levels is one of the most effective ways of preventing headaches, and reducing the severity of any headache attacks that do occur.

Stress is a key factor in the Integrated Headache Model, where emotional stress acts like a 'pain volume control', intensifying or reducing the impact of the sum of pain signals from musculoskeletal and neurovascular sources. Suppose both musculoskeletal and neurovascular pain don't alter. As stress levels increase the total pain signal reaching the pain relay centre will increase. At a certain level, we will start to experience a mild headache. As stress levels increase further the headache will become more severe.

Emotional stress contributes to headaches in other ways, including:

- Altering blood flow to and within the brain – mental stress causes the carotid artery to dilate and blood flow to the meninges to increase118
- Instigating the release of histamine, a potent vasodilator and inflammatory substance
- Increasing musculoskeletal pain by making muscular trigger points more painful and increasing muscle tension
- Instigating teeth clenching and grinding, often during sleep.

On-going emotional stress can lower your headache threshold, making headache attacks more likely. For example, some headache sufferers will recall that their headaches first began or became much more frequent during a particularly stressful period of their lives.

Specific short-term stressful episodes may trigger a headache attack or worsen an existing headache. Stress can also be a hidden trigger for headaches. In early studies on migraine, it was noted that stress caused the temporal artery to dilate up to three days in advance of an attack, but stress on the day of the attack had no effect on the temporal artery. In other words, a migraine attack can be due to a three to four-day delayed effect of stress.[119,120]

A recent study, unrelated to headache, confirmed that mental stress causes the carotid artery to dilate in healthy volunteers.[121] Subjects were studied before and after short tests, including reading, arithmetic and anger recall. Dilation of the carotid artery was accompanied by increased blood flow in the main artery that supplies the meninges (the three membranes that line the skull and vertebral canal and enclose the brain and spinal cord.)

This delayed effect of stress on the carotid artery could explain why many people experience headache and migraine pain on the weekend or when they go on holidays. If you think about it, we're often stressed in preparation for a holiday or gearing up for the weekend. Working to meet a deadline, travelling more in traffic, juggling a budget, extra shopping and organisation – all of this happens in the days leading up to period of relaxation. When you stop, although you are resting and doing everything 'right', you get hit with a headache, which may well be the effect of stress from earlier in the week. A headache diary will help determine if a stress headache always happens on a day off, or is just more memorable for having ruined the start of a holiday.

And of course, the headache experience itself can be a source of stress. If this stress is not properly handled, it is easy to get stuck in a self-perpetuating cycle of more stress and more headaches that impacts on your health and quality of life.

Recognising the Symptoms of Stress and Stress Overload

Stress which is long term, repeated or severe can overwhelm our ability to cope and seriously affect our health and wellbeing, as well as our relationships, work and general enjoyment of life. If we have been under stress for a long time, it may start to feel familiar, even normal.

When people feel overloaded by stress, they normally respond in one of three ways that parallel the fight, flight and freeze responses of animals when under threat:

- They become angry, and are often agitated, overly emotional, restless and unable to sit still.
- They withdraw and distance themselves. They tend to shut down, and often show very little energy or emotion.
- They freeze under pressure and feel like they can't do anything. They look paralysed, but under the surface they are extremely agitated.

If you regularly respond to stressful situations in one of the three ways described, then it's important to reduce your stress levels. Self-help techniques like those outlined in this chapter will assist, however they may not be enough. You may need to seek professional help from a qualified psychologist or counsellor.

If you can, it's best to act in the early stages to prevent stress overload. To do this, you need to learn how to recognise the symptoms of stress. There are many different symptoms of stress that affect our physical body, our emotions, cognitive (thinking) processes and behaviour. Everyone experiences stress differently. The lists on the following page give some of the common symptoms. The more you notice, the closer you might be to stress overload.

Please note: The symptoms of stress can also be caused by various medical or psychological conditions that require treatment. If you're experiencing any of the warning signs of stress, don't assume that your symptoms are just due to stress, you should have them evaluated by a doctor.

Some Common Symptoms of Stress – Part 1

Physical	Emotional
Muscle tension	Feeling moody, tearful
Headaches	Anger, irritability, short temper
Neck, shoulder and back pain	Agitation, restlessness, inability to relax
Excessive tiredness, fatigue	Impatience
Shortness of breath	Frustration
Chest pain, heart palpitations	Resentment
Difficulty sleeping	Nervousness, anxiety
Diarrhoea or constipation	Depression or general unhappiness
Upset stomach, abdominal pain, nausea	Sudden attacks of panic
Urinary problems	Feeling lonely or isolated
Missed periods	Lack of motivation or focus
Loss of appetite	Feeling overwhelmed and out of control
Loss of sex drive	Apathy
Dizziness	
Frequent colds	
Skin problems, e.g. eczema	
Cold hands and feet	

Some Common Symptoms of Stress – Part 2

Cognitive (Thinking)	Behavioural
Memory problems	Jaw clenching, teeth grinding
Inability to concentrate	Crying spells
Short attention span	Nervous habits (e.g. nail biting, pacing)
Poor judgment	Being argumentative, bossy, inflexible
Indecisiveness	Over-reacting to petty annoyances
Seeing only the negative	Using alcohol, cigarettes, drugs to relax*
Anxious or racing thoughts	Comfort eating*
Easily confused, disorganised	Over-eating or under-eating*
Misinterpreting what people tell you	Sleeping too much*
Taking things personally	Neglecting responsibilities*
Constant worrying	Procrastinating*
Continuing to re-run the same thoughts	Isolating yourself from others*
Thoughts of escaping, running away	Taking inappropriate risks*
Less interest in previous leisure activities	Excessive gambling or impulse buying*
	Finding excuses to avoid going to work*
	Working long hours to delay going home*
	Zoning out for hours in front of the TV*

* Some behaviours, such as those marked with an * in the table, represent unproductive, unhealthy ways of coping with stress. Reducing stress by using these strategies has only short-term benefits as in time, these behaviours often become major stressors in their own right.

Common Stressors

It's important to identify your personal stressors so you can start to work out what to do about them. Just having a plan can give you a greater sense of control over how you feel, which will reduce stress.

Sometimes there are practical solutions which eliminate some stressful situations, or at least reduce our exposure to them. If we can't change the situation, we can at least change our reaction to it by altering the way we think about it. We can also calm ourselves with various relaxation techniques when (or preferably before) we encounter it.

And if we look after ourselves, making time for rest and leisure, we will be better able to adjust to life changing events and handle the stress of daily hassles.

External Stressors

Although people differ greatly in what they find stressful, there are several situations and events that most people consistently report are significant sources of stress. Researchers who study the negative effects of stress on physical and mental health group these stressors into three broad categories:

- Catastrophes, such as floods, storms, car accidents, physical assault
- Significant life events[122,123], which can be both positive and negative – starting a new job, birth of a baby, divorce, death of a partner
- Daily hassles[124,125], traffic jams, arguments with co-workers or neighbours, losing your keys, not having enough money to cover regular bills.

Internal Stressors

Not all stress is caused by external events and situations. Some is self-generated by our thoughts, beliefs (rules for living), fears, personality traits and habitual behaviour patterns. Internal stressors can include:

- Chronic worrying
- All-or-nothing thinking
- Rigid, inflexible thinking
- Negative self-talk
- Pessimistic outlook, focussing more attention on negative events and outcomes than on positive ones
- Unrealistic or perfectionist expectations. (Note that a perfectionist is not the same as a high achiever. A high achiever is happy if they do their best and get a good result. For a perfectionist, nothing less than perfect will do.)

- Trying too hard to please everybody, failing to be assertive, inability to say no, putting your own needs last
- Procrastination and/or failing to plan
- Fears, e.g. of flying, heights, public speaking.

Managing Stress

For stressors, you can do something about, the best strategy is to target and remove the root cause of stress, rather than to try and cope with its effects. This is known as problem-focused coping. If you check your list of stressors, you'll probably recognise certain daily hassles that fit into this category. For example, if you're always misplacing your keys, make a designated place in clear view, where you can train yourself to always leave your keys.

Cognitive Behavioural Therapy

When we can't change the situation, we can change the way we think about it. Cognitive Behavioural Therapy (CBT) is a common type of therapy which helps you become aware of inaccurate or negative thinking, and to challenge that thinking so you can respond to events in a more effective way.

In addition to its role in stress management, CBT has been used to treat a wide range of conditions including severe anxiety, phobias, depression, addiction and chronic pain. It is one of several psychological methods that are used to prevent and stop headaches and to treat headache pain. The most useful source of professional help for changing thought patterns and self-talk is a psychologist who practices CBT.

The Power of Relaxation

The body's stress (fight-or-flight) response is automatic, but we can intentionally replace it with the relaxation (rest-and-digest) response. All the bodily changes caused by the stress response are reversed: heart rate slows, blood pressure falls, breathing slows and muscles relax. Fingers and feet get warmer as blood flow returns to more normal patterns. Our mind also becomes calmer as feelings of fear and anxiety subside. Other unpleasant symptoms, such as our heart pounding in our throat and our stomach tying itself in knots, gradually subside.

A range of formal techniques can be used to initiate the body's relaxation response. Most of these techniques take some time to learn, and, to be effective, they need to be practiced regularly, preferably daily.

By far the simplest and the most important technique to master is slow, relaxed diaphragmatic (belly) breathing. It also forms the starting point for many other relaxation techniques. There are also lots of informal, common sense ways of 'turning down' the body's stress response which are easy to apply in our everyday lives. You will probably find some of these techniques suit you better than others.

These methods, both formal and informal, are discussed below. Whilst they are great for lowering stress when you feel it, it's also important to be proactive, not just wait until something happens. A selection of the same methods can help reduce our overall levels of stress before they get too high.

Initiating the Body's Relaxation Response

Relaxed Diaphragmatic Breathing

We've already discussed relaxed diaphragmatic breathing, so this is just a recap on the important points here:

- Your belly must be relaxed
- Breathe in and out slowly through your nose. (One commonly recommended timing is to breathe in for 4 seconds, hold for 2 seconds and breathe out for 6 seconds.)
- Your belly should move outwards as you breathe in and move inwards when you breathe out. These movements should be relaxed, not forced or exaggerated.
- Your chest shouldn't move very much
- It is very important to prolong the exhalation phase. Only then does the brain signal the body to replace the stress response with the relaxation response. Ideally exhalation should take one and half to two times as long as inhalation. If necessary, breathe out through pursed lips to slow down the exhalation.

You are likely to encounter many minor variations on these instructions. These include different timings for each breath in and out, whether you should hold your breath for a short time before you exhale, pause for a moment before you inhale again and whether you should breathe out through your nose or your mouth.

Provided you are following the general guidelines in the dot points above, I think these types of details are less important than how you feel. You should start to feel some sense of relaxation. The most important thing is to be comfortable with whatever method you are following. If you feel anxious when holding your breath, don't do it as part of your practice. It will be more relaxing if you can turn your focus to something like the air flowing in and out of your nostrils or your belly rising and falling whenever distracting thoughts come into your mind, as they inevitably will. If you can do this, you are on your way to learning how to meditate.

Listening to Calming Music

Listening to calming music has a relaxing effect on body and mind that can be quite profound.[126] It has also been shown to reduce pain.[127] You can very easily combine it with relaxed diaphragmatic breathing. Other relaxation methods may also incorporate calming music. These include meditation, where it helps prevent our thoughts from wandering back into stressful or negative patterns.

But just what is calming music? After all, individual tastes in music differ widely, as do responses to it. Calming music is sometimes called sedative music to distinguish it from music intended to be stimulating.

It needs to have a slow underlying tempo (around or below 80 beats per minute) that stays steady. The melody should be free of sudden changes in pitch and without extreme high or low notes. The volume should also be constant. It is usually best to avoid vocals as these can be distracting, and certain words in the lyrics may have unwanted emotional effects that you didn't anticipate.

Certain pieces of classical music and easy listening music fit these requirements. Even if you don't normally listen to these types of music it may be worth giving them a trial when trying to find the most calming type of music for you.

Music promoted for relaxation and meditation may also be suitable. This is typically slow paced, modern, instrumental music. It often includes sounds from nature, such as the sound of water running in a mountain stream or birdsong, to conjure up peaceful, relaxing images. This type of music doesn't work for everyone. Some people find the lack of structure unsettling or even irritating.

If you are keen to follow this strategy, you might consider making an appointment with a music therapist. A music therapist is a university-trained allied health professional, who can help you select music that you will find relaxing. They will consider the sorts of music you like. A music therapist can also produce a playlist for you which includes suitable background music together with spoken instructions for muscle relaxation of different types or meditation. Each track may conclude with an extended period of music so you can prolong the relaxation session.

Progressive Muscle Relaxation

Progressive muscle relaxation is a two-stage process. You slowly tense and then relax each muscle group, while you focus on the sensations that accompany tension and relaxation. This helps you learn what tensed and relaxed muscles feel like in different parts of the body. You can then identify when and where you feel muscle tension when you are in a stressful situation.

Progressive muscle relaxation starts with relaxed diaphragmatic breathing. You then systematically tense and relax the different muscle groups of your body, typically beginning at your feet and working your way up to your face. With practice, you can relax these tense muscles on command. As the muscles relax, the brain tells the body to initiate the relaxation response.

Although you can learn to do progressive muscle relaxation on your own, it is a lot easier if you follow spoken instructions, preferably from a therapist or from a self-help recording. Most therapists will make you a recording so you can practice at home. If you want to get started straight away, you can make your own recording. There are lots of free examples of progressive muscle relaxation scripts online.

Once you have been practising progressive muscle relaxation for a couple of weeks and have become familiar with it, you can start to practice a shortened version. This tenses and relaxes larger groups of muscles at the same time.

When doing this shortened version, it can be helpful to say a certain cue word or phrase to yourself as you slowly exhale, such as 'relax', 'let go', 'peace', 'calm', etc. Gradually your mind will associate this word or phrase with a relaxed state. Eventually, just saying this cue word when you feel stressed can make you feel calmer.

Passive Progressive (Body Scan) Relaxation

Once you've learnt to recognise what tense and relaxed muscles feel like, and are reasonably confident with the progressive muscle relaxation technique, you may want to move on to relaxing your muscles without tensing them first.

In fact, if you have a lot of muscle tension, it might even be better to start with this method, as tightening muscles that are already tight can cause them to cramp.

As before, start with relaxed diaphragmatic breathing. You continue to breathe slowly, deeply and steadily as you progressively scan each muscle group looking for the areas of muscle tension in your body. When you notice any tension, you imagine the tension letting go as you exhale, perhaps while saying your cue word.

It is common to start with your scalp and face, trying to imagine relaxation flowing downwards through your body with each breath out. Again it is a lot easier to follow spoken instructions from a therapist or CD.

Spoken instruction often includes a variety of suggestions to help you stay focused and assist the relaxation process, such as feeling the weight of your feet on the floor, your back sinking into the chair or your arms becoming warm and heavy.

Guided Imagery for Relaxation

Guided imagery, or visualisation, is a series of thoughts and suggestions designed to help your imagination transport you to a place which is special for you, a place where you feel calm, peaceful and relaxed.

For some people, this could be lying on a tropical beach, sitting beside a waterfall in the forest, floating on an air mattress in a pool, or sitting beside an open fire while the cold rain beats at the windows.

As usual, you begin with slow diaphragmatic breathing. Once you have begun to relax, you imagine you are in your special place. Use not only your visual sense, but also your sense of taste, touch, smell, and sound to recreate the scene in your own mind as vividly as possible. With practice your body will respond as if you are there.

For example, in the forest scene, you not only see the many shades of green, you hear the splash of the waterfall, the wind rustling the leaves of the trees, and the songs of different birds. You smell the wet earth, taste the fine spray of the waterfall on your tongue and feel the temperature around you.

You can learn to visualise your relaxing place on your own in silence or while listening to calming music. However, initially it is probably easiest for a therapist (or a CD made by the therapist for home practice) to help guide you through the process.

You can also purchase a commercial CD. However, it's important you feel safe and none of the images used inadvertently cause you stress. For example, if you can't swim, imagining floating in a pool would be stressful.

To be able to imagine you are in a calm relaxing place is a very useful skill to be able to call on quickly when you are in the middle of a stressful situation. If you sometimes think, 'I wish I was out of here', then you can be, without even leaving the room.

Meditation for Relaxation

Most of us spend a major part of each day submerged in an overload of information, busily doing things whilst on autopilot. We pay little attention to our thoughts, emotions or what is happening around us from one moment to the next. While our minds are off wandering, we're not present in our lives.

We may miss the beautiful sunset, fail to notice what our body is telling us about the tension in our jaw muscles, or inadvertently slip into fruitless worrying about future events, many of which we can do nothing about.

Meditation helps us become aware of our transient thoughts and emotions as they come and go but without getting caught up in them. It's a way of training our thoughts so we can gain better control over them and focus our attention on whatever we choose, free of distraction.

This mental focus combined with diaphragmatic breathing has a calming effect on body and mind. Even a five-minute mini meditation will be beneficial.

There are many different forms of meditation and types of meditation practice. In fact, there are so many, it's difficult to come up with an all-encompassing definition of meditation or to make sense of the confusing variety of approaches. This is partly due to meditation's long history. It has been practiced for thousands of years by people from many different cultures, usually as a way of finding inner peace.

Meditation is still an important spiritual practice in many religious traditions around the world. Meditation practices can be as varied as the contemplation of Christian meditation, the Buddhist practice of sitting meditation and emptying the mind of thoughts, and the whirling of the Sufi dervishes.

These days, meditation is part of complementary medicine and is used as a method of psychological treatment. Meditation can be practiced by anyone (irrespective of their religious or cultural background) to relieve stress and pain and improve mental and physical health.

Most meditation courses, especially those taught by psychologists, make no mention of religion or spiritual values. If the spiritual aspects of meditation are important to you, it should be possible find a suitable course. Your local community information office or religious centre is probably the best place to go for advice. If you don't want to take a course, you will find instructions for different types of meditation in books, on the web and on CDs.

Some people like to be still while they meditate, but others prefer to be moving or doing some type of repetitive movement activity, accompanied, where possible, by relaxed diaphragmatic breathing. When their thoughts wander, it is the repetitive movement they return to.

Some suitable movement activities for meditation include walking, swimming, jogging and simple dance steps. The activity doesn't have to be aerobic. Just going for a gentle stroll in nature and focusing on the sights, smells and sounds around you, letting any distracting thoughts pass by, can be an effective form of meditation and stress reduction.

Some sorts of repetitive tasks can become mini meditations, provided you pay attention to them and perform them in a slow rhythmic manner. You also need to do relaxed diaphragmatic breathing. Examples include the circular movements you make when stirring a pot of soup or polishing the car, or the to-and-fro movements of vacuuming. Even knitting has been suggested as a meditation activity!

Biofeedback

Biofeedback is not itself a relaxation method. It is an instrumental teaching method to help you learn various relaxation methods discussed above more effectively.

It wasn't until the 1960s that scientists realised we can exert some control over the bodily reactions involved in the stress response. Before that, these reactions were thought to be completely automatic.

Since then, various electronic devices have been developed which can continuously monitor a range of bodily reactions. These give immediate feedback about how stressed you are and how much progress you are making in becoming more relaxed.

The most commonly monitored parameters are:

- Heart rate (shown in the photo)
- Blood pressure
- Muscle tension
- Skin temperature.

Signals from sensors on the skin (specific to the parameter being measured) are converted into a simple audio or visual form that is easy to detect. This could be a series of beeps, a sound of varying pitch, flashes of light or a simple varying display on a screen.

During a biofeedback session, a therapist will guide you through relaxation methods, such as progressive muscle relaxation or visualisation, which you will also be expected to practice at home.

Suppose your aim is to reduce muscle tension. Sensors will detect electrical signals from your muscles. The two frontalis muscles in the middle of the forehead are the muscles most commonly monitored. They are highly responsive to stress. As your muscles relax, the beeps, flashes of light, or other feedback will slow down. With sufficient practice, you will learn to relax your muscles without the assistance of the equipment.

Biofeedback provides a very convincing demonstration of just how quickly a stressful thought can increase muscle tension or other bodily responses to stress and why we can't consider the brain and body separately. Biofeedback is particularly useful for people who find it hard to recognise that they are stressed, or whether various relaxation procedures are effective or not. Normally about ten sessions are required to become proficient.

Cognitive Methods and Relaxation to Prevent, Abort and Relieve Headaches

For almost 40 years a variety of mind-body techniques have been extensively used in preventing headaches, particularly migraines.[128]

Current clinical practice guidelines to prevent both tension headaches and migraines recommend the following techniques:[129]

- Cognitive Behavioural Therapy (CBT) (as related to headaches)
- Biofeedback to reduce muscle tension
- Relaxation methods

For migraines, the guidelines additionally recommend biofeedback to raise finger temperature. This technique can also be used to abort a migraine in its early stages. Migraine sufferers typically have colder hands and feet than those who don't get migraines, even between attacks.

Stress causes the temperature of our extremities to drop as blood is re-routed towards the brain, heart and large muscles. The blood vessels of migraine sufferers are particularly reactive to stress and the temperature drop is larger than usual. Noticing that hands and feet are unusually cold is a common warning sign that a migraine attack is approaching.

If you are a migraine sufferer you can make your own crude finger warming biofeedback device for use at home. All you need to do is to tape a thermometer to the index finger of your dominant hand and record the temperature before and after you do each relaxation session.

These simple measurements can be useful to supplement the instantaneous temperature feedback you get in the therapist's office. It generally takes more practice sessions (and hence costs more) to learn finger warming than muscle relaxation.

Relaxation and biofeedback reduce the body's physical responses to stress which may provoke a headache attack, such as increased muscle tension and blood flow changes.

CBT counteracts stress generating beliefs and the self-talk which follows and hence reduces the size of the initial stress response. It also helps overcome counter-productive behaviour that is likely to make headaches occur more often.

Relaxation and CBT are more effective in preventing headaches if used together, as many headache researchers advise.

Relaxation (preferably learnt through biofeedback so you know it is having the desired effect) is best practised daily. Try also to be attuned to any negative automatic thoughts about headaches as they come into your mind and replace them with the positive alternatives that you have developed.

If you are keeping records, I think you will be pleasantly surprised by the reduction in frequency and severity of your headache attacks.

Relaxation and CBT can also be used as required to stop an impending headache and to ease headache pain. Stress is well known to make any sort of pain worse. The pain and disability caused by headaches are themselves important stressors which can precipitate a headache attack.

It's possible to get stuck in an escalating cycle of more pain and more headaches, which will affect your relationships, work and quality of life. Relaxation and CBT are two powerful tools to help you break free of this cycle. Knowing there are actions you can take to regain some control over your headaches, rather than being at their mercy, will allow you to cope better with the stress that headaches cause.

CBT can also treat the fear of headache pain that can lead some people to take pain-killers in case they get a headache. As we have seen, this is a fast track towards a developing medication overuse headache on top of their original headache.

Learning to cope with the fear rather than escaping from it will help you avoid this danger.

Active Ways to Reduce Stress

Exercise

Regular aerobic exercise is a very effective way of lowering stress levels. In our past, the stress response provided our muscles with extra energy so we could flee from a predator or fight an intruder.

In the modern world, these responses are seldom appropriate, but we are still left like a coiled spring, with our muscles tensed ready for action. This is why we often automatically pace the floor or tap our fingers and feet when we feel under stress.

Exercise is the one of the best ways to use up this 'stress energy'. It reduces levels of the body's stress hormones, such as adrenaline and cortisol, and stimulates the release of endorphins (the body's natural painkillers and mood elevators). It improves circulation, warms and relaxes cold tight muscles and provides a welcome distraction from regular activities. About 30 minutes of moderate aerobic exercise most days of the week is recommended. This could include walking, jogging, swimming, riding your bike or doing an aerobics or cycling class at the gym.

If you are in the middle of a stressful situation and can't take much time out, just getting out of your chair and taking a brisk walk to the water cooler or down the corridor will help to reduce your stress levels.

Stretching

Slow controlled stretching accompanied by relaxed diaphragmatic breathing will not only loosen tense muscles it will also relax the mind. The stretching movement is performed when you breathe out. Concentrating on your breathing and on the sensation of stretching will help keep worrying thoughts at bay.

Develop a Social Support Network

Having close and positive relationships with others is a powerful antidote to stress.[130] Just knowing you have trusted friends and family members you can talk to when you need to can make stressful events seem less overwhelming. Sometimes all you need is a shoulder to cry on or to feel that you have been listened to and understood. Talking about your problems can also help you see them in a new way and start looking for solutions.

Laughter and Humour

Laughter is one of the quickest ways of reducing stress.

It distracts you from your stressful thoughts, promotes physical relaxation, and helps defuse conflicts with other people. It also has a range of other longer term beneficial effects on our physical and mental health.[131]

So how can you add more humour to your life?

Here are a few tips.

- Watch a funny movie or TV show. Keep a few funny DVDs on hand for when you need some quick relief of stress.
- Put a few photos or comic strips you find funny on your wall or inside a cupboard door.
- Be on the lookout for funny or whimsical situations in everyday life. Pets and children are good sources. Sometimes, if you look at it in the right way, you can even see a humorous side to some of your own stressful situations.
- Seek out people who make you laugh. Shared laughter helps strengthen relationships.
- Look in the humour section of your local bookshop or library. Check out some humour sites on the web.

You may even want to consider joining a laughter club. These began in India in 1995, and there are now over 3000 clubs world-wide.

Get in Contact with Nature

Seeing green spaces, trees and other plants, through gardening or being out in natural environments has long been known to have a calming effect and improve mood.[132,133] 'Nature therapy' has been used in treating work-related stress and burnout.[134]

If you are going for a walk, whenever possible go to a park rather than just walking around a city block – it will be more effective in reducing stress. Even in winter, walking in an urban park in which most of the trees had lost their leaves has been shown to have a relaxing effect.[135]

If you often drive or walk between the same two points you could try varying your route a little, so you go through more streets lined with street trees. But what can we do about the highly artificial indoor environment where we now spend most of our time? Contact with nature is minimal at best, but we can bring nature inside in various ways.

Looking at potted plants[136] and flowers[137] has been shown to reduce stress. A view through a window over trees or some other natural landscape is ideal, but failing that, looking at a large nature photograph will help.

These principles are starting to be put into practice inside large public buildings such as hospitals and offices.

A Few Extra Tips

- Pat a dog or cat.
- Soak in a warm bath or take a warm shower.
- Try inhaling the vapours of essential oils. Add a few drops of oil to your bathwater. In the shower, put a few drops on your washcloth, place it on your chest and let the heat of the shower water release the vapours. Other methods include using a diffuser or putting a few drops on a handkerchief. You may like to experiment first with lavender oil. Inhalation of lavender oil vapour has been found to have a calming effect and to relieve migraines and tension headaches.
- Get a friend or partner to give you a neck massage.
- Take a quick nap. Sleeping for 10 – 30 minutes is very refreshing and helpful in reducing stress. More than 30 minutes and you will probably wake up groggy. Depending on your circumstances, a nap may not be so easy to arrange but is probably still possible, even if you just sit back in your chair or find an empty room where you can put your head down on the desk.
- Take several short breaks during the day. Make sure you get out of your chair and walk around to stretch your legs and rest your eyes.
- Consider turning off violent, frightening or distressing news items. These types of stories tend to give the impression that the world is a much more dangerous place than it is and add to your stress levels.
- Be selective in the movies and TV programs you choose to watch. The more neutral or positive scenes and the less negative scenes, the lower your stress

levels will be. The effects can be quite significant. For example, one study found that watching a funny movie segment versus a stressful one caused a 50% difference in blood flow in the upper arm. Violent computer games are another source of stress (and aggression).[138]

- Make time each day for relaxing activities you enjoy, like reading or listening to music.
- Look after yourself so you can handle stressful situations better. Eat a well-balanced healthy diet with regular meal times and drink plenty of water. Make sure you always eat breakfast and avoid sugary snacks. Get plenty of sleep. Hunger, sugar sags, dehydration and tiredness can stop us thinking clearly before we are aware of it and make us less able to handle stress.
- Can you delegate some tasks?
- Can you say no to additional tasks? Every extra task you take on leaves less time for the remainder.
- Are some of your tasks not really your responsibility – you are doing them because you like to be nice and helpful? It is important to set firm boundaries about what you will and will not do.
- Plan your day – don't just respond to interrupts. Make a 'to do' list and cross off items as you complete them. Your list shouldn't be too long or you will feel overwhelmed. Schedule some time for yourself and for regular breaks.
- Prioritise your tasks. Set aside plenty of time in the early part of the day when you are freshest for working on what you think is important. Cut back on 'busy busy' work and activities others think are urgent but are not important.
- Break-up large projects into smaller, more manageable parts and focus on one part at a time. You will gradually reach your target.
- Minimise distracting interruptions. Interruptions from co-workers in open-plan offices, from endless meetings and from the technology we rely on are reaching epidemic proportions – see below for some practical suggestions.
- Turn off the pings – the distracting audible prompts for email, instant messages, text messages and so on. Put your mobile phone on silent and direct your office phone through to your message machine.
- Set aside several specific times each day to read and where necessary reply to email (it often isn't necessary) and to reply to phone messages. Discipline yourself to avoid checking your phone or computer at other times.
- Avoid checking social media at work or searching the internet on personal matters even in during your lunch break. You are far better getting away from your desk and the office and going for a walk.
- If your work colleagues continually interrupt you politely but firmly end the conversation with something like 'I am sorry I can't spend any more time talking at the moment. I have to get a report finished.'
- In an open plan office use headphones to block out conversations from other workers. Some people don't actually play music, but if you do, experiment with different genres so that the music doesn't become a distraction in itself.

Key Points

- Stress is part of everyday life but if prolonged stress hormones stay elevated, it can have significant effects on our physical and mental health.
- Stress is a key factor in the Integrated Headache Model, where emotional stress acts like a 'pain volume control', intensifying or reducing the impact of the sum of pain signals from the musculoskeletal and neurovascular sources.
- The body's stress (fight-or-flight) response is automatic, but we can intentionally replace it with the relaxation (rest-and-digest) response.
- Relaxation techniques can offer significant relief from the effects of stress. It is an effective way of preventing headaches, and reducing the severity of any headache attacks that do occur.
- The most important relaxation technique to master is slow, relaxed diaphragmatic breathing.

21

Life

In this chapter, we discuss diet, exercise, sleep, air quality and the magic of house plants.

Diet

Search for information about diet and headaches, especially for migraines, and you're likely to be overwhelmed by the number of self-help books, magazine articles and websites offering advice.

Unfortunately, much of this advice is about avoiding long lists of potential 'trigger' foods and beverages, which I think is the wrong approach. For most headache sufferers, avoiding foods will do very little to prevent headache attacks or reduce their severity. Restricting your diet can even be counter-productive – fear of developing a headache if you aren't careful enough may be all that is needed to provoke an attack. Often, total avoidance of problem food components is not necessary. Just reduce your intake.

Instead of leaving things out, the emphasis in this chapter is on what you should include so that you have a healthy, varied diet. This is the type of diet that health authorities advise to lower your risk of developing cardiovascular disease, type 2 diabetes and certain cancers. As a bonus, I believe it will help to prevent headache attacks.

As well as maintaining a healthy diet, headache sufferers also need to pay more attention to:

- Maintaining constant eating patterns and avoiding hunger by eating regularly spaced, balanced meals
- Staying well hydrated
- Avoiding excessive caffeine intake and caffeine withdrawal
- Closely monitoring their intake of alcoholic beverages.

Dehydration, caffeine and alcohol are the most common and powerful dietary headache triggers.

Finally, headache sufferers should maintain a healthy body weight and work towards reducing excess fat around their waist-line.

Abdominal fat deposits lead to low grade inflammation[139,140], which increases the risk of both cardiovascular disease and migraine attacks.[141]

How Can a Healthy Diet Help Prevent Headaches?

A healthy diet will help to prevent headaches by raising your headache threshold and reducing your exposure to several potential dietary headache triggers. A healthy diet, full of fresh fruit and vegetables, is rich in key vitamins and minerals needed for optimal functioning of nerves and muscles. Vitamin and mineral deficiencies perpetuate muscular trigger points and increase the excitability of the central nervous system, making a headache attack more likely to occur. Eating well keeps your blood vessels healthier, including major vessels such as the carotid arteries, which supply the brain. It makes it easier for your body to keep your blood glucose levels stable – a rapid rise and fall in blood glucose levels may trigger a headache attack.

Headache sufferers (and, for that matter, anyone concerned for their long-term health) should avoid meals that are high in fat, salt or added sugar. This rules out most fast food and pre-prepared or convenience foods. It's best if you prepare as many meals as possible using fresh and minimally processed ingredients. And it is not just meals. Watch out for times when you are feeling stressed. When we reach for comfort food, it is likely to be something like chips, chocolate or cake. Try to reduce how much of these foods you eat, while you work on finding alternative ways of dealing with your stress, like taking a short walk, phoning a friend or doing some relaxation.

Four Key Dietary Considerations

Hunger

The brain needs a steady supply of glucose for fuel, so don't skip or delay meals and don't go on crash diets or fasts – if you are trying to lose weight, it's best to proceed at a slow, steady pace. Headaches from delaying and skipping meals can be quite severe and are sometimes accompanied by mild nausea. They are thought to be due to blood glucose levels falling too low. The longer the delay in eating, the more likely a headache attack is to occur. Even people who rarely suffer from headaches can be affected. Religious fasts, such as for Yom Kippur[142] in Judaism and Ramadan[143] in Islam, are well known to increase both headache frequency and severity.[144]

A good breakfast is especially important and the foods you choose for breakfast matter. Most breakfast cereals and commercial fruit juice drinks are loaded with added sugar. Steer well clear of these – they will cause your blood glucose levels to rise rapidly and then fall, and this may trigger a headache attack. Alternatives such as homemade porridge, natural muesli, whole grain toast, avocado, fruit salad or an egg are much better for you.

Hydration

Studies on hydration status normally focus on water balance over a 24-hour period. For water balance to be maintained, water intake must equal water losses. The tricky part is working out how much water is required to maintain your water balance.

It is difficult to make universal recommendations. People vary widely in their water needs depending on many different factors, including age, gender, body size and composition, health, level of physical activity and the temperature and humidity of their environment. Working in a dry air-conditioned office can lead to water losses we're not aware of.

There are two conflicting points of view on how much fluid (including water) you should consume per day to stay well hydrated.

One view is to let thirst be your guide. This is based on defining mild dehydration as starting at 3% loss of body weight.[145] This method may work for people who sweat a lot, such as athletes or those doing physical activity in hot climates. But it doesn't seem to work so well for the average person going about their everyday activities, where water loss is less and more gradual.

Part of the problem is that we don't sense thirst until we've lost 1% to 2% of our body mass as water.[146] By that stage, you're already mildly dehydrated. Water has been transferred from within and between the cells of your body and into your blood-stream. In addition, some people get used to ignoring thirst signals. In others, such as the elderly, the thirst mechanism is less effective.

The other problem is that the brain is 80% water. Recent research has shown that a loss of just 1.6% of body mass impaired cognitive performance and mood in healthy young men.[147] It seems reasonable to assume that a similar minor water loss can trigger a headache attack.

The alternative view on maintaining water balance is to offer specific guidelines for an average non-exercising person in a temperate climate (20°C, 68°F). It's commonly assumed about 20% of our water intake comes from food.[148] That leaves about 1700 ml to be made up by water and other beverages. It fits reasonably well with what in the US is referred to as the 8 x 8 rule –drink eight 8oz glasses of water per day, which comes to a bit less than 2 litres.

What is generally not emphasised is the need to spread fluid intake evenly throughout the day. It takes time for water to be absorbed from the gut, enter the blood-stream and rehydrate the cells.

Drink too much too quickly and a lot of it will pass straight through. It can also be dangerous to drink a lot under some circumstances, especially when a lot of salts have been lost in sweat and not replaced in the fluid.

In the absence of any better evidence, I suggest you aim to drink roughly 1.5 litres of water evenly spread out over the whole day, giving a total fluid intake of about two litres.

Even if you don't like water, this is an achievable target, especially if you gradually replace some of your other beverages with water. You could try filtering tap water (this is a lot cheaper than bottled water) and adding a slice of lemon, or drinking herbal tea.

As a habit, you should drink water regularly during the day – how much water per person per day is a surprisingly controversial subject, but a good indicator of hydration is the colour of your urine. The volume should be much the same as usual and the colour should be a very pale yellow, almost but not completely colourless.

Caffeine

Caffeine acts as a vasoconstrictor and nervous system stimulant. Large amounts (greater than 600 mg) can cause headaches, along with anxiety, restlessness, rapid heart-beat and insomnia. However, most caffeine related headaches are symptoms of caffeine withdrawal, due to rebound vasodilation, which occurs when blood caffeine levels fall. Typically, the symptoms begin between 12 to 24 hours after the last caffeine intake.

Other symptoms of caffeine withdrawal can include fatigue, depressed mood, nausea and muscle pain and stiffness and these can last for up to nine days. You may feel like you have got the flu.[149]

People vary in their sensitivity to caffeine but generally, the larger the regular daily dose of caffeine, the more severe these withdrawal symptoms will be. For some, regular consumption of caffeine in amounts as small as 100 mg per day can lead to physical dependence and hence withdrawal symptoms when the next dose is missed.

Caffeine is found in coffee, tea, cocoa, and various carbonated soft drinks, as well as in many over-the-counter and prescription painkillers and other medications. For example, Excedrin pain relievers promoted for tension headaches and migraines contain 130 mg of caffeine in the standard dose of two tablets.

The amount of caffeine in coffee and tea is highly variable. The table below gives some typical ranges.[150] (I haven't included decaffeinated coffee as it only contains small residual amounts of caffeine.) Regulations governing the maximum permissible amount of caffeine in various drinks and other products also vary between countries.

Table of Caffeine Contents

Caffeine Source	Caffeine Content	Serve
Instant coffee	60–80 mg	250 ml cup
Café coffee (e.g. latte or cappuccino)	113–282 mg	250 ml cup
Espresso / short black	107 mg (25–214 mg)	1 shot
Starbucks Breakfast Blend brewed coffee	415 mg (300–564 mg)	600 ml (Venti)
Iced coffee	30–200 mg	500 ml bottle
Black tea	25–110 mg	250 ml cup
Green tea	30–50 mg	250 ml cup
Cola soft drinks	36–48 mg	375 ml can
Energy drinks	80 mg	250 ml can
Milk chocolate	20 mg*	100 g bar
OTC and prescription medications	20–200 mg	Usual dose

* Values for caffeine in chocolate and other cocoa products generally include compounds related to caffeine which have similar but weaker effects.

The amount of caffeine in instant coffee depends on how much coffee is in your cup. For fresh coffee, additional factors are important including the type of beans (the more expensive, more flavoursome Arabica beans contain less caffeine than the cheaper Robusta varieties), how the coffee beans are prepared and how the coffee is made. This is also true for tea.

All this variability makes it difficult to calculate your total daily caffeine consumption. However, if you start to get a headache after delaying your morning cuppa, you're probably dependent on caffeine. If you also notice that having caffeine eases that headache, then it's even more likely you're dependent on caffeine. It is important to cut back on the amount of the different caffeinated products you typically consume, but do it very gradually.

Alcohol

As a group, headache sufferers tend to be more sensitive to alcohol than those not prone to headaches. Headaches may develop anywhere from 30 minutes to 24 hours after drinking a modest amount of alcohol.[151] Although a hangover almost always comes with a headache, for most headache sufferers, one standard size serving of an alcoholic drink shouldn't cause problems. The key is to have food with any alcoholic drink and sip it slowly.

A standard drink is defined as containing 10 g of alcohol. For table wine this corresponds to 100 ml (although note that the typical serving size is 150 ml – in other words 1.5 standard drinks).

Sufficient Vitamins and Minerals in Your Diet is Important

Adequate levels of certain key vitamins and minerals are essential for the proper functioning of the nervous and muscular systems.

Sub-optimal levels can lower your headache threshold and lead to the formation of muscular trigger points. They can also cause secondary headaches in people not ordinarily prone to headaches.

Vitamin D is one of these key nutrients[152,153]. Others include:

- Vitamin C
- Several B vitamins – vitamin B1 (thiamine), B6, B12, and folic acid
- The minerals calcium, magnesium, iron and potassium.

Sub-optimal levels of these and other vitamins and minerals in the body are generally the result of a poor diet.

However, they may also be due to poor absorption from the diet. Medical conditions which impair digestion may be responsible for this. Examples include chronic diarrhoea, insufficient stomach acid and coeliac disease which damages the surface of the small intestine.

Other causes include smoking (vitamin C deficiency) and excessive alcohol consumption (deficiencies of vitamin B1 and B6).

See Chapter 22 for more information.

General Guidelines for a Headache Friendly Diet

- Minimise how much fast food, pre-prepared or convenience foods you eat.
- Check the labels of pre-prepared foods and ingredients for their energy content, added salt, added sugar and the amount of total, saturated and trans fats.
- Avoid fatty or salty meals. Meals high in fat or salt can cause platelets to clump together,[154] triggering a headache attack. Even one salty meal temporarily reduces blood flow.[155]
- Prepare your own meals using fresh and minimally processed ingredients.
- Store produce promptly in the refrigerator and cook and eat it soon after purchase.
- Meals should be balanced (with respect to carbohydrates, protein, fat and fibre)
- Vegetarians need to combine foods with complementary proteins to optimise the balance of essential amino acids.
- Eat plenty of different coloured vegetables and fruits as well as whole grains. These will supply vitamins, minerals, fibre and phytochemicals. While fresh is best, frozen or canned vegetables and fruit are a good way to increase your intake.
- Look for cereal products made with wholemeal (whole-wheat) rather than refined flour.
- Reduce the amount of salt in your diet.
- Replace some saturated fat with unsaturated fat.
- Include some healthy sources of omega-3, such as nuts and fish.
- Minimise the amount of trans fats in processed foods you eat.
- Avoid frying your food, whether it's shallow or deep.
- Try steaming or microwaving vegetables.
- You may want to consider a multi vitamin / mineral supplement 'for insurance' against sub-optimal levels of vitamins and minerals. Vegans will need vitamin B12 supplements.
- It is worthwhile having your vitamin D levels checked. You may need an additional vitamin D supplement.

Keep Your Blood Glucose Levels Stable

- Maintain constant eating patterns and avoid hunger.
- Eat regularly spaced meals. Don't skip or delay meals.
- Always have breakfast.
- Don't go on crash diets or fasts.
- Have plenty of fibre in your meals.
- Most carbohydrates should be in the form of slowly digested starch (grains and vegetables containing starch, like potatoes, should be minimally processed).
- Get almost all your sugars from fruit and vegetables. Minimise the amount of added sugar you consume (check the labels of pre-packaged foods).
- Avoid sugary snacks and sugary drinks, particularly on an empty stomach.

Stay Well Hydrated

- Aim to drink roughly 1.5 litres of water for a total fluid intake of about 2 litres.
- Space the drinking of water evenly over the whole day.

Monitor Your Caffeine Intake

- Avoid excessive caffeine intake.
- Watch out for signs of caffeine withdrawal – signs are headaches when you delay having caffeine and which caffeine quickly relieves.
- If you are dependent on caffeine, reduce your intake very gradually.

Monitor Your Intake of Alcoholic Beverages

- Avoid excessive alcohol consumption.
- Always eat food when you have an alcoholic drink.
- Cap your intake at one standard drink and drink it slowly.

Reduce Excess Fat Around the Waist-Line

- Reduce the size of the portions you eat.
- Check the energy and nutrient content of packaged foods. Weigh and possibly reduce your usual serving of foods that are high in fat, like chips.
- Alcohol has almost as much energy as fat. Alcoholic beverages are one source of empty calories you can cut back on.
- Avoid other sources of empty calories like sugary drinks, snack foods and most fast foods.
- Eat more fruit and vegetables which are high in fibre and water and so are filling.
- Use up more energy by moving about more and doing some moderate exercise each day.

Exercise

Most of us are aware of the benefit of regular exercise. Regular, moderate, aerobic exercise reduces the risk of developing chronic diseases like diabetes, cardiovascular disease and some cancers.[156,157]

The long-term health benefits of regular moderate exercise are thought to be due to the effect of reduced weight gain and especially deposition of deep abdominal fat, more stable blood glucose levels, better circulation and improved health of blood vessels and reduced stress.

Moderate Exercise as a Headache Preventative

These same four factors above can also explain why regular moderate exercise helps prevent migraine and tension headaches.

Physical inactivity is a risk factor for headaches, but many headache sufferers, especially those who get migraines, tend to avoid exercise[158] for fear it may provoke an attack. While intense exercise is known to trigger headaches in some people[159,160], this is not true of moderate exercise.

For example, a controlled study published in 2011 showed that exercise was effective in reducing the number of migraine attacks and improving quality of life as preventative medication and relaxation.[161]

Moderate exercise is something like brisk walking, dancing, mowing the lawn, swimming or cycling at a medium pace. It's an activity that's vigorous enough to cause a small but noticeable increase in your breathing and heart rate, but not so much that you can't easily carry on a conversation with a companion.

It's important that whatever types of exercise you choose, you can do them at a moderate level, and you enjoy doing them, so you stay motivated and embrace exercise as part of your life.

It is also important that you:

- Begin your exercise program gradually – slowly increasing the intensity over several weeks. Short, frequent sessions are probably best
- Make sure your blood sugar doesn't drop – eat something before exercising (but not a sugary snack) and allow at least an hour and a half for your food to digest
- Stay hydrated – drink water before, during and after exercise. (Sports drinks aren't necessary for short, moderate exercise sessions. What's more, many contain a lot of sugar which can cause blood glucose levels to surge and then fall, possibly even triggering a headache attack.)
- Include a warm up, cool down and stretching.

If you already have a migraine, the last thing you should do is exercise. Moving your head will only make the pain and nausea worse. You need to rest in a dark, quiet room. If you have a tension headache, however, a brisk walk may relieve tension.

Don't Sit for Too Long

As well as doing regular exercise, we also need to move more. Most of us spend far too much time each day sitting – in our jobs, while travelling between home and work and during our leisure time. It is important to take regular breaks from sitting and divide the total sitting time up into smaller chunks.

This is as true for the person who jogs each morning as for the person who does no exercise at all. No matter how fit you are, too much sitting is bad for your long-term health. It will also lead to worsening head and neck posture and muscle overuse. This in turn will aggravate headaches.

You need to get out of your seat at least once an hour. Occupational health and safety organisations recommend that you have a 5–10 minute break for every 40–50 minutes of sitting while at work and this is a useful guide elsewhere.

During each break, spend some time walking around to help restore circulation, exercise heart, lungs and muscles and reduce muscle tension. Do several of the exercises from the stretching and strengthening routine.

It's a good idea to measure how many steps you take during a day. You could buy a simple pedometer or use an App on your phone. The numbers may be a real eye opener. If you are very sedentary you may only average 1000 – 3000 steps per day, whereas the ideal stated goal is 10,000 steps per day.

This target is something you can gradually build up to, one week at a time. It would be realistic to aim for a 500 step per day increase each week. Even if you don't quite make it to 10,000 steps per day any increase over your usual baseline amount of activity will be beneficial.

There are many ways you can increase the number of steps you take, for example:

- Use the stairs instead of the lift or escalator
- Walk to a colleague's desk instead of phoning or emailing
- Go to the water cooler
- Make sure you eat lunch away from your desk and go for a walk during your lunch-break
- Park further away from your destination and walk the extra distance
- Get off the train or bus one stop earlier and walk the rest of the way.

Just getting out of your chair and standing for a short time is a healthy move. You use your muscles much more to stand than to sit and you often move from one leg to the other. Here are a few tips:

- Stand up to make phone calls and answer the phone
- If you work at a computer a lot, consider asking your employer for a sit-stand desk. These can be quickly adjusted in height so you can easily swap between sitting and standing
- Sit on a fit ball (Swiss ball, physio ball) as a break from sitting on a chair. The fit ball will help you move around more while sitting. Once you get used to it you can pedal your feet up and down, do small bounces and hip circles
- Move the bin further from your desk so you have to get up more regularly
- Get up to change the TV channel
- Get up and move around during the ad breaks.

Sleep

Sleep and Headaches

We've discussed the importance of sleeping posture (remember – do not sleep on your stomach). The role of poor sleep posture in provoking headache attacks is generally ignored. The quality of your sleep is also important. Poor quality sleep is strongly linked to triggering headaches. Conversely, sleep can terminate a headache attack.

Lack of sleep is the most important sleep-related trigger for both tension headaches and migraines,[162,163,164] whether this is the result of staying up too late or insomnia (difficulty in falling asleep or staying asleep). It also makes it more likely that an episodic headache will transform into a chronic one.[165]

How a lack of sleep triggers a headache is not known. However, experiments have shown that sleep deprivation reduces the threshold at which healthy volunteers feel pain of different sorts.[166]

Disturbed or interrupted sleep and changes in sleep patterns (late nights, sleeping in) can also trigger a headache attack. Headache sufferers are best to keep to a regular sleep schedule, going to bed and getting up at the same time each day, including weekends.

In a small study on women with chronic migraine, improving sleep habits led to a decrease in headache severity. Headaches also reverted from a chronic to an episodic pattern. No such improvements were seen in the control group.[167]

But how much sleep do we need? This is not an easy question to answer. It depends on the individual and varies as we age. The recommended duration of sleep is 7–8 hours for adults, but some people may need up to 9 hours. Teenagers need 9–10 hours (most don't get this much during the week).

There is also some evidence that headache sufferers on average need more sleep than the general population. They may be relatively sleep deprived even when their sleep duration falls within the recommended range.[168]

If you wake up feeling refreshed most mornings and don't get sleepy during the day, you are probably having about the right amount of sleep. If not, you should experiment to see how much sleep you need. Try going to bed a half hour earlier for at least a week and test how you feel.

If this doesn't help and you are still sleepy during the day, and especially if you snore, you should be checked by your doctor for obstructive sleep apnoea. Obstructive sleep apnoea is a relatively common (and health-threatening) condition, but most people who have it are unaware of it. It causes sufferers to temporarily stop breathing many times during the night, leading to daytime sleepiness and morning headaches.

On the other hand, if you often wake up with a sore jaw and aching jaw muscles, you may be unconsciously clenching and grinding your teeth during sleep. This is normally a sign of stress and a potent headache trigger. If you think this is the case, first have your jaw checked and treated by a manual therapist. To break the cycle, you will also need to do some work on reducing your stress levels.

There are lots of things you can do to help you get a better night's sleep. Here are a few simple suggestions:

- Start to wind down with relaxing activities an hour or so before bed-time. For example, take a bath, read, listen to calming music, practice some relaxation exercises
- Refrain from stimulating activities like using the computer, playing video games or exercising close to bed-time
- Dim the lights. Bright light at night, especially the blue component of the light from electronic screens, tends to reset your body clock so you start feeling sleepy later. Some people are more sensitive to this effect than others. It can be like living with a mild case of jet lag
- Avoid caffeine (found in coffee, tea, chocolate and some pain relievers) within 4–6 hours of bed-time. It can keep you awake and lead to lighter, less restful sleep. Again, some people are more sensitive to caffeine than others
- Avoid alcohol within a few hours of bed-time. It will make you fall asleep faster but it causes lighter, more fragmented sleep in the second half of the night
- Don't have a large meal too late at night, especially high fat foods like pizza, or spicy foods. Finish dinner several hours before bed-time
- Restrict napping to before 5 pm
- Your bedroom should be cool, dark and quiet.

Air Quality

Oxygen

Reduced availability of oxygen in the air will often trigger headaches even among those who seldom get them. There are three ways it commonly occurs.

Firstly, the oxygen in the air inside a room or building is used up faster than it can be adequately replaced from fresh air coming in from the outside. Going for a walk outside and taking a few slow, deep diaphragmatic breaths may help.

Using a gas cooker, or some form of fuel burning internal heating, e.g. a gas heater, open fire or slow combustion stove, will also cause a large extra drop in oxygen levels. It is important to let in a little outside air to replace stale inside air.

Ascending too quickly from sea level to a higher altitude where air pressure is lower will result in less oxygen being available. It could involve driving over a mountain pass or travelling to a ski village or mountain resort. Altitudes as low as 1500 m (5000 feet) can trigger a headache attack in those who are prone to them. More people begin to develop headaches at 2000 m (6500 feet) and above 2500 m (8200 feet), everyone is at risk. There's nothing easy you can do to prevent these headaches except break your journey so you ascend more slowly. Headaches and other symptoms usually abate over a couple of days as your body adapts to the higher altitude.

Headaches triggered by airline travel are very common. Flying in the pressurised cabin is equivalent to rapidly ascending from sea level to an altitude of around 2400 m (8000 feet). This produces blood oxygen levels that are only about 93% of normal values.

The only thing you can do about the reduced oxygen supply during a flight is to maintain correct posture so you can breathe deeply and practice slow diaphragmatic breathing so you get more air into your lungs. You should also pay attention to counteracting the various other headache triggers associated with flying – dehydration, stress, fatigue, uneven spacing of meals and restricted movement.

Carbon Monoxide

Carbon monoxide is a poisonous, odourless gas produced when fossil fuels are incompletely burnt. It also occurs in cigarette smoke and in car exhaust gases.

Carbon monoxide preferentially attaches to the red blood cells, displacing oxygen. This reduces the amount of oxygen the blood can carry. At low concentrations, carbon monoxide causes a range of symptoms including headaches. At higher concentrations, it can be fatal.

Some of the sources of carbon monoxide in the indoor air in our homes include gas stoves, unvented gas and kerosene space heaters (these put the combustion products back into the room air – vented heaters are much safer), gas water heaters and clothes dryers, open fireplaces and wood heaters and leaking or blocked chimneys.

It's important to let in outside air to prevent carbon monoxide and other exhaust gases from accumulating. Gas stoves should be used in conjunction with a range hood or at least an exhaust fan to vent exhaust gases to the outside world.

Other Indoor Air Pollutants

Without sufficient ventilation, a range of indoor pollutants can build up to levels where they start to cause health effects such as eye, nose, and throat irritation, asthma, and headaches.

Some people are more sensitive to these effects. They begin to have symptoms when levels are still well inside occupational health and safety standards and the pollutants are unable to be smelt.

Common types of indoor air pollutants include:

- Tobacco smoke – a complex, toxic and irritating mixture of vapours and particles. Although second hand smoke is becoming less of a problem as more public and common places become smoke free, it can still be a problem in homes and cars
- By-products of combustion of fossil fuels – these include nitrogen and sulphur oxides (in addition to carbon monoxide), irritating gases which are formed even when the combustion appliance is working perfectly
- Volatile organic compounds (VOCs) – these are a wide variety of synthetic organic chemicals that are gases at ordinary room temperature and so can be breathed in. They are released into room air from a diverse range of home and industrial products, including synthetic building materials, foam insulation, furniture and shelving made from veneered particle board, adhesives, carpets, drapes, upholstery, photocopiers, paper tissues and towels, cleaning products, cosmetics, permanent press fabrics, dry cleaning, varnishes and paints
- Formaldehyde (HCHO), which is emitted from many of these products, is one of the most common and highly irritating indoor pollutants. Formaldehyde is also a by-product of incomplete combustion of fossil fuels and is present in tobacco smoke

The Power of the House Plant

Even in the office, where you probably don't have much control over the ventilation, there is something you can do to reduce the levels of VOCs in your area. Introduce some house plants.

In the late 1980s, NASA discovered that house-plants could purify the air in enclosed living compartments, like the International Space Station.

Plants absorb VOCs from the room air into their leaves and then transport them to their root zone, where microbes break them down. Soil microbes in the potting mix and processes in the plant's roots also assist in the break-down process.[169]

Plants also improve indoor air quality by increasing local humidity. This helps to remove dust particles, which may have various allergens and irritating substances adsorbed on their surfaces. House-plants have also been shown to reduce stress.

Suitable plants are ones demonstrated to be effective in removing VOCs, suit your taste and the growing conditions you have available (usually low light) and are easy to maintain.[170] Three suitable plants which cope with semi-shade to low light are Peace lily (Spathiphyllum varieties), English ivy (Hedera helix) and Dracaena deremensis 'Janet Craig'.

The Weather

The weather and changes in the weather are commonly reported to trigger headaches, particularly migraines, although the mechanisms are mostly unclear. Some of the weather variables implicated are a drop in barometric pressure, high humidity, both high and low temperatures, and dry, windy and dusty conditions.

Dust particles are irritating. They also carry plant and animal allergens on their surfaces. Both factors will lead to histamine release from nose and throat membranes and this may provoke a headache.

There is obviously not much you can do to avoid a drop in barometric pressure, although you can limit your exposure to most other potential weather triggers by staying indoors. Before you start restricting your activities (which may be unnecessary), try to verify any suspected weather triggers using your headache diary.

Intense Sensory Stimuli

Several environmental headache triggers can be grouped under the general category of intense stimuli to the senses of vision, hearing and smell. These stimuli may initiate the headache process by provoking a larger than normal response from the headache sufferer's excitable brain. They appear to be most important for those who suffer migraine with aura.

It may be possible to avoid some of these stimuli, or else reduce their effect. Here are a few common examples:

- Sun glare, especially from water or snow. Sunglasses will help, especially wrap-around designs which cut light entering your peripheral vision. Polarising lenses are the most effective for reducing sun glare
- Glare from overhead indoor lighting, particularly if there is a detectable slow flicker from fluorescent lighting. You probably don't have much control over the level of your office lighting, but some people have been known to wear a sunshade like those worn by tennis players to protect against glare from above. Not exactly a fashion statement, but it does help to reduce one source of glare
- Glare or flicker from your computer screen. To minimise this, you could:
    - Close the drapes or blinds to prevent glare from bright outside light and reflections making the problem worse
    - Position your screen so that windows are to the side of it, not in front or behind
    - Tilt the top of the screen slightly backwards to eliminate reflections
    - Install an anti-glare screen filter
    - Reduce the brightness of your screen to a level similar to your surroundings. If there's still too much contrast between the brightness of your screen and a darker desk, a small desk lamp may help
- Loud and irritating noise – in some situations, ear plugs or noise cancelling earphones may be useful
- Strong odours, both pleasant, such as perfume and strongly scented flowers, and unpleasant, including chemical solvent odours. Strong odours can be difficult to avoid in a shared office environment – about all you can do is ask your co-workers not to use perfumes or after-shave.

Some strongly smelling substances are nasal irritants and so may also provoke headaches by leading to histamine release. This may be the same mechanism by which environmental triggers such as traffic fumes and outdoor pollution which lack a strong odour provoke an attack.

The good news in all this: headache triggers are accumulative – you don't have to fix them all, just target some of them and stay underneath your headache threshold.

Key Points

- Eating regular meals (without skipping or delaying meals), maintaining hydration, avoiding excessive amounts of caffeine and alcohol are the crucial elements of a headache-free diet.
- Aim to drink 1.5 litres of water evenly spread out over the whole day.
- Intense exercise can trigger headaches in some people, but this is not true of moderate exercise. Moderate exercise should be a regular feature in your week.
- Whether at work or home – don't sit still for too long.
- Make sure you are getting enough sleep (remember – do not sleep on your stomach).
- Air quality can affect the frequency and severity of your headaches.
- House plants can improve air quality and reduce stress.

22

Vitamins and Minerals

Vitamins and minerals are a hot topic in health and headache management and are worth considering as part of your headache prevention program.

Insufficient levels of certain key vitamins and minerals can contribute to developing muscular trigger points. The most important vitamins for healthy muscle function are the C, B1, B6, B12, folic acid and D, and the minerals calcium, magnesium, iron and potassium. Sub-optimal levels of vitamins and minerals can also lower your headache threshold and cause secondary headaches in people not ordinarily prone to headaches.[171,172]

Like medication, if you are going to use vitamins and/or minerals as part of your headache management strategy, you should know what you're taking and why.

Vitamin D – A Special Case

Because natural dietary sources of vitamin D are so limited, if you're unable to synthesise enough vitamin D through exposure of the skin to sunlight, you have to rely on stores of vitamin D in fat tissues. If this keeps happening, it can result in vitamin D deficiency. We often think of people who live in colder climates and higher latitudes (further away from the equator) as being susceptible to vitamin D deficiency, but people who live close to the equator need to monitor their vitamin D intake. Many people who live in sunny climates limit their exposure to the sun because of the detrimental effects of over exposure to sunlight. That's a good thing, but sub-optimal levels of vitamin D, and even vitamin D deficiency, are much more common than would be expected from people living in sunny climates.[173]

Important Vitamins and Minerals for Headache Prevention

All vitamins and minerals are essential, but sub-optimal levels of the water-soluble vitamins C, B1, B6, B12, folic acid, fat soluble vitamin D and the minerals calcium, magnesium, iron and potassium can contribute to headache attacks.

Sub-optimal levels of vitamins and minerals are generally the result of an inadequate diet. However, before you start eating bags of spinach, it's worth noting that sometimes, lower levels of these nutrients may be due to poor absorption. Medical conditions such as chronic diarrhoea, insufficient stomach acid and coeliac disease, which all impair digestion, can affect your ability to absorb nutrients. Other causes of poor absorption include smoking (vitamin C deficiency) and excessive alcohol consumption (deficiencies of vitamin B1 and B6).

Blood tests are designed to pick up significant nutrient deficiencies, so if your results are within the normal range, it's not a guarantee your nutrition is optimal. If any of your values are close to the low end of the range, it might be worthwhile consulting a dietician.

The best way to get sufficient vitamins and minerals is to eat a wide variety of foods, including lots of fruits, vegetables and whole grains, that have been prepared from fresh or minimally processed ingredients. To see if you're in the ballpark with your diet, it can be helpful to check the vitamin and mineral content of what you're eating – there are lots of reference sites online.

When you're calculating your vitamin and mineral intake, remember, the information about the percentage of RDI (recommended daily intake) in each food is a guide only. Different samples of the same food will contain different amounts of vitamins and minerals, the recommended dietary intake varies with gender and age and you will also find slightly different values quoted by health authorities in different countries.

Detailed numerical comparisons between foods can be misleading. The values listed don't take into account bioavailability – the proportion of a nutrient that is taken up by the cells of the body.

Let's take spinach as an example. Spinach is certainly good for you – it's an excellent source of folic acid, magnesium and vitamin B2 (riboflavin), which has been suggested as a migraine preventative. It also appears to have more iron than red meat. However, less than 2% of the iron and 5% of the calcium in spinach is absorbed, although iron absorption can be increased by adding vitamin C. We absorb iron and calcium much better from animal foods like meat and milk.

Just as some foods work better when they are eaten together, various substances in food can interfere with absorption of particular nutrients. For example, calcium in milk and the tannins in tea can reduce the absorption of iron, especially the iron in plant foods like spinach. Deficiency in one nutrient can also create deficiencies in others. For example, a deficiency in vitamin B6 reduces the absorption and storage of vitamin B12, increases excretion of vitamin C, and blocks synthesis of vitamin B3 (niacin).

Vitamin and Mineral Supplements

Supplements can't compensate for a poor diet and if you have a healthy, varied diet you shouldn't need supplements. The best source of vitamins and minerals is food, rather than from supplements. We absorb nutrients better from food, they are in the chemical form we need, and we also get other benefits, such as fibre and phytochemicals.

If you want to take a supplement 'for insurance' get a multivitamin that contains all the necessary vitamins and minerals in the correct proportions. Don't take more than the recommended amount – certain vitamins and minerals are toxic in high doses.

Enrichment and Fortification of Processed Foods

Vitamins and minerals are often added to processed foods.

Enrichment involves replacing vitamins and minerals lost through food processing. On the other hand, fortification involves adding vitamins and minerals that were never present in the original food.

Fortification is often done as a public health measure. The aim is to prevent diseases caused by nutrient deficiencies which result from an inadequate diet, whether this is due to poverty or just poor eating habits.

The foods that are normally fortified are frequently eaten staples, like bread, milk and flour. Two of the B vitamins, thiamine (vitamin B_1) and folic acid, and vitamin D are the most commonly added nutrients.

Where possible, it is better to obtain your vitamins and minerals from unprocessed foods rather than from foods which have been artificially enriched or fortified. The reasons are the same as for preferring unprocessed foods over supplements.

Vitamin D Supplements

In the United States manufacturers voluntarily fortify a wide range of foods with vitamin D, but this is not true of many countries. Hence vitamin D supplements may be necessary.

It's very important to test vitamin D levels in the blood first to determine the necessary dose and to assess the results of treatment. High doses of vitamin D can be toxic. If they are required, it is best to take supplements which contain vitamin D_3 as this form is identical to that manufactured in the skin.

Salt and Headaches

Sodium is an essential mineral which comes mainly from ordinary salt (sodium chloride). Throughout most of human history, when we consumed the sodium which occurred naturally in our food, our estimated daily intake was approximately 0.2 gram. Salt has only been added to food for about 5000 years.

Today, the recommended upper limit is 2.3 grams of sodium per day, which corresponds to about 6 grams of salt or a bit over 1 teaspoon, more than sufficient to replace salt lost in sweat. Most people eat a lot more salt than this.

Processed foods are the main source of salt in our diet – bread and ready-made sauces are two of the items that contain the highest salt levels. Soy sauce is particularly salty with a 15 ml serve of one popular brand containing almost 1000 mg (1 gram) of salt. And processed foods, such as canned baked beans and breakfast cereals, contain added salt as well as added sugar.

Too much salt has several harmful effects on health, particularly on the health of the cardiovascular system. High salt intake makes arteries stiffer[174], restricting blood flow and making headaches more likely. A salty meal can cause platelets to clump together which may trigger a headache attack.[175] Even one salty meal has been shown to temporarily restrict blood flow 30 minutes after eating.[176]

Reducing the amount of salt in your diet and avoiding salty meals will certainly benefit your health. It's also likely to improve your headaches.

Minimising Loss of Vitamins and Minerals from Your Food

The vitamins in food can be destroyed by exposure to heat, air, water and light during storage, transport and cooking. The water-soluble vitamins, and especially vitamin C, are the least stable. To minimise losses, fresh produce should be stored in a cool, dark place and used as soon as possible. Avoid cooking for a prolonged time at high temperatures.

For vegetables, it's best to use cooking methods which require less water, like steaming or microwaving, rather than boiling. Preferably cook vegetables whole with the skin on. These steps also minimise losses of minerals into the cooking water.

Adding frozen or canned vegetables or fruit to different dishes can be an easy way of getting more nutrients in your diet. They are not necessarily inferior in nutrient content to fresh vegetables bought at the supermarket – often, fresh produce has undergone prolonged storage and transport before even arriving at its destination.

Treatment of Migraines with Vitamin and Mineral Supplements

Several dietary supplements have been tested as migraine preventatives. The two with the best scientific support (placebo controlled clinical trials) are high dose vitamin B2 (riboflavin)[177,178] and magnesium[179]. Broadly speaking, results have been similar to the results with migraine preventative medication, where a reduction of 50% in frequency, severity and duration of attacks is considered a good result. The main adverse effect was diarrhoea in the case of magnesium.

Many headache sufferers have lower than normal levels of magnesium ions in their blood and brain[180] and intravenous magnesium can quickly relieve a headache attack.[181] Intravenous magnesium has also been used successfully in hospital emergency departments to abort severe migraine attacks and relieve migraine symptoms.[182]

Menstrual migraines are associated with low free magnesium levels in the blood much more often than migraines unrelated to the menstrual cycle. One placebo controlled study demonstrated that magnesium supplements taken on the last 15 days of the menstrual cycle could reduce the number of days with menstrual migraine and the severity of the pain experienced.[183]

Before trying vitamin B2 or magnesium supplements for your migraines, you should first improve your diet. Leafy green vegetables are a good source of both vitamin B2 and magnesium. It's worth remembering however, that it will take several months for any beneficial effects to be felt. A similar time delay was also seen in the clinical trials involving supplements.

If you do decide to trial supplements, it's best to do so under the supervision of your doctor and after you have had blood tests. Remember, supplements won't help if your levels aren't low.

Epsom Salts

Adding Epsom salts to your bath is an old home remedy for easing muscle pain, still widely used today and there are good reasons for thinking it will help your muscles and your headaches.

Epsom salts act as a source of magnesium ions, which play an essential role in body chemistry, including the maintenance of normal functioning of nerves and muscles. Magnesium ions can enter the bloodstream by absorption across the skin. A small study showed that soaking in an Epsom salt bath for 12 minutes two times a week should be sufficient to restore normal levels.[184] The effects on headaches have not been studied, but it seems well worth trying – at the very least, you'll get to relax in a warm bath twice a week! You will need two cups of Epsom salts in a standard sized bathtub.

Key Points

- Sub-optimal levels of vitamins and minerals can lower your headache threshold.
- The most important vitamins for healthy muscle function are the C, B1, B6, B12, folic acid and D, and the minerals calcium, magnesium, iron and potassium.
- The best way to get optimal levels of vitamins and minerals is to eat a wide range of healthy foods, including lots of fruit, vegetables and whole grains, that have been prepared from fresh or minimally processed ingredients.
- B2 and magnesium supplements are associated with migraine preventatives and treatment.
- Supplements can't compensate for a poor diet. Improve your diet before you start taking any kind of vitamin and/or mineral supplement.

23

Strategies for Female Hormones

Hormonal changes can't be avoided, only managed. Natural methods of treatment and prevention for headaches initiated by changes in hormone levels mostly revolve around reducing your exposure to other known triggers to help you stay below your headache threshold.

You should also pay extra attention to your overall spinal posture and especially the posture of your head and neck. Women of all ages are more likely to suffer from headaches related to head and neck posture than men. Women's necks are thinner and less muscular, and their shoulder and neck muscles must support the weight of breasts. Women tend to have a larger curve in their lower back so their head and neck is held further forward in compensation. A supportive bra and manual therapy will help, plus stretching and strengthening exercises. The guidelines for a healthy lifestyle apply here too – do some regular gentle to moderate exercise, get adequate sleep, reduce stress, stay hydrated and eat regular meals.

Strategies for Menstrual Headaches

There is no doubt that rapid drops in estrogen can either trigger a headache or make you more sensitive to your other headache triggers by lowering your headache threshold.

To verify you are suffering from menstrual headaches, whether migraines or tension headaches, you will need to keep a headache calendar for at least 3 complete menstrual cycles.

The same natural methods of treatment and prevention can be applied to menstrual headaches as for headaches that aren't related to the menstrual cycle. You need to lower your total exposure to your known headache triggers and look after yourself so you don't reduce your headache threshold further.

In the week before your period is due:

- Pay extra attention to maintaining good head and neck posture
- Reduce stress
- Have regular meals
- Maintain constant sleep patterns
- Although you may feel bloated, drink water regularly so you don't get dehydrated.

If you suffer menstrual migraines, don't forget that there can sometimes be a delay of 3-4 days between becoming stressed and the start of a migraine attack.

Some additional specific natural remedies for menstrual headaches are:

- Wear a supportive bra with wide straps. This will relieve the strain on shoulder and neck muscles. Pre-menstrual water retention leads to enlargement of the breasts and the extra weight can make you round your shoulders and project your neck – a real no-no if you want to avoid headaches of any sort
- Get some remedial massage for tight neck and shoulder muscles
- Get a manipulation of the lumbar spine before your period. You could trial this for several cycles to see if it helps. There is anecdotal evidence supporting the effectiveness of manipulation of the lumbar spine for menstrual migraine, including for pure menstrual migraine[185,186]
- Magnesium supplementation – brain levels of magnesium appear to be low during migraine attacks. Menstrual migraines are associated with low free magnesium levels in the blood much more often than are migraines unrelated to the menstrual cycle.[187] This may also be worth trialling for several cycles.

Strategies for Headaches During Pregnancy

Pregnancy is an important time to avoid the use of headache medications. Sometimes, however, the stress hormones released in response to severe pain and the dehydration due to excessive vomiting can be harmful to the unborn baby and medication may be necessary in the short-term.

Similarly, while breast-feeding, if possible, avoid the use of headache medications, as these pass into the breast milk. It's essential that you check with your doctor before you take any medications or herbal remedies while pregnant or breast-feeding.

Most of the remedies in this book, such as manual therapy and relaxation, are equally applicable to headaches during pregnancy as at other times.

This includes moderate exercise such as walking, swimming, aqua-aerobics and supervised gentle to moderate exercise classes. You need to be more careful than usual during pregnancy to avoid injury. The forward shift in your centre of gravity affects your balance, ligaments soften due to high levels of the hormone relaxin,[188] and weight gain puts extra strain on joints and muscles. Check with your doctor to ensure the exercise you are doing is suitable.

Some simple specific tips that may be useful for headache during pregnancy include:

- Drink plenty of water – in early pregnancy nausea can lead to reduced fluid intake and vomiting can lead to fluid loss. Dehydration is an important headache trigger. You may tolerate water better if you drink frequent small amounts
- Eat small, frequent snacks containing carbohydrates, such as a piece of wholemeal toast or some fruit, to stop blood sugar getting too low – another likely consequence of nausea. Avoid sugary snacks as these cause a peak followed by a dip in your blood sugar – another common headache trigger
- Have adequate rest to counteract overtiredness, particularly in the first and third trimesters. With the postural changes that occur to accommodate the developing baby, especially during the third trimester, it can be hard to maintain good posture.

Manual therapy can help the headaches that occur during pregnancy. It may incorporate massage, mobilisation and manipulation, as well as stretching and strengthening exercises that you can continue for yourself at home.

Strategies for (Peri) Menopausal Headaches

To help prevent headaches during perimenopause and menopause, focus on:

- Reducing stress
- Improving overall spinal posture
- Exercising regularly.

Because stress is such an important contributor to both tension headaches and migraines, it's important to practice some relaxation and stress reduction techniques. Declining estrogen levels increase the tendency to put on weight around the middle and cause muscles to weaken. With age, the height of the discs which separate the spinal vertebrae gradually decrease. The result of these changes is worsening spinal posture, especially of the head and neck, and stiffening neck joints.

These physical changes may help explain the relatively high rate of tension headache after menopause, even when estrogen levels have stabilised. As you know, spinal posture can be improved by manual therapy, stretching and specific exercises to strengthen postural muscles.

Exercise is important to maintain muscular strength to support the spine, improve circulation, assist with weight control, reduce stress and improve mood.

You should also review with your doctor any hormonal medication you are taking. External sources of estrogen and progesterone from hormone replacement therapy

(HRT) and hormonal contraceptives can have a major effect on headaches, especially migraines.[189,190,191,192]

Hormonal Contraceptives and Headaches

There are two types of hormonal contraceptives:

- Combinations of estrogen and progesterone, taken for three weeks, followed by a one week break. These contraceptives often trigger an estrogen withdrawal headache during the week off
- Progesterone only contraceptives, especially the 'mini pill' which is taken continuously without a break. They may cause headaches, especially at higher doses.

Migraine sufferers should discuss the pros and cons of hormonal contraceptives with their doctor. Generally, migraine sufferers are advised to avoid a combination contraceptive if they:

- Get aura
- Don't get aura but are over the age of 35
- Have previously suffered severe menstrual headaches – estrogen withdrawal can sometimes trigger a severe form of migraine known as status migrainosus which requires emergency medical attention.

Some of the strategies your doctor may recommend for minimising your headaches are:

- Use monophasic pills – these have the same dose of estrogen and progesterone in all 21 active pills. They lead to the most stable hormonal levels and so would be expected to be less likely to provoke headaches
- Treat / prevent estrogen withdrawal headache by supplying low doses of estradiol from a skin patch during days 22 to 28 of the treatment cycle
- Use a low dose pill – the aim is to minimise the size of the estrogen drop at the end of the treatment cycle, and to avoid triggering a migraine aura.

Your doctor may also suggest that you trial the mini pill. It doesn't contain estrogen, so it won't cause an estrogen drop prior to menstrual bleeding. Alternatively, your doctor may recommend that you use the pill for four consecutive cycles without taking any days off (discard the dummy pills). This should reduce the number of headaches due to estrogen withdrawal by reducing the number of estrogen free intervals from 13 per year to 4.

Hormonal contraceptives don't appear to have much effect on tension headaches in women.

HRT and Headaches

The effect of Hormone Replacement Therapy (HRT) on headaches is highly variable. Overall, HRT appears to have little effect on tension headaches,[193] it worsens migraine with aura and, provided the dose is sufficient, improves migraine without aura.

To optimise HRT medication to minimise headache attacks, you should consult with your doctor to find a dosing regimen which keeps estrogen levels reasonably constant and above the threshold necessary to avoid an estrogen withdrawal headache.

Key Points

- Hormonal changes can't be avoided, only managed.
- Manual therapy can help with hormonal headaches.
- Posture is an important consideration during menopause.
- Reducing stress can help manage the impact of hormonal headaches
- Consult with your doctor before taking any sort of hormonal medication if you already suffer from migraine headaches.

24

Botox, Surgery

Botox

Botox is the trade name for one form of botulinum toxin, a neurotoxin produced by bacteria, and the most poisonous substance known. It destroys nerve terminals causing muscle paralysis. If it happens to get into a blood vessel by mistake it can spread through the body causing difficulty with breathing, swallowing and vision.

Botox has been used 'off-label' to treat headaches since the late 1990s, after plastic surgeons noticed patients having injections for frown lines were getting fewer headaches. When Botox is used to treat headaches, it's injected in tiny doses to temporarily paralyse or weaken muscles in the head and neck region. After two to three months, the effect wears off and muscle strength, and the headaches, return.

Botox injections were approved for use as a migraine preventative for adult sufferers of chronic migraines in the United States in October 2010, following earlier approval in the UK.

Despite the hype, Botox isn't a cure-all for headaches. Headache specialists believe sub-groups of patients may benefit from Botox treatment, but it's not yet clear how to predict who they are. This is partly because there's no accepted understanding for how Botox acts to prevent migraine.

In 2008, prior to its approval, a review of all published studies (involving a total of over 3000 patients) concluded that Botox 'should not be considered in patients with episodic migraine and chronic tension-type headaches'. In the case of chronic daily headache (mainly migraine), there was not enough reliable information to make a recommendation either way.[194]

Injections of a placebo were found to be almost as effective as Botox in headache patients.[195] High placebo response rates also characterised the two manufacturer-funded studies[196] on which the approval of Botox was based.

I think the main reason Botox sometimes works is related to muscular trigger points. If the Botox injection happens to target the right place in the injected muscle, it will allow taut bands to relax and fresh blood to enter. This restores depleted energy reserves, ending the local hypercontraction of the muscle. It would also flush out pain-producing metabolic wastes and natural inflammatory substances. Muscular trigger points would be deactivated.

A second possibility involves the effect of the needle itself. Depending on where in the muscle it is inserted, the needle used for the injection may unintentionally disrupt some taut bands or possibly even some muscular trigger points, reducing pain further.

When dry needling was first discovered it was found that it didn't matter if the syringe contained a local anaesthetic, salt solution or nothing at all.[197] It was the action of the needle that deactivated the muscular trigger points and supplied pain relief. Even just inserting the needle into the taut band relieved pain somewhat.

This 'needle effect', leading to the accidental treatment of muscular trigger points, may help explain why migraines improve almost as much following an injection with a placebo as with Botox.

However, these types of explanations are not accepted by scientists who discount the role of muscle pain in provoking headache attacks. It is common to read statements such as:

> *Researchers are unsure why Botox relieves head pain. For its other uses, including alleviating wrinkles... the purified protein relaxes the overactive muscle ... For migraines, there is no muscle component.*[198]

Yet in those patients with a one-sided migraine, the muscles of the scalp and facial expression and the temporalis muscles on both sides of the head are injected. If they are not, the headaches may shift to the side which was not affected before.[199]

This comment is made without any explanation. However, to me, it is further evidence of the importance of trigger points in the migraine process. As we have seen, the temporalis muscle is both an important chewing muscle and commonly involved in producing migraine-like pain. If the muscle on one side of the head is weakened by Botox, the other side will be overloaded and will develop trigger points. Pain is the result.

It's unlikely that the medical practitioners who treat headache with Botox injections are familiar with muscular trigger points. Nor is it likely they are aware headache pain can be referred pain from muscles. The decision about which muscles to inject is mainly influenced by the type of headache the patient is thought to have and the site of the pain.

In other words, Botox injections don't treat the source of pain – they treat the area the pain is referred to. The practitioner may use a 'follow-the-pain' approach, which includes palpating the muscles for tenderness, but not for muscular trigger points, or they may use pre-determined injection sites where many patients have previously reported they feel pain. Sometimes a mixture of both approaches is used.

The muscles that are commonly injected include[200]:

- Several superficial muscles of the scalp and facial expression (frontalis, occipitalis, procerus and corrugator)
- The outer jaw muscles – the temporalis and (infrequently) the masseter
- The deeper muscles of the back of the neck (splenius and semispinalis)
- The upper trapezius muscle.

Each muscle will receive multiple injections in different locations, usually making a total of 30–39 injections in a single treatment.

Notice that only one of our 'big three' headache pain producers, the upper trapezius, has made it onto this list. The SCM and the sub-occipital muscles are absent.

For a few migraine sufferers who have frequent attacks or a lengthy migraine history, the frontalis, occipitalis, corrugator and procerus muscles may be a source of pain.[201,202] This group of people may obtain short-term relief from Botox injections into the facial and scalp muscles. Removing just one of several sources of pain referred to the same area will make headaches less severe. It may even be sufficient to reduce the total input to the headache pain centre below the threshold needed to provoke a headache attack in the first place.

I believe a far more effective and much safer way of achieving the same result is to treat the 'big three' muscular trigger point sites with manual therapy, which also removes satellite muscular trigger points in the facial and jaw muscles. If necessary, muscular trigger points in the scalp and facial muscles can be treated by manual therapy, just like any other muscle. If they are an important source of pain for you, it is relatively easy to learn how to treat them yourself.

The Risks of Botox Treatment

Like pain-killers in tablet form, Botox aims to mask the pain, rather than understand the causes and treat them. And Botox isn't really very effective for headache pain.

A recent review of the evidence for Botox, the Drug and Therapeutics Bulletin (a well-respected British journal) stated that it could not 'see a place' for giving Botox to sufferers of chronic migraine.[203] They also reported that Botox actually made headache symptoms worse in about 1 in 10 people and caused a similar number to develop side effects such as itching, rash, pain, stiffness and muscle spasms.

For the splenius and semispinalis muscles at the back of the neck, practitioners have to be particularly cautious about the dose, depth and sites of injection. Otherwise patients can end up with neck pain or excessive muscle weakness which can require them to wear a surgical collar until the effects of the Botox wear off.[204]

Experiments with animals have also raised concerns that repeated Botox injections reduce muscle strength, not just in the muscles injected, but in other muscles far from the injection site. Muscles atrophied and muscle tissue was replaced by fat.[205]

Why Botox Treatment Isn't More Effective

- Muscular trigger points are not recognised as a source of headache pain. They are not palpated. If they are injected it is only by luck.
- Because of this, the source of pain is not treated. Injections are made into pre-determined locations in specific muscles or into sites which are tender – in other words into the areas where pain is referred but not its source.
- Of the 3 most important muscles to treat for headache pain, the sternocleidomastoid, upper trapezius and sub-occipital muscles, only the upper trapezius receives treatment (sometimes).
- Almost all trigger points that by good luck happen to be injected will be satellites. Key trigger points are not treated so these satellites will soon recur.
- Factors which perpetuate trigger points, such as forward head posture or teeth grinding, are not corrected, so again any treated trigger points will recur.
- Pain in the forehead and eye areas is very likely to contain a major contribution from untreated trigger points in the sternocleidomastoid. These are also responsible for the autonomic symptoms that characterise migraines.
- Muscles of the scalp and facial expression are always injected. Yet trigger points in these muscles are an uncommon source of headache pain, so this won't help most headache sufferers.

Surgery

Nerve Decompression Surgery

Patients whose headaches show 50% improvement in either frequency or severity in response to Botox are considered suitable candidates for nerve decompression surgery. This involves the surgical removal or weakening of particular muscles. All surgery has risks, and, unlike Botox, the effects on muscles are permanent.

Surgeons who perform nerve decompression surgery reason that if Botox injections into a muscle improves migraines, that muscle must be causing migraines by compressing nerves, however this has not been proven.

Vascular Surgery for Migraines

In a migraine attack, the arteries that lie outside the skull beneath the scalp are enlarged and pulsate with every heartbeat, which stretches the fine network of nerves wrapped around them, causing pain.

The main arteries involved are the temporal artery, which lies just under the skin of the temple near the ear, and the superficial part of the occipital artery which lies beneath the scalp at the back of the head, near the base of the skull (Figure 24.1). Both are downstream branches of the common carotid artery, one of the two main arteries that supply blood to the brain.

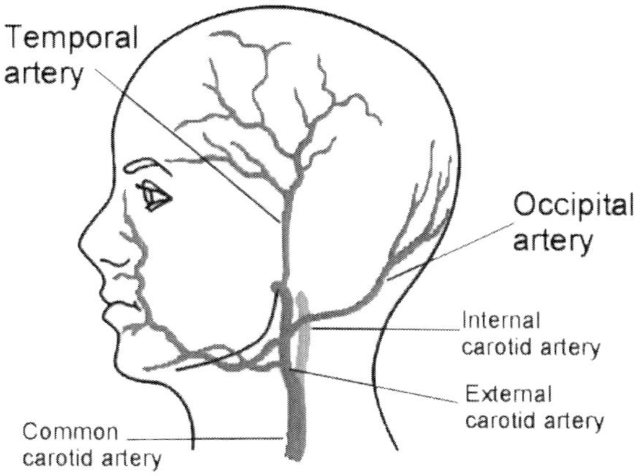

Figure 24.1 – The main arteries of the scalp

When a migraine attack is in progress, compressing the various sub-branches of these arteries can identify which of the arteries are causing pain.

Finger pressure stops blood flow to the area. If the pain decreases with pressure and then increases again as the pressure is released (usually within a few seconds) then this part of the artery is a source of pain.[206] Injection of saline around the pressure sensitive arteries, particularly around the temporal artery, can relieve the pain of a migraine attack.[207]

In vascular surgery for chronic migraine, the arterial segments that are causing pain are identified and then surgically removed. This type of operation has a very long history, being first performed by the renowned Moorish surgeon, Al Zahrawi, who lived in 10th century Spain.

Why the scalp arteries dilate during migraine has been debated for many decades. However, it is known that the fine network of nerves which surround all blood vessels can be irritated by inflammation of the surrounding tissues.

I think the inflammatory soup present in muscular trigger points is the most likely explanation for the pain that is observed in the scalp arteries of migraine sufferers between attacks.

The effect of applying sustained pressure to painful parts of the temporal artery or injecting saline into areas surrounding it, will be to deactivate at least some of the muscular trigger points in the temporalis muscle. Using saline, the effect of the needle and washing away some of the inflammatory soup may both contribute to pain relief.

Actions like clenching the teeth, which cause the temporalis muscle to remain contracted for a prolonged period, will make muscular trigger points in the muscle more irritable. The contracted muscle will also compress small branches of the painful temporalis artery that pass through it. This combination may well be sufficient to provoke a migraine attack.

Once again, I don't think surgery is called for. Far better to begin with seeing a good manual therapist for muscular trigger point treatment!

Key Points

- When Botox is used to treat headaches, its aim is to temporarily paralyse or weaken muscles in the head and neck region.
- Botox injections for headaches treat the site of the pain, not the source.
- After two or three months, the effects wear off and muscle strength, and headaches return.
- Like painkillers in tablet form, Botox aims to mask the pain, rather than understand the causes and treat them.
- Surgery for migraines should be a last resort.

Conclusion

This is the exciting part! It's time for you to begin your journey to fewer headaches, less pain, better health and genuine, measurable, positive improvements to your life. It's time to take charge.

It's time to end your reliance on pain killers as a solution to headache pain. As a society, we are pre-occupied with the short-term, quick-fix – it's one of the main reasons we have an over-reliance on painkillers. Marketing campaigns might promise 'rapid relief' for headache pain, but pain killers only ever mask your symptoms and, in the end, can make your headaches worse, cause rebound headaches and damage your overall health. Now you know there's a new way to manage headache pain, it's time to start practising the strategies that will bring you significant, long-lasting relief.

So much of this book is common sense. Whilst headaches can feel mysterious, in the end, I believe managing your headaches comes down to a few simple instructions, suggestions and guidelines: drink more water, breath more deeply, stretch regularly, reduce stress, improve and monitor your posture and find a manual therapist who can treat possible muscular trigger points.

None of it is especially glamorous, high tech or immediate, but this method of tackling the sources of headache pain and raising your headache threshold will deliver significant and lasting improvement. Most importantly, it puts you back in charge. Headaches are not all in your head. They are a real, debilitating condition that deserves more attention than continually taking a pain killer to mask the symptoms. Taking a pain killer for your headaches is like turning up the radio to cover a strange sound in your car. You might not be able to hear the sound anymore, but you haven't solved the problem.

Headaches are a sign that something is not working as it should somewhere in your body. Knowing you need to track down the source of the pain somewhere in your body is a big step in the right direction. As a bonus, the simple, accessible, inexpensive strategies I have suggested to reduce the intensity and frequency of your headaches will have a huge impact on your quality of life.

The most vital aspect of your treatment is to find what works for you. Keeping a headache diary, talking to people about what works and considering the impact of any medication will help you find a set of strategies that work best for you.

As you begin your headache diary*, you should:

- Have at least 3–5 professional manual therapy treatments that focus on:
    - Deactivation of active muscular trigger points, especially those in neck, shoulder and jaw muscles
    - Making stiff neck joints more mobile with gentle techniques such as joint mobilisation, muscle energy technique and stretching
    - Correction of overall spinal posture by treating muscle imbalances
- Improve your ergonomic set-up to eliminate forward head posture, especially when sitting. Check your head and neck posture when you are using a computer, laptop, smart phone, tablet, reading in bed, watching TV, driving
- Stop sleeping on your stomach and improve your sleeping posture if necessary
- Don't carry bags over one shoulder
- Work on improving your head and neck posture by doing stretching and strengthening exercises for neck and shoulder muscles
- Stop sitting for prolonged periods. Take regular breaks and move around.
- Reduce stress where possible
- Stay well hydrated by drinking water throughout the day
- Eat regularly spaced meals at about the same time each day and eat a varied, healthy, balanced diet. Avoid sugary drinks and snacks. Monitor caffeine and alcohol intake. Don't worry too much about avoiding other foods. This is less important than you might think for most headache sufferers
- Do regular, moderate aerobic exercise
- Get enough sleep so that you don't feel sleepy during the day. Keep a regular sleep pattern – go to bed and get up at about the same time each day
- Don't smoke or take illicit drugs.

Small steps, completed consistently over time, will accumulate to create a big, positive difference. Your journey will be gradual and steady – this is all about being the tortoise, not the hare. Be kind to yourself if you wander off track – lapses, restarts, resets, rests and adjustments are all part of the process. For some people, the lack of immediate improvement can be dispiriting. They might quit after the eighth day of stretching because they're still tight, stop exercising after three weeks because they still feel stressed, or stop making remedial massage appointments because they only experienced short-term pain relief. Remember, small, smart choices and consistency over time lead to less headaches, less stress and a healthier lifestyle.

Your commitment to making progressive, lasting change will make all the difference. Friends and family can be a great support for you, especially early on as you establish new habits, and re-reading relevant chapters can also help keep you focused and committed to your new path. I hope you keep this book close by and refer to it often as a guide and reminder of the profound benefits of your new practice. Every tortoise needs a support team!

As part of your new practice, I urge you to investigate muscular trigger point therapy. It is the key to managing headaches successfully. Time and again, I have seen people whose lives have been transformed for the better after several sessions of manual therapy that treats their muscular trigger points. If it doesn't work, at worst, you've had a massage, but if it does work, I predict it will feel like a magical revelation – one you're very welcome to share with me and this growing community.

I have dedicated my professional life to helping others. Nothing makes me feel better than when I can see the improvements I have helped someone make in their own life. That's one of the main reasons I wrote this book and one of the main reasons I would encourage you to gift a copy to a friend or colleague if you feel they would benefit from the strategies and advice here. One of my driving motivations is to share this message as far and wide as I can – slowly and steadily – and there is no better endorsement than from someone who has lived the journey and felt the benefits.

If you'd like to share your story, or have any questions, please contact me at info@pablotymoszuk.com

Yours gratefully and in health – Pablo

* **A printable PDF of the Headache Diary** can be downloaded from:

https://newapproachtoheadaches.com/headache-diary-download/

Acknowledgements

Clive Edington – thank you for your generous and on-going support with the computer aspects of this book, for patiently reading multiple drafts and for your feed-back.

Liz Tymoszuk – my gorgeous, supportive and loving wife. Thank you for demonstrating the stretches and numerous methods of self-treatment of headaches.

Carolyn Tetaz – thank you for your patience, word mastery and editing.

Gregory and Ana Tymoszuk - I am honoured and blessed to have you as my parents.

Friends and patients – I would like to express my appreciation to the various friends and patients who agreed to let us tell their stories in our headache case histories.

Reviewers – thank you for taking the time to read and write such encouraging and insightful reviews of my book – I am truly humbled.

Photo Credits

Photos of Liz are by Aaron Stott Photography © Copyright 2013.
Illustrations throughout the book are by the author unless otherwise noted.
Credits for stock photos are listed below.
(PD means Public Domain)

Chapter 13

Figure 13.2, Muscle structure, adapted from National Cancer Institute PD.

Chapter 15

Figure 15.3, Adapted, Back of male head and neck, © TheSupe87 Fotolia.com.
Figure 15.6, Adapted, Body builder with large shoulders, © Shakzu Fotolia.com.
Figure 15.13, Adapted, Muscle layers, neck and face, © York Fotolia.com.
Figure 15.14, Adapted, Muscles of neck, front view, © CLIPAREA.com Fotolia.com.
Figure 15.15, Adapted, Muscle layers, neck and face, © York Fotolia.com.
Figure 15.16, Adapted, Muscle layers, neck and face, © York Fotolia.com.
Figure 15.17, Adapted, Muscles of neck, front view, © CLIPAREA.com Fotolia.com.

Chapter 18

Man with forward head posture, © snaptitude Fotolia.com.
Figure 18.1, Adapted, spine Gray Wikimedia commons & skull WPClipart PD.
Figure 18.2, Adapted, Male rear view line drawing, © Anna Rassadnikova Fotolia.com.
Adapted, Young man in shorts side view, © Ljupco Smokovski Fotolia.com.
Adapted, People waiting in a queue, © Yuri Arcurs Fotolia.com.
Figure 18.3, Extract from people waiting in a queue, © Yuri Arcurs Fotolia.com.
Adapted, Girl in high heels, curved spine, © Ljupco Smokovski Fotolia.com.
Figure 18.4, Adapted, Waiting businessman 9 am, © biker3 Fotolia.com.
Waiting businessman 10 am, © biker3 Fotolia.com.
Adapted, Slumped businessman, © magann Fotolia.com.
Adapted, Businessman leaning on thighs, © Roman White Fotolia.com.
Adapted, Man with forward head posture, © snaptitude Fotolia.com.
Adapted, Young woman lying on couch with book, © stokkete Fotolia.com.
Adapted, Young man asleep under paper, © Yuri Arcurs Fotolia.com.
Young man playing video game, © Crashoran Fotolia.com.
Monk in scriptorium, © William Blades Wikimedia Commons PD.
Head rest position, © gemenacom Fotolia.com.

Adapted, Young man asleep arms crossed, © Yuri Arcurs Fotolia.com.
Adapted, Young man asleep on stomach, © Monkey Business Fotolia.com.
Illustration, orthopedic mattress, © germina Fotolia.com.
Woman asleep on couch-1, © djma Fotolia.com.
Woman asleep on couch-2, © Tomasz Trojanowski Fotolia.com.
Adapted, Businessman sitting on fit ball, © Blend Images Fotolia.com.
Adapted, Woman phoning & typing, © WavebreakmediaMicro Fotolia.com.

Chapter 19

Adapted, Young man with laptop on couch, © beatrice prève Fotolia.com.
Young people texting, © Andres Rodriguez Fotolia.com.
Smart phone for internet, © bloomua Fotolia.com.
Ideal computer posture, Safety & Health, Uni WA (with permission)
Correct chair adjustment, Dept Labor & Industries, Wash State PD.
Correct keyboard height, © Alexey Klementiev Fotolia.com.
Young boy using computer-1, © Jacek Chabraszewski Fotolia.com.
Adapted, Young boy using computer-2, © Jacek Chabraszewski Fotolia.com.
Adapted, Woman, laptop on kitchen bench, © Ambro freedigitalphotos.net.

References

[1] BB Vargas (2008). "Tension-type headache and migraine: Two points on a continuum?" Curr Pain Headache Rep 12(6) 433-436.
[2] See discussion in E Loder and VT Martin (2004). "Chapter 5: Tension-type Headache", p80-83, *Headache: a guide for the primary care physician*, ACP Press.
[3] F Mongini (1999), "Chapter 9: Factor interplay. Interplay between migraine and tension-type headache", p100, *Headache and facial pain*, Thieme.
[4] Olesen (1991). "Clinical and pathophysiological observations in migraine and tension-type headache explained by integration of vascular, supraspinal and myofascial inputs". J Pain 46(2): 125-132.
[5] Travell & Simons, Myofascial Pain and Dysfunction: The Trigger Point Manual. Volume 1. Upper half of body, Edition 2, Lippincott, Williams and Wilkins, p.57
[6] GD Hack, RT Koritzer, WL Robinson, RC Hallgren and PE Greenman (1995). "Anatomic relation between the rectus capitis posterior minor muscle and the dura mater". Spine (Phila Pa 1976) 20(23):2484-2486.
[7] C F Fernández-de-Las-Peñas, L Arendt-Nielsen and RD Gerwin (2009). "Chapter 7: Suboccipital Muscle Contribution to TensionType Headache", p86-87, Tension- Type and Cervicogenic Headache: Pathophysiology, Diagnosis, and Management, Jones and Bartlett.
[8] GD Hack and RC Hallgren (2004). "Chronic Headache Relief After Section of Suboccipital Muscle Dural Connections: A Case Report". Headache 44(1):84-89.
[9] JD Loeser, JJ Bonica, SH Butler, CR Chapman, DC Turk (2001). "Basic Concepts in Biomechanics and Rehabilitation", p1819, Bonica's Management of Pain, Edition 3, Lippincott, Williams and Wilkins.
[10] K Khan and P Brukner (2001), "Chapter 3: Pain: Where is it coming from", p32, Clinical Sports Medicine, Edition 2, Mcgraw-Hill.
[11] J Holzhammer and C Wöber (2006). "Alimentary trigger factors that provoke migraine and tension-type headache." *Schmerz* 20(2): 151-159.
[12] FC Rockett, VR de Oliveira, K Castro, MLF Chaves, A da S Perla and IDS Perry (2012). "Dietary aspects of migraine trigger factors." Nutr Rev 70(6): 337-356.
[13] PB Prince, A Rapoport, FD Sheftell, S Tepper and M Bigal (2004). "The Effect of Weather on Headache", *Headache* 44(6): 596-602.
[14] RA Purdy and AM Rapoport (2005). "Chapter 10: The women with multiple trigger factors." p56, *Advanced therapy of headache*, Edition 2, PMPH-USA.
[15] Sleep Apnoea, Better Health Channel, Government of Victoria, Australia.
[16] "Sinus Headache: A Neurology, Otolaryngology, Allergy, and Primary Care Concensus on Diagnosis and Treatment." Mayo Clinic Proceedings 2005;80(7):908-916
[17] C Rondón, G Canto and M Blanca (2010). "Local allergic rhinitis: a new entity, characterization and further studies." *Curr Opin Allergy Clin Immunol* 10(1): 1-7.

[18] MG Spigt, EC Kuijper, CP van Schayck, J Troost, PG Knipschild, VM Linssen and JA Knottnerus (2005). "Increasing the daily water intake for the prophylactic treatment of headache: a pilot trial "*Eur J Neurol* 12(9): 715-718.
[19] RA Purdy and AM Rapoport (2005). "Chapter 10: The women with multiple trigger factors" p54, *Advanced therapy of headache,* Edition 2, PMPH-USA. And RA Davidoff (2002). "Chapter 5: Initiators, precipitators and triggers", p99, *Migraine: manifestations, pathogenesis, and management*, Edition 2, Oxford University Press.
[20] The International Classification of Headache Disorders." 2nd edition, The International Headache Society (IHS).
[21] RHM Kwok (1968). "Chinese restaurant syndrome". *N Engl J Med,* 278: 796.
[22] Monica Singh (2005). "Fact or Fiction? The MSG Controversy" Harvard Law School.
[23] JM Borkum (2012). Chronic Headaches: Biology, Psychology, and Behavioral Treatment, p235-236, Psychology Press
[24] RA Davidoff (2002). "Migraine: Manifestations, Pathogenesis and Management." Contemporary Neurology, Volume 65, p101-102, Oxford University Press
[25] BT Daniel (2010). Migraine, p154-155, AuthorHouse
[26] JO Lundberg, E Weitzberg and MT Gladwin (2008). "The nitrate–nitrite–nitric oxide pathway in physiology and therapeutics". *Nat Rev Drug Discov*, 7(2):156-167.
[27] SB Miller. "IgG Food Allergy Testing by ELISA/EIA. What Do They Really Tell Us?". Gives a simple overview.
[28] S Gavura (2012). Science-Based Medicine. Exploring issues and controversies in the relationship between science and medicine. This reference gives the position statements of major national immunology groups on IgG tests.
[29] A Hougaard, F Amin, AW Hauge, M Ashina and J Olesen (2013). "Provocation of migraine with aura using natural trigger factors." *Neurology* **80**(5): 428-431.
[30] AH Calhoun (2004). "Chapter 9: Women's issues in headache", p157-167. "*Headache: a guide for the primary care physician*", Editors E Loder and VT Martin, ACP Press.
[31] Reported in CA Warfield and ZH Bajwa (2004). "Chapter 18: Historical features in primary headache syndromes", p199-201, *Principles and Practice of Pain Medicine*, Edition 2, McGraw-Hill.
[32] AH Calhoun (2004). "Chapter 9: Women's issues in headache", p157-167. "*Headache: a guide for the primary care physician*", Editors E Loder and VT Martin, ACP Press.
[33] ibid.
[34] ibid.
[35] ibid.
[36] ibid.
[37] DA Marcus (2001). "Estrogen and tension-type headache". *Curr Pain Headache Rep* 5(5):449-453.
[38] CD Bushnell, M Jamison and AH James (2009). "Migraines during pregnancy linked to stroke and vascular diseases: US population based case-control study". *BMJ* 338:b664.
[39] RE Nappi, A Cagnacci, F Granella, F Piccinini and FF Facchinetti (2001). "Course of primary headaches during hormone replacement therapy". *Maturitas* 38(2):157-163.
[40] Cited in the review article by FV Abbott and MI Fraser (1998). "Use and abuse of over-the-counter analgesic agents". *J Psychiatry Neurosci.* **23**(1):13-34.
[41] ibid.
[42] American Headache Society, "Information for patients, Commonly Used Acute Migraine Treatments".

[43] American Headache Society, "Information for patients, Commonly Used Acute Migraine Treatments."
[44] American Academy of Neurology (2008). "Overuse Of Codeine, Oxycodone And Barbiturates Increases Risk Of Chronic Migraine". *ScienceDaily*, April 27, 2008.
[45] SD Silberstein (2005)."Chronic Daily Headache". *JAOA* **105** (4): 23-29.
[46] Cited in the review article by FV Abbott and MI and Fraser (1998). "Use and abuse of over-the-counter analgesic agents". *J Psychiatry Neurosci.* **23**(1):13-34.
[47] RA Moore, S Derryl and HJ McQuay (2008). "Faecal blood loss with aspirin, nonsteroidal anti-inflammatory drugs and cyclo-oxygenase-2 selective inhibitors: systematic review of randomized trials using autologous chromium-labelled erythrocytes". *Arthritis Res Ther.* 10(1) :R7.
[48] RA Moore, S Derryl and HJ McQuay (2008). "Faecal blood loss with aspirin, nonsteroidal anti-inflammatory drugs and cyclo-oxygenase-2 selective inhibitors: systematic review of randomized trials using autologous chromium-labelled erythrocytes". *Arthritis Res Ther.* 10(1) :R7.
[49] PB Watkins, N Kaplowitz, JT Slattery, CR Colonese, SV Colucci, PW Stewart and SC Harris (2006). "Aminotransferase Elevations in Healthy Adults Receiving 4 Grams of Acetaminophen Daily. A Randomized Controlled Trial" *JAMA* 296(1):87-93.
[50] KA Kobak, DJ Katzelnick, G Sands, M King, JJ Greist and M Dominski M (2005). "Prevalence and burden of illness of migraine in managed care patients". *J Manag Care Pharm.* **11**(2):124-136.
[51] V Di Piero, M Altieri, G Conserva, B Petolicchio, L Di Clemente and J Hettiarachchi J (2007). "The effects of a sensitisation campaign on unrecognised migraine: the Casilino study". *J Headache Pain* **8**(4):205-208.
[52] N Karli, M Zarifoglu, N Calisir and S Akgoz (2005). "Comparison of pre-headache phases and trigger factors of migraine and episodic tension-type headache: do they share similar clinical pathophysiology?" *Cephalalgia* **25**(6):444-451.
[53] CP Schreiber, S Hutchinson, CJ Webster, M Ames, MS Richardson and C Powers (2004). "Prevalence of migraine in patients with a history of self-reported or physician-diagnosed "sinus" headache." *Arch Intern Med* **164**(16):1769-1772.
[54] DM Biondi (2005). "Cervicogenic Headache: A Review of Diagnostic and Treatment Strategies." *JAOA* **105**(4):16-22.
[55] N. Bogduk (2001). "Cervicogenic headache: anatomic basis and pathophysiologic mechanisms."*Curr Pain Headache Rep.***5**(4):382-386.
[56] DG Simons, JG Travell and LS Simons (1999). "Chapter 5: Overview of Head and Neck Region", p247-248, 255-256, *Travell & Simons' Myofascial Pain and Dysfunction: The Trigger Point Manual. Volume 1. Upper half of body,* Edition 2, Lippincott, Williams and Wilkins.
[57] LW Ferguson and R Gerwin (2004). "Chapter 1: Headache", p3, *Clinical mastery in the treatment of myofascial pain*, Lippincott, Williams and Wilkins.
[58] Travell and Simons' Volume 1, p246-247, 248-253.
[59] JI Ingle, LK Bakland, JC Baumgartner, Teton Data Systems (Firm) (2008). "Chapter 11: Non-endodontic toothache and chronic head and neck pain," p428, *Ingle's Endodontics*, Edition 6, PMPH-USA.
[60] S Haldeman (2004). "Chapter 24: Headaches of Spinal Origin", p458, *Principles and Practice of Chiropractic*, McGraw-Hill.
[61] SS. DeRossi, ET Stoopler and TP Sollecito (2005). "Temporomandibular Disorders And Migraine Headache: Comorbid Conditions?" *The Internet Journal of Dental Science* **2**(1).

[62] "The International Classification of Headache Disorders." 2nd edition, The International Headache Society (IHS).
[63] ibid.
[64] JK Roth, RS Roth, JR Weintraub and DG Simons (2007). "Cervicogenic headache caused by myofascial trigger points in the sternocleidomastoid: a case report." *Cephalalgia* 27(4): 375–380.
[65] DG Simons, JG Travell and LS Simons (1999). "Part 2: Head and Neck Pain", Chapters 5 to17, *Travell & Simons' Myofascial Pain and Dysfunction: The Trigger Point Manual. Volume 1. Upper half of body*, Edition 2, Lippincott, Williams and Wilkins.
[66] J Travell, S Rinzler and M Herman (1942). "Pain and disability of the shoulder and arm: Treatment by intramuscular infiltration with procaine hydrochloride." *JAMA* **120**(6): 417–422.
[67] O Steinbrocker (1944). "Therapeutic injections in painful musculoskeletal disorders. With special reference to the saline-procaine test." *JAMA* **125**(6): 397-401.
[68] K Lewit (1979). "The needle effect in the relief of myofascial pain." *Pain* **6**(1):83-90.
[69] CZ Hong (1994). "Lidocaine injection versus dry needling to myofascial trigger point: The importance of the local twitch response." *Am J Phys Med Rehabil* 73(4): 256-263.
[70] DG Simons, JG Travell and LS Simons (1999). "Part 1: Introduction", Chapter 3, p151, *Travell & Simons' Myofascial Pain and Dysfunction: The Trigger Point Manual. Volume 1. Upper half of body*, Edition 2, Lippincott, Williams and Wilkins.
[71] JP Shah, TM Phillips, JV Danoff and LH Gerber (2005). "An in vivo microanalytical technique for measuring the local biochemical milieu of human skeletal muscle". J Appl Physiol 99(5): 1977-1984.
[72] TS Issa, PA Huijbregts (2006). "Physical Therapy Diagnosis and Management of a Patient with Chronic Daily Headache: A Case Report." *J Man Manip Ther* **14**(4): E88 - E123.
[73] Travell and Simons, Volume 1, p150, 151.
[74] K Khan and P Brukner (2001), "Chapter 8: Principles of treatment", p155, *Clinical Sports Medicine*, Edition 2, Mcgraw-Hill.
[75] CZ Hong, TS Kuan, JT Chen and SM Chen (1997). "Referred pain elicited by palpation and by needling of myofascial trigger points: a comparison." *Arch Phys Med Rehabil* **78**(9): 957-960.
[76] J Dommerholt (2006). "Trigger Point Dry Needling." *J Man Manip Ther* **14**(4): E70 - E87
[77] E Schultz, DL Jaryszak and CR Valliere (1985). "Response of satellite cells to focal skeletal muscle injury." *Muscle Nerve* **85**(8): 217-222.
[78] H Teravainen (1970). "Satellite cells of striated muscle after compression injury so slight as not to cause degeneration of the muscle fibres." *Z Zellforsch Mikrosk Anat* **103**(3): 320-327. Cited in reference 18.
[79] J Chu and I Schwartz (2002). "The muscle twitch in myofascial pain relief: effects of acupuncture and other needling methods." *Electromyogr Clin Neurophysiol* **42**(5):
[80] A Moraska and C Chandler (2008). "Changes in Clinical Parameters in Patients with Tension-type Headache Following Massage Therapy: A Pilot Study." *J Man Manip Ther* **16**(2): 106–112.
[81] H Mori, H Ohsawa, TH Tanaka, E Taniwaki, G Leisman and K Nishijo (2004). "Effect of massage on blood flow and muscle fatigue following isometric lumbar exercise." *Med Sci Monit* **10**(5): CR173-178.
[82] C Geoffrey and C Goats (1994). "Massage - the scientific basis of an ancient art: part 2. Physiological and therapeutic effects." *Br J Sp Med* **28**(3) 153 – 156.

[83] G Fryer, CM Morse and JC Johnson (2009). "Spinal and sacroiliac assessment and treatment techniques used by osteopathic physicians in the United States." *Osteopath Med Prim Care* **3**(4).
[84] SM. Johnson and ME. Kurtz (2003). "Osteopathic Manipulative Treatment Techniques Preferred by Contemporary Osteopathic Physicians." *J Am Osteopath Assoc* **103**(5) 219 -224.
[85] T Grant and K Niere (2000). "Techniques used by manipulative physiotherapists in the management of headaches." *Aust J Physiother* **46**(3):215-222.
[86] S Jensen (2005). "Neck related causes of headache." *Aust Fam Physician* **34**(8):
[87] J van Duijn, AJ. van Duijn and W Nitsch (2007). "Orthopaedic Manual Physical Therapy Including Thrust Manipulation and Exercise in the Management of a Patient with Cervicogenic Headache: A Case Report." *J Man Manip Ther* **15**(1): 10–24.
[88] T Grant and K Niere (2000). "Techniques used by manipulative physiotherapists in the management of headaches." *Aust J Physiother* **46**(3):215-222.
[89] S Jensen (2005). "Neck related causes of headache." *Aust Fam Physician* **34**(8):
[90] T Grant and K Niere (2000). "Techniques used by manipulative physiotherapists in the management of headaches." *Aust J Physiother* **46**(3):215-222.
[91] CY Hsieh, CZ Hong, AH Adams, KJ Platt, CD Danielson, FK Hoehler and JS Tobis (2000). "Interexaminer reliability of the palpation of trigger points in the trunk and lower limb muscles." *Arch Phys Med Rehabil* **81**(3): 258-264.
[92] LE Armstrong (2012). "Hydration Biomarkers During Daily Life: Recent Advances and Future Potential." *Nutrition Today* **47**(4) Supplement 1: S3 - S6. http://www.nursingcenter.com/lnc/journalarticle?Article_ID=1411155#TT1
[93] JN Blau, CA Kell and JM Sperling (2004). "Water-Deprivation Headache: A New Headache With Two Variants." *Headache* **44**(1): 79–83.
[94] JN Blau and SL Dexter (1980). "Hyperventilation during migraine attacks." *Br Med J* **280**(6226): 1254.
[95] LA Bobeĭko, IV Moldovanu and OA Kolosova (1994). "The role of hyperventilation and neuromuscular excitability in the clinical picture and pathogenesis of migraine headaches." Zh Nevrol Psikhiatr Im **94**(5): 10-12. [Article in Russian]
[96] P Sarchielli, G Coata, C Firenze, P Morucci, G Abbritti and V Gallai (1992). "Serum and salivary magnesium levels in migraine and tension-type headache. Results in a group of adult patients." *Cephalalgia* **12**(1): 21-27.
[97] BM Altura and BT Altura (1996). "Role of magnesium in patho-physiological processes and the clinical utility of magnesium ion selective electrodes." *Scand J Clin Lab Invest Suppl* **224**: 211-234.
[98] A Mauskop, BT Altura, RQ Cracco and BM Altura (1993). "Deficiency in serum ionized magnesium but not total magnesium in patients with migraines. Possible role of ICa2+/IMg2+ ratio." *Headache* **33**(3): 135-138.
[99] A Mauskop and BM Altura (1998). "Role of magnesium in the pathogenesis and treatment of migraines." *Clin Neurosci* **5**(1): 24-27.
[100] A Mauskop, BT Altura, RQ Cracco and BM Altura (1996). "Intravenous magnesium sulfate rapidly alleviates headaches of various types." *Headache* **36**(3): 154-160.
[101] H Laudańska, A Lemancewicz, M Kretowska, T Reduta and T Laudański (2002). "Permeability of human skin to selected anions and cations--in vitro studies." *Commun Mol Pathol Pharmacol* **112**(1-4): 16-26.
[102] Dr RH Waring (2009). "Report on Absorption of magnesium sulfate (Epsom salts) across the skin."

[103] S Diamond and FG Freitag (1986). "Cold as an adjunctive therapy for headache." *Postgrad Med* **79**(1): 305-309.
[104] S Ucler, O Coskun, E Levent E and Y Kanatli (2006). "Cold Therapy in Migraine Patients: Open-label, Non-controlled, Pilot Study." *Evid Based Complement Alternat Med* **3**(4): 489–493.
[105] MH Friedman, SJ Peterson, CF Behar and Z Zaidi (2001). "Intraoral chilling versus oral sumatriptan for acute migraine." *Heart Dis* 3(6): 357-361.
[106] JW Lance (1988). "The controlled application of cold and heat by a new device (Migra-lief apparatus) in the treatment of headache." *Headache* 28(7): 458-461.
[107] E Shevel (2007). "Chapter VII: The role of the external vasculature in migraine", p165-171, *Migraine Disorders Research Trends*, Editor: LB Clarke, Nova Publishers.
[108] Y Hmaidan and C Cianchetti (2006). "Effectiveness of a prolonged compression of scalp arteries on migraine attacks." *J Neurol* 253(6): 811–812.
[109] SA Lipton (1986). "Prevention of classic migraine headache by digital massage of the superficial temporal arteries during visual aura." *Ann Neurol* 19(5):515-6.
[110] SJ Gordon, KA Grimmer and P Trott (2004). "Self reported versus recorded sleep position: an observational study". *Internet Journal of Allied Health Sciences and Practice* 2(1).
[111] See references in JM Ebben (2003). "Improved Ergonomics for Standing Work" Occ Health and Safety (Apr)
[112] CE Matthews, KY Chen, PS Freedson, MS Buchowski, BM Beech, RR Pate and RP Troiano (2008). "Amount of Time Spent in Sedentary Behaviors in the United States, 2003–2004". *Am. J. Epidemiol.* **167**(7): 875-881.
[113] Use of Fitballs at UWA, The University of Western Australia, Safety and Health.
[114] D Fishman (2010). "Forward Head Posture Caused by Texting, Tell Your Patients: Your Body Is Sending You a Message". *Dynamic Chiropractic* 28(9).
[115] A Lenhart (2010). "Adults, Cell Phones and Texting", Pew Internet & American Life Project, Pew Research Center Publications.
[116] JG Young, M Trudeau, D Odell, K Marinelli and JT Dennerlein (2012). "Touch-screen tablet user configurations and case-supported tilt affect head and neck flexion angles." *Work* **41**(1): 81-91.
[117] JM Nash and RW Thebarge (2006). "Understanding Psychological Stress, Its Biological Processes, & Impact on Primary Headache". *Headache* **46**(9):1377-1386.
[118] TZ Naqvi and HK Hyuhn (2009). "Cerebrovascular mental stress reactivity is impaired in hypertension". *Cardiovascular Ultrasound* **7**: 32.
[119] PR Martin (1996). "Chapter 3: Psychophysiological Mechanisms of Headaches", p30, *Psychological management of chronic headaches*, Guilford Press.
[120] JM Borkum (2007). "Chapter 5:Psychophysiology of Migraine" p138, *Chronic Headaches: Biology, Psychology, and Behavioral Treatment*, Routledge.
[121] TZ Naqvi and HK Hyuhn (2009). "Cerebrovascular mental stress reactivity is impaired in hypertension". *Cardiovascular Ultrasound* **7**: 32.
[122] TH Holmes and RH Rahe (1967). "The Social Readjustment Rating Scale".*J Psychosom Res.* **11**(2):213-218.
[123] BP Dohrenwend (2006). "Inventorying Stressful Life Events as Risk Factors for Psychopathology: Toward Resolution of the Problem of Intracategory Variability." *Psychol Bull.* **132**(3): 477–495.
[124] JE Holm and KA Holroyd (1992). "The Daily Hassles Scale (Revised): Does it Measure Stress or Symptoms?" *Behavioral Assessment* **14**: 465-482, Pergamon Press.

[125] AD Kanner, JC Coyne, C Schaefer and RS Lazarus (1981). "Comparison of Two Modes of Stress Measurement: Daily Hassles and Uplifts Versus Major Life Events" *Journal of Behavioral Medicine* **4**(1): 1-39.

[126] See refs in Music Therapy Association of BC: Stress Management.

[127] JA Vossemail, M Good, B Yates, MM Baun, A Thompson and M Hertzog (2004). "Sedative music reduces anxiety and pain during chair rest after open-heart surgery." *Pain* **112**(1): 197-203.

[128] PJ McGrath, D Penzien and JC Rains (2006). "Chapter 48: Psychological and Behavioural Treatments of Migraines", p441-443. The Headaches, Editor J Olesen, Edition 3, Lippincott Williams and Wilkins.

[129] JM Nash and RW Thebarge (2006). "Understanding Psychological Stress, Its Biological Processes, & Impact on Primary Headache". *Headache* **46**(9):1377-1386.

[130] E Pastorino and S Doyle-Portillo (2012). What is Psychology? Essentials. See refs on p441. Cengage Learning.

[131] E Pastorino and S Doyle-Portillo (2012). What is Psychology? Essentials. See refs on p442. Cengage Learning.

[132] B Grinde and GG Patil (2009). "Biophilia: Does Visual Contact with Nature Impact on Health and Well-Being?" *Int J Environ Res Public Health* **6**(9): 2332–2343.

[133] M Townsend and R Weerasuriya (2010). "Beyond Blue to Green: The Benefits of contact with nature for mental health and well-being." Beyond Blue Ltd.

[134] E Sahlin, G Ahlborg Jr, JV Matuszczyk and P Grahn (2014). "Nature-Based Stress Management Course for Individuals at Risk of Adverse Health Effects from Work-Related Stress—Effects on Stress Related Symptoms, Workability and Sick Leave". *Int J Environ Res Public Health* **11**(6): 6586–6611.

[135] C Song, D Joung, H Ikei, M Igarashi, M Aga, BJ Park, M Miwa, M Takagaki and Y Miyazaki (2013). "Physiological and psychological effects of walking on young males in urban parks in winter." *J Physiol Anthropol.* **32**(1): 18.

[136] B Grinde and GG Patil (2009). "Biophilia: Does Visual Contact with Nature Impact on Health and Well-Being?" *Int J Environ Res Public Health* **6**(9): 2332–2343.

[137] H Ikei, M Komatsu, C Song, E Himoro and Y Miyazaki (2014). "The physiological and psychological relaxing effects of viewing rose flowers in office workers." *J Physiol Anthropol.* **33**(1): 6.

[138] M Miller, C Mangano, Y Park, R Goel, GD Plotnick and RA Vogel (2006). "Impact of cinematic viewing on endothelial function." *Heart* **92**(2):261–262.

[139] RW Evans, MA Williams, AM Rapoport and BL Peterlin (2012). "The Association of Obesity With Episodic and Chronic Migraine". *Headache*, **52**(4):663-671.

[140] L Fontana, JC Eagon, ME Trujillo, PE Scherer and S Klein (2007). "Visceral fat adipokine secretion is associated with systemic inflammation in obese humans". *Diabetes*, **56**(4):1010-1013.

[141] BL Peterlin, AL Rosso, MA Williams, JR Rosenberg, JA Haythornthwaite, KR Merikangas, RF Gottesman, DS Bond, JP He and AB Zonderman (2013). "Episodic migraine and obesity and the influence of age, race, and sex". *Neurology*, **81**(15):1314-1321.

[142] A Mosek and AD Korczyn (1995). "Yom Kippur headache". *Neurology*, **45**(11): 1953-1955.

[143] A Awada and M Jumah (1999). "The first-of-Ramadan headache". *Headache*, **39**(7): 490-493.

[144] A Mosek and AD Korczyn (1995). "Yom Kippur headache". Neurology, 45(11): 1953-1955 and A Awada and M Jumah (1999). "The first-of-Ramadan headache". *Headache*, **39**(7): 490-493.

[145] H Valtin (2002). "Drink at least eight glasses of water a day." Really? Is there scientific evidence for "8 x 8"?" *Am J Physiol Regul Integr Comp Physiol*, 283(5): R993–R1004.
[146] LE Armstrong (2012). "Hydration Biomarkers During Daily Life: Recent Advances and Future Potential." *Nutrition Today*, 47(4): Supplement 1: S3 - S6.
[147] MS Ganio, LE Armstrong, DJ Casa, BP McDermott, EC Lee, LM Yamamoto, S Marzano, RM Lopez, L Jimenez, L Le Bellego, E Chevillotte and HR Lieberman (2011). "Mild dehydration impairs cognitive performance and mood of men". *Br J Nutr*, 106(10): 1535-1543.
[148] E Perrier, S Vergne, A Klein, M Poupin, P Rondeau, L Le Bellego, LE Armstrong, F Lang, J Stookey and I Tack (2013). "Hydration biomarkers in free-living adults with different levels of habitual fluid consumption". *Br J Nutr*; 109(9): 1678–1687.
[149] LM Juliano and RR Griffiths (2004). "A critical review of caffeine withdrawal: empirical validation of symptoms and signs, incidence, severity, and associated features". *Psychopharmacology (Berl)*, 176(1):1-29.
[150] Food Standards, Australia and New Zealand; Australian Institute of Sport, Caffeine Fact Sheet.
[151] A Panconesi (2008). "Alcohol and migraine: trigger factor, consumption, mechanisms. A review." J Headache Pain, 9(1): 19-27.
[152] M Kjærgaard, AE Eggen, EB Mathiesen and R Jorde (2012). "Association between headache and serum 25-hydroxyvitamin D; the Tromsø Study: Tromsø 6". *Headache*, **52**(10): 1499–1505.
[153] S Prakash and ND Shah (2009). "Chronic tension-type headache with vitamin D deficiency: casual or causal association?" *Headache*, **49**(8): 1214-1222.
[154] P Borgdorff and GJ Tangelder (2012). "Migraine: Possible Role of Shear-Induced Platelet Aggregation With Serotonin Release". *Headache*, **52**(8):1298-1318.
[155] KM Dickinson, PM Clifton and JB Keogh (2011). "Endothelial function is impaired after a high-salt meal in healthy subjects". *Am J Clin Nutr*, **93**(3): 500-505.
[156] DER Warburton, CW Nicol and SSD Bredin (2006). "Health benefits of physical activity: the evidence" *CMAJ* **174**(6): 801 – 809.
[157] SS Dhaliwal, TA Welborn and PA Howat (2013). "Recreational Physical Activity as an Independent Predictor of Multivariable Cardiovascular Disease Risk." *PLOS ONE* **8**(12): e83435 1 – 6.
[158] E Varkey, K Hagen, JA Zwart and M Linde (2008). "Physical activity and headache: results from the Nord-Trondelag Health Study (HUNT)." *Cephalalgia* **28**(12): 1292–1297.
[159] A Hougaard, FM Amin, AW Hauge, M Ashina and J Olesen (2013). "Provocation of migraine with aura using natural trigger factors." *Neurology* **80**(5):428 -431.
[160] H Koppen and PLJ van Veldhoven (2013). "Migraineurs with exercise-triggered attacks have a distinct migraine". *J Headache Pain* **14**(1):99.
[161] E Varkey, A Cider, J Carlsson and M Linde (2011). "Exercise as migraine prophylaxis: A randomized study using relaxation and topiramate as controls." *Cephalalgia* 31(14):1428–1438.
[162] M de Tommaso, M Delussi, E Vecchio, V Sciruicchio, S Invitto and P Livrea (2014). "Sleep features and central sensitization symptoms in primary headache patients." *J Headache and Pain* **15**(1):64.
[163] P Barbanti, G Fabbrini, C Aurilia, N Vanacore and G Cruccu (2007). "A case–control study on excessive daytime sleepiness in episodic migraine." *Cephalalgia* **27**(10):1115–1119.
[164] HF Boardman, E Thomas, DS Millson and PR Croft (2005). "Psychological, sleep, lifestyle, and comorbid associations with headache." *Headache* **45**(6): 657–669.

[165] M de Tommaso, M Delussi, E Vecchio, V Sciruicchio, S Invitto and P Livrea (2014). "Sleep features and central sensitization symptoms in primary headache patients." *J Headache and Pain* **15**(1):64.
[166] S Schuh-Hofer, R Wodarski, DB Pfau, O Caspani, W Magerl, JD Kennedy and RD Treede (2013). "One night of total sleep deprivation promotes a state of generalized hyperalgesia: a surrogate pain model to study the relationship of insomnia and pain." *Pain* 154(9):1613–1621.
[167] AH Calhoun and S Ford (2007). "Behavioral Sleep Modification May Revert Transformed Migraine to Episodic Migraine." *Headache* 47(8):1178–1183.
[168] M Engstrøm, K Hagen, MH Bjørk, LJ Stovner and T Sand (2014). "Sleep quality and arousal in migraine and tension-type headache: the headache-sleep study." *Acta Neurol Scand Suppl* (198):47-54.
[169] KD Kobayashi, AJ Kaufman, J Griffis and J McConnell (2007). "Using Houseplants To Clean Indoor Air." *Ornamentals and flowers*, December OF –39.
[170] ibid.
[171] M Kjærgaard, AE Eggen, EB Mathiesen and R Jorde (2012). "Association between headache and serum 25-hydroxyvitamin D; the Tromsø Study: Tromsø 6". *Headache*, **52**(10): 1499–1505.
[172] S Prakash and ND Shah (2009). "Chronic tension-type headache with vitamin D deficiency: casual or causal association?" *Headache*, **49**(8): 1214-1222.
[173] CA Nowson and C Margerison (2002). "Vitamin D intake and vitamin D status of Australians". *Med J Aust*; **177** (3): 149-152.
[174] HE de Wardener and GA MacGregor (2002). "Harmful effects of dietary salt in addition to hypertension". *J Hum Hypertens*, **16**(4): 213-223.
[175] P Borgdorff and GJ Tangelder (2012). "Migraine: Possible Role of Shear-Induced Platelet Aggregation With Serotonin Release". *Headache*, **52**(8):1298-1318.
[176] KM Dickinson, PM Clifton and JB Keogh (2011). "Endothelial function is impaired after a high-salt meal in healthy subjects". *Am J Clin Nutr*, **93**(3): 500-505.
[177] J Schoenen, J Jacquy and M Lenaerts (1998). "Effectiveness of high-dose riboflavin in migraine prophylaxis. A randomized controlled trial". Neurology, 50(2): 466-470.
[178] C Boehnke, U Reuter, U Flach, S Schuh-Hofer, KM Einhäupl and G Arnold (2004). "High-dose riboflavin treatment is efficacious in migraine prophylaxis: an open study in a tertiary care centre". *Eur J Neurol*, **11**(7): 475-477.
[179] A Peikert, C Wilimzig and P Köhne-Volland (1996). "Prophylaxis of migraine with oral magnesium: results from a prospective, multi-center, placebo-controlled and double-blind randomized study". *Cephalalgia*, 16(4): 257-263.
[180] P Sarchielli, G Coata, C Firenze, P Morucci, G Abbritti and V Gallai (1992). "Serum and salivary magnesium levels in migraine and tension-type headache. Results in a group of adult patients." *Cephalalgia* 12(1): 21-2 and BM Altura and BT Altura (1996). "Role of magnesium in patho-physiological processes and the clinical utility of magnesium ion selective electrodes." *Scand J Clin Lab Invest Suppl* 224: 211-234.
[181] A Mauskop and BM Altura (1998). "Role of magnesium in the pathogenesis and treatment of migraines." *Clin Neurosci* 5(1): 24-27 and A Mauskop, BT Altura, RQ Cracco and BM Altura (1996). "Intravenous magnesium sulfate rapidly alleviates headaches of various types." *Headache* 36(3): 154-160.
[182] S Demirkaya, O Vural, B Dora and MA Topçuoğlu (2001). "Efficacy of intravenous magnesium sulfate in the treatment of acute migraine attacks". *Headache*, 41(2): 171-177.

[183] F Facchinetti, G Sances, P Borella, AR Genazzani and G Nappi G (1991). "Magnesium prophylaxis of menstrual migraine: effects on intracellular magnesium". *Headache*, 31(5): 298-301.
[184] Dr RH Waring (2009). "Report on Absorption of magnesium sulfate (Epsom salts) across the skin."
[185] J Greeves (2000). "Circamensal Rhythmicity and Muscle Function: The Role of Reproductive Hormones in the Regulation of Strength". *Biological Rhythm Research*. **31**(1): 15–28.
[186] DR Stewart, AC Celniker, CA Taylor, JR Cragun, JW Overstreet and BL Lasley (1990). "Relaxin in the peri-implantation period". *J Clin Endocrinol Metab* **70**(6):1771-1773.
[187] F Facchinetti, G Sances, P Borella, AR Genazzani and G Nappi (1991). "Magnesium prophylaxis of menstrual migraine: effects on intracellular magnesium". *Headache* **31**(5):298-301.
[188] AH Calhoun (2004). "Chapter 9: Women's issues in headache", p157-167. *"Headache: a guide for the primary care physician"*, Editors E Loder and VT Martin, ACP Press.
[189] ibid.
[190] H Massiou and EA MacGregor "Chapter 35: Influence of female hormones on migraines", p337-339. *The Headaches*, Editor J Olesen, Edition 3, Lippincott Williams and Wilkins.
[191] RW Evans (2004). "Chapter 11: Headaches in Women", p230-235. *Handbook of Headache*, RW Evans and NT Mathew, Lippincott Williams and Wilkins.6
[192] EW Loder, DC Buse and JR Golub (2005). "Headache and Combination Estrogen-Progestin Oral Contraceptives: Integrating Evidence, Guidelines, and Clinical Practice". *Headache* **45**(3):224-231.
[193] RE Nappi, A Cagnacci, F Granella, F Piccinini and FF Facchinetti (2001). "Course of primary headaches during hormone replacement therapy". *Maturitas* **38**(2):157-163.
[194] M Naumann, Y So, CE Argoff, MK Childers, DD Dykstra, GS Gronseth, B Jabbari, HC Kaufmann, B Schurch, SD Silberstein and DM Simpson (2008). "Assessment: Botulinum neurotoxin in the treatment of autonomic disorders and pain (an evidence-based review). Report of the Therapeutics and Technology Assessment Subcommittee of the American Academy of Neurology." *Neurology* **70**(19):1707-1714.
[195] WJ Schulte-Mattler and E Leinisch (2008). "Evidence based medicine on the use of botulinum toxin for headache disorders". *J Neural Transm* **115**(4):647-651.
[196] SK Aurora, DW Dodick, CC Turkel, RE DeGryse, SD Silberstein, RB Lipton, HC Diener and MF Brin. PREEMPT 1 Chronic Migraine Study Group. (2010). "OnabotulinumtoxinA for treatment of chronic migraine: results from the double-blind, randomized, placebo-controlled phase of the PREEMPT 1 trial." *Cephalalgia* **30**(7):793-803.
[197] O Steinbrocker (1944). "Therapeutic injections in painful musculoskeletal disorders. With special reference to the saline-procaine test." *JAMA* **125**(6): 397-401.
[198] T Robert (2006). "Report: Botox for Head Pain, Largest Study Yet. A report from the American Headache Society Annual Scientific Meeting." About.com 9 July 2006.
[199] RW Evans and A Blumenfeld (2003). "Botulinum toxin injections for headache."
Headache **43**(6): 682-685.
[200] A Blumenfeld, SD Silberstein, DW Dodick, SK Aurora, CC Turkel and WJ Binder (2010). "Method of Injection of OnabotulinumtoxinA for Chronic Migraine: A Safe, Well-Tolerated, and Effective Treatment Paradigm Based on the PREEMPT Clinical Program." *Headache* **50**(9):1406-1418.

[201] EP Calandre, J Hidalgo, JM Garcia-Leiva and F Rico-Villademoros (2006). "Trigger point evaluation in migraine patients: An indication of peripheral sensitization linked to migraine predisposition?" *Eur J Neurol* **13**(3): 244-249.
[202] JM García-Leiva, J Hidalgo, F Rico-Villademoros, V Moreno and EP Calandre (2007). "Effectiveness of Ropivacaine Trigger Points Inactivation in the Prophylactic Management of Patients with Severe Migraine." *Pain Medicine* **8**(1):65-70.
[203] H Briggs (2011). "Botox 'little help' for migraines." BBC News 9 February 2011.
[204] A Blumenfeld, SD Silberstein, DW Dodick, SK Aurora, CC Turkel and WJ Binder (2010). "Method of Injection of OnabotulinumtoxinA for Chronic Migraine: A Safe, Well-Tolerated, and Effective Treatment Paradigm Based on the PREEMPT Clinical Program." *Headache* **50**(9):1406-1418.
[205] R Fortuna, MA Vaz, AR Youssef, D Longino and W Herzog (2011). "Changes in contractile properties of muscles receiving repeat injections of botulinum toxin (Botox)." *J Biomech* **44**(1):39-44.
[206] E Shevel (2007)."Vascular surgery for chronic migraine." *Therapy* **4**(4): 451-456.
[207] C Cianchetti, Y Hmaidan, G Finco and MG Ledda (2009). "Scalp periarterial saline efficacy in migraine and relation to exploding and imploding headache." *J Neurol* **256**(7): 1109-1113.

Made in United States
North Haven, CT
05 November 2026

21763432R00193